Managing Instabilities of the Foot and Ankle

Editor

ANDREA VELJKOVIC

FOOT AND ANKLE CLINICS

www.foot.theclinics.com

Consulting Editor
MARK S. MYERSON

December 2018 • Volume 23 • Number 4

ELSEVIER

1600 John F. Kennedy Boulevard • Suite 1800 • Philadelphia, Pennsylvania, 19103-2899

http://www.theclinics.com

FOOT AND ANKLE CLINICS Volume 23, Number 4
December 2018 ISSN 1083-7515, ISBN-978-0-323-64217-0

Editor: Lauren Boyle
Developmental Editor: Meredith Madeira

Foot and Ankle Clinics (ISSN 1083-7515) is published quarterly by Elsevier, Inc., 360 Park Avenue South, New York, NY 10010-1710. Months of issue are March, June, September, and December. Periodicals postage paid at New York, NY, and additional mailing offices. Subscription price per year is $326.00 (US individuals), $519.00 (US institutions), $100.00 (US students), $367.00 (Canadian individuals), $623.00 (Canadian institutions), $215.00 (Canadian students), $460.00 (international individuals), $623.00 (international institutions), and $215.00 (international students). To receive student/resident rate, orders must be accompanied by name of affiliated institution, date of term, and the *signature* of program/residency coordinator on institution letterhead. Orders will be billed at individual rate until proof of status is received. Foreign air speed delivery is included in all *Clinics* subscription prices. All prices are subject to change without notice. **POSTMASTER:** Send address changes to *Foot and Ankle Clinics*, Elsevier Health Sciences Division, Subscription Customer Service, 3251 Riverport Lane, Maryland Heights, MO 63043. **Customer Service: 1-800-654-2452 (US and Canada). From outside of the United States and Canada, call 314-447-8871. Fax: 314-447-8029. E-mail: JournalsCustomerService-usa@ elsevier.com (for print support); JournalsOnlineSupport-usa@elsevier.com (for online support).**

Reprints. For copies of 100 or more, of articles in this publication, please contact the Commercial Reprints Department, Elsevier Inc., 360 Park Avenue South, New York, NY 10010-1710. Tel.: 212-633-3874; Fax: 212-633-3820; E-mail: reprints@elsevier.com.

Contributors

CONSULTING EDITOR

MARK S. MYERSON, MD
Medical Director, The Foot and Ankle Association, Inc, Baltimore, Maryland, USA

EDITOR

ANDREA VELJKOVIC, MD, MPH(Harvard), BComm, FRCSC
Associate Clinical Professor, Department of Orthopaedics, St. Paul's Hospital, The University of Brtish Columbia, Fellowship Director, UBC Foot and Ankle, Research Director, UBC Orthopaedic Residency Program, Research Director, Canadian Foot and Ankle Society, Footbridge Clinic, Vancouver, British Columbia, Canada

AUTHORS

JORGE I. ACEVEDO, MD
Director, Foot and Ankle Center, Department of Orthopedics, Southeast Orthopedic Specialists, Jacksonville, Florida, USA

CRAIG C. AKOH, MD
Orthopaedic Department, University of Iowa Hospital and Clinics, Iowa City, Iowa, USA

MESHAL ALHADHOUD, MD
Division of Orthopedic Surgery, Department of Surgery, Dalhousie University, Queen Elizabeth II Health Sciences Center, Halifax, Nova Scotia, Canada

YOUSEF ALRASHIDI, MD
Assistant Professor, Orthopaedic Foot and Ankle Surgeon, Orthopaedic Department, College of Medicine, Taibah University, Medina, Saudi Arabia

SAUD ALSHALAWI, MD
Consultant of Orthopaedic Surgery, Foot and Ankle Surgeon, Prince Sultan Military Medical City, Riyadh, Saudi Arabia

CLAUDIA ASTUDILLO, MD
Department of Radiology, Clinica Las Condes, Santiago, Chile

ALEXEJ BARG, MD
Assistant Professor, Department of Orthopaedics, University of Utah, Salt Lake City, Utah, USA

GONZALO F. BASTIAS, MD
Department of Orthopedic Surgery, Clinica Las Condes, Foot and Ankle Unit, Complejo Hospitalario San José, Department of Orthopedic Surgery, Universidad de Chile, Santiago, Chile

JEAN BRILHAULT, MD, PhD
Service de Chirurgie Orthopédique, C.H.R.U. Tours, Université François-Rabelais de Tours, Tours, France

TIM M. CLOUGH, BSc (Hons), FRCS (Tr&Orth)
Consultant Orthopaedic Surgeon, Department of Foot and Ankle Surgery, Wrightington Hospital, Wrightington, Lancashire, United Kingdom

MARK E. CRESSWELL, MBBCh, BSc (Hon), FRCR, FRCPC
Clinical Associate Professor, Department of Radiology, St. Paul's Hospital, The University of British Columbia, Vancouver, British Columbia, Canada

MIKI DALMAU-PASTOR, PhD, PT, DPM
Human Anatomy and Embryology Unit, Experimental Pathologies and Therapeutics Department, Universitat de Barcelona, Health Sciences Faculty of Manresa, Universitat de Vic-Central de Catalunya, Barcelona, Spain; Groupe de Recherche et d'Etude en Chirurgie Mini-Invasive du Pied, Merignac, France

MOHAMMAD EID, MSc, MD, MRCS
Division of Orthopedic Surgery, Department of Surgery, Dalhousie University, Queen Elizabeth II Health Sciences Center, Halifax, Nova Scotia, Canada

MARIO I. ESCUDERO, MD
Department of Orthopedics, Division of Distal Extremities, The University of British Columbia, Vancouver, British Columbia, Canada

AHMED E. GALHOUM, MD, MRCS (England)
Consultant of Orthopaedic Surgery, Department of Orthopedics, Nasser Institute for Research and Treatment, Cairo, Egypt

MARK GLAZEBROOK, MSc, MD, PhD, FRCSC
Division of Orthopedic Surgery, Department of Surgery, Dalhousie University, Queen Elizabeth II Health Sciences Center, Halifax, Nova Scotia, Canada

STEPHANE GUILLO, MD
Doctor, Clinique du Sport, Bordeuax-Mérignac, France

GREGORY P. GUYTON, MD
Department of Orthopaedic Surgery, MedStar Union Memorial Hospital, Baltimore, Maryland, USA

MARIO HERRERA, MD
Professor, Head Foot and Ankle Unit, Orthopaedic Department, University of La Laguna, Tenerife, Spain

KREIGH A. KAMMAN, MD
Resident, Department of Orthopedics, Indiana University, Indianapolis, Indiana, USA

FABIAN KRAUSE, MD
Head of Foot and Ankle Surgery, Department of Orthopaedic Surgery, Inselspital, University of Berne, Freiburgstrasse, Berne, Switzerland

VU LE, MD, FRCSC
Clinical Fellow, Department of Orthopaedics, St. Paul's Hospital, The University of British Columbia, Vancouver, British Columbia, Canada

HAROON MAJEED, MRCS, MSC, FEBOT, FRCS (Tr&Orth)
Senior Fellow, Department of Foot and Ankle Surgery, Wrightington Hospital, Wrightington, Lancashire, United Kingdom

PETER G. MANGONE, MD
Department of Orthopedics, Blue Ridge Division of Emergeortho, Co-Director, Foot and Ankle Center, Asheville, North Carolina, USA

KENTARO MATSUI, MD, PhD
Department Manager, Department of Orthopaedic Surgery, Teikyo University School of Medicine, Itabashi, Tokyo, Japan

JOSEPH T. O'NEIL, MD
Department of Orthopaedic Surgery, MedStar Union Memorial Hospital, Baltimore, Maryland, USA

ROBERT C. PALMER, MD
Resident, Department of Orthopedics, University of Florida, Jacksonville, Florida, USA

MANUEL J. PELLEGRINI, MD
Department of Orthopedic Surgery, Universidad de Chile, Hospital Clinico Universidad de Chile, Clinica Universidad de los Andes, Santiago, Chile

PHINIT PHISITKUL, MD
Orthopaedic Surgeon, Tri-State Specialist, LLC, Sioux City, Iowa, USA

DAVID A. PORTER, MD, PhD
Orthopedic Foot and Ankle Consultant Indianapolis Colts, Purdue University, Methodist Sports Medicine, Volunteer Clinical Faculty, Department of Orthopedics, Indiana University, Indianapolis, Indiana, USA

PETER SALAT, MD, FRCPC
Clinical Assistant Professor, Department of Radiology, University of Calgary, Mayfair Diagnostics, Calgary, Alberta, Canada

ANDREW SANDS, MD
Section Chief, Foot and Ankle Surgery, Downtown Orthopedic Associates, Clinical Associate Professor of Orthopedic Surgery, Weill Cornell Medical College, Chairman, AO Foot and Ankle Expert Group, New York, New York, USA

ANGELA SEIDEL, MD
Senior Resident, Department of Orthopaedic Surgery, Inselspital, University of Berne, Freiburgstrasse, Berne, Switzerland

KIM SLATER, MB BS, FRACS, FaORTHA
Consultant Orthopaedic Surgeon, Mater Hospital, North Sydney, New South Wales, Australia

JAMES STONE, MD
Orthopedic Surgery, Medical College of Wisconsin, Milwaukee, Wisconsin, USA

MICHAEL SWORDS, DO
Chair, Department of Orthopedic Surgery, Michigan Orthopedic Center, Director of Orthopedic Trauma, Sparrow Hospital, Lansing, Michigan, USA

MICHAEL SYMES, MD
Department of Orthopedics, Division of Distal Extremities, The University of British Columbia, Vancouver, British Columbia, Canada

MASATO TAKAO, MD, PhD
Departments of Orthopaedic Surgery, and Sport and Medical Science, Teikyo Institute of Sports Science and Medicine, Tokyo, Japan

JOÃO TEIXEIRA, MD
Doctor, Department of Orthopaedics and Traumatology, Centro Hospitalar de Entre o Douro e Vouga, Santa Maria da Feira, Portugal

VICTOR VALDERRABANO, MD, PhD
Professor, Chairman, Orthopaedic Department, Swiss Ortho Center, Swiss Medical Network, Schmerzklinik Basel, Basel, Switzerland

ANDREA VELJKOVIC, MD, MPH(Harvard), BComm, FRCSC
Associate Clinical Professor, Department of Orthopaedics, St. Paul's Hospital, The University of Brtish Columbia, Fellowship Director, UBC Foot and Ankle, Research Director, UBC Orthopaedic Residency Program, Research Director, Canadian Foot and Ankle Society, Footbridge Clinic, Vancouver, British Columbia, Canada

MARTIN WIEWIORSKI, MD
Head Foot and Ankle Unit, Orthopaedic and Trauma Department, Kantonsspital Winterthur, Winterthur, Switzerland

ALASTAIR S.E. YOUNGER, MB,ChB, ChM, MSc, FRCSC
Professor, Department of Orthopedics, Division of Distal Extremities, The University of British Columbia, Vancouver, British Columbia, Canada

Editorial Advisory Board

Contents

This article reviews the imaging aspects relevant to ligamentous instabilities of the foot and ankle with a focus on MRI and ultrasound imaging. A pictorial review of the anatomy of the medial and lateral ankle ligaments, syndesmosis, spring ligament, Lisfranc complex, hallux sesamoid complex, and lesser toe plantar plate as seen on MRI is presented. Selected cases of ligamentous pathology relevant to foot and ankle instability are presented. The value of imaging in the assessment of foot and ankle instability is reviewed.

Acute injuries to the lateral ankle complex remain common and account for 20% to 25% of musculoskeletal injuries. Initial assessment should use the Ottawa ankle rules, and grading should take into account degree of mechanical instability. Nonoperative measures are preferable for all grades of injury; however, mechanical instability is a predictor for resprains. Functional treatment after a short period of relative immobilization gives satisfactory results, and residual chronic ankle instability can be managed by repair or reconstruction. Delayed physical examination in elite athletes, along with 3T MRI, may be helpful in making a case for early surgical stabilization.

 Video content accompanies this article at http://www.foot.theclinics.com.

Open surgical reconstruction for chronic lateral ankle instability is a proven and effective means of providing renewed stability. Ankle arthroscopy is recommended before reconstruction to address intra-articular pathology. The open procedure discussed is well researched and proven to restore stability and the ability to return to sport and daily activity. Anatomic shortening with reattachment into a bony trough allows return to full motion, reliable stability, and return to an active lifestyle without sacrificing any tendons or requiring a tenodesis. The authors' aggressive rehabilitation protocol is provided; the approach to athletes/patients with ligament laxity or cavovarus alignment is also addressed.

Over the last 10 years, significant advances have been made and successful techniques have now been developed that effectively treat ankle instability via the arthroscope. Currently arthroscopic lateral ligament repair techniques can be grouped into "arthroscopic-assisted techniques," "all-arthroscopic techniques," and "all-inside techniques." Recent studies have proven these arthroscopic techniques to be a simple, safe, and biomechanically equivalent, stable alternative to open Brostrom Gould lateral ligament reconstruction.

Inversion ankle sprains represent one of the most common traumatic injuries in the active sports population. Although most respond well to conservative treatment, some hide important lesions. Lateral ankle ligament injuries occur in more than 80% of all ankle sprains, with one-third of these developing chronic ankle instability (CAI). Lateral ankle ligament repair or reconstruction procedures aim to restore normal ankle anatomy and function in patients with CAI. Arthroscopic reconstruction techniques allow the surgeon to reach surgery objectives with minimal soft tissue injury. When the indications and surgical steps are respected, this arthroscopic technique seems to be safe and reproducible.

Chronic ankle instability following ankle sprains causes pain and functional problems such as recurrent giving way. Within the 3 ligaments of the lateral ligament complex, 80% of patients tear the anterior talofibular ligament (ATFL), whereas the other 20% of patients tear the ATFL and calcaneofibular ligament (CFL). Rarely, the posterior talofibular ligament is involved. An incidence of 10% to 30% of patients will fail conservative treatment and result in chronic ankle instability that may require surgical treatment. To date, numerous open surgical procedures for anatomic repair or reconstruction of ATFL and/or CFL provide good clinical results.

A lower leg or hindfoot varus malalignment is a frequently encountered but underestimated cause of chronic ankle instability and ankle arthritis in the long term. When evaluating patients with ankle instability, a high index of clinical suspicion for tibia and hindfoot malalignment and subsequent biomechanics should be maintained. Management of lateral ankle instability in the presence of varus malalignment must comprise a generous indication for accurate hindfoot realignment. In young and active patients, realignment should be combined with formal lateral ligamentous repair.

Ankle sprains continue to be among the most common musculoskeletal injuries, most of which never require surgical treatment. Surgical treatment has traditionally been successful for those patients whose symptoms do not improve with nonoperative care. However, recurrent instability, although rare, can occur early or late after a stabilization procedure, as the result of an acute traumatic event or chronic repetitive minor injury. A complete workup of patients with recurrent ankle instability should be completed before revision surgery and should include evaluation for generalized joint hypermobility as well as anatomic variations, such as hindfoot varus, first ray plantarflexion, and midfoot cavus.

Ankle injuries are a common traumatic injury. Rupture to the syndesmosis may occur as a result of these injuries. Strategies for the treatment of both acute and chronic syndesmotic repair are reviewed in detail. Significance of Chaput, Wagstaffe, and posterior malleolus fractures on syndesmotic stability are reviewed. Treatment considerations for total ankle arthroplasty are discussed, and correction of coronal plane deformity as a result of late syndesmotic injury at the time of ankle arthroplasty is outlined.

Diagnosis and treatment of medial ankle instability (MAI) are still controversial and poorly discussed in literature. The purpose of this review is to highlight different clinical presentations of MAI and develop a guide for its management. The deltoid ligament complex is injured more commonly than expected, because deltoid ligament injuries may either be isolated or occur in combination with other lesions, such as lateral ankle ligament injury, posterior tibial tendon insufficiency, osteochondral lesion, and others. The presence of a pes planovalgus deformity in a patient without posterior tibial tendon insufficiency may indicate MAI.

The crucial role of the spring ligament complex within the pathologic process that leads to flatfoot deformity has evolved recently. There has been improvement in the anatomic knowledge of the spring ligament and understanding of its complex relationship to the deltoid complex and outstanding advances in biomechanics concepts related to the spring ligament. Optimization of flatfoot treatment strategies are focused on a renewed interest in the spring ligament and medial soft tissue reconstruction in concert with bony correction to obtain an adequate reduction of the talonavicular deformity and restoration of the medial longitudinal arch.

Tarsometatarsal (TMT) joint complex injuries can be caused by either direct or indirect injuries. The Lisfranc joint represents approximately

0.2% of all fractures. Up to 20% of these injuries are misdiagnosed or missed on initial radiographic assessment; therefore, a high index of suspicion is needed to accurately diagnose TMT joint injuries and avoid the late sequelae of substantial midfoot arthrosis, pain, decreased function, and loss of quality of life. This review discusses the anatomy, diagnosis, and management of athletic Lisfranc injuries, including a description of the preferred minimally invasive surgical techniques used by the senior author of this article.

Tim M. Clough and Haroon Majeed

Turf toe injuries can be a disabling if not recognized and treated early. A high index of suspicion, based on the mechanism of injury and appropriate imaging, helps in the timely diagnosis. These injuries are frequently known to occur on artificial playing surfaces, because of the increased traction at the shoe-surface interface. Stress and instability testing are key components to assess the need for surgical intervention. Accurate timely diagnosis and treatment can allow full return to physical activities for most athletes, back to their pre-injury level.

Craig C. Akoh and Phinit Phisitkul

Lesser toe plantar plate injuries at the metatarsophalangeal (MTP) joint are a common source of metatarsalgia. The second MTP joint is the most commonly affected digit. The fibrocartilaginous plantar plate is the most important static stabilizer of the MTP joint; high loading with weight bearing can lead to attritional plantar plate injuries. Chronic pain with weight bearing is the common presentation of lesser toe instability. Untreated plantar plate instability can lead to hammer toe and mallet toe deformities. Combined Weil osteotomy and plantar plate repair yields favorable pain relief and angular deformity correction for patients who fail conservative treatment.

FOOT AND ANKLE CLINICS

RELATED INTEREST

Clinics in Podiatric Medicine and Surgery, April 2017 (Vol. 34, No. 2)
Achilles Tendon Pathology
Paul Dayton, *Editor*

THE CLINICS ARE NOW AVAILABLE ONLINE!
Access your subscription at:
www.theclinics.com

Preface

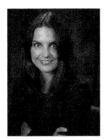

Andrea Veljkovic, MD, MPH(Harvard), BComm, FRCSC
Editor

Injuries of the lateral ankle ligaments are among the most common musculoskeletal problems in humans. They account for 40% of sports-related injuries and are prevalent in sports requiring changes of direction. In addition to lateral ankle instability, instabilities of the medial ankle, syndesmosis, and foot are coming to the forefront of orthopedic literature, improving our understanding of the subtleties of presentation and degree of diagnostic suspicion required in the recognition of these injuries.

It is interesting to note the continued evolution and increasing complexity of our treatment strategies related to the instabilities of the foot and ankle. Of course, we have learned a great deal about the intricacies of these problems over the past decades while concurrent technological advances have enabled us to continue perfecting and individualizing our nonoperative and surgical management. A more profound understanding of foot and ankle anatomy and mechanics have enabled elucidation of causes of failed primary treatment of foot and ankle instability and have improved the success of revision procedures.

This issue of the *Foot and Ankle Clinics of North America* is devoted to a discussion of the latest developments and knowledge advances in the treatment of the various flavors of foot and ankle instability. Our expert contributors present the most up-to-date treatments for acute and open chronic lateral ankle instability initially with most of the issue devoted to state-of-the-art percutaneous and arthroscopically guided procedures. An entire article is devoted to the often forgotten topic of malalignment as it pertains to lateral ankle instability. Finally, individual articles on medial ankle, spring ligament, plantar plate, and syndesmotic instability round out this issue on the management of foot and ankle instabilities. I hope

Foot Ankle Clin N Am 23 (2018) xv–xvi
https://doi.org/10.1016/j.fcl.2018.09.001
1083-7515/18/© 2018 Published by Elsevier Inc.   **foot.theclinics.com**

you enjoy this interesting collection of articles from some of the top experts in the world as much as I have.

Andrea Veljkovic, MD, MPH(Harvard), BComm, FRCSC
Department of Orthopaedics
St. Paul's Hospital
The University of Brtish Columbia
UBC Foot and Ankle
UBC Orthopaedic Residency Program
Canadian Foot and Ankle Society
Footbridge Clinic
221-181 Keefer Place
Vancouver, British Columbia V6B6C1, Canada

E-mail address:
docveljkovic@yahoo.com

Imaging in Foot and Ankle Instability

Peter Salat, MD, FRCPC[a,b,*], Vu Le, MD, FRCSC[c],
Andrea Veljkovic, MD, MPH(Harvard), BComm, FRCSC[c],
Mark E. Cresswell, MBBCh, FRCR, FRCPC[d]

KEYWORDS

- Ankle instability • Ligament tear • Flat foot • Pes planus • Turf toe • Spring ligament
- Lateral ankle ligament • Deltoid ligament

KEY POINTS

- Imaging of ligaments in the foot and ankle is readily achieved with MRI and ultrasound.
- Other imaging modalities have a role in the work-up of foot and ankle instability.
- Ligament pathology in the setting of foot and ankle instability is readily assessed on MRI and ultrasound.

INTRODUCTION

Ankle injuries are a common presenting concern to the emergency department, accounting for up to 10% of emergency room visits.[1] Up to 1 in 5 patients suffering an acute ankle sprain develops chronic ankle instability.[2] Assessment of foot and ankle instability is optimized by appropriately selected imaging tests. Imaging of osseous and soft tissue structures important for stability of the foot and ankle can be achieved with several modalities, each of which has a specific role in the treatment algorithm of foot and ankle instability. In general, the initial imaging investigation of suspected foot or ankle instability is weight-bearing radiography. Depending on the clinical scenario, MRI or ultrasound may be the next imaging modality of choice (**Table 1**). Although both modalities have well described roles in the assessment of foot and ankle ligamentous instability, the method of choice is often a reflection of local availability

Disclosure Statement: The authors have nothing to disclose.
[a] Department of Radiology, University of Calgary, 2500 University Drive Northwest, Calgary, Alberta T2N 1N4, Canada; [b] Mayfair Diagnostics, 6707 Elbow Drive Southwest 132, Calgary, Alberta T2V 0E3, Canada; [c] Department of Orthopaedics, St. Paul's Hospital, University of British Columbia, 1081 Burrard Street, Vancouver, British Columbia V6Z 1Y6, Canada; [d] Department of Radiology, St Paul's Hospital, University of British Columbia, 1081 Burrard Street, Vancouver, British Columbia V6Z 1Y6, Canada
* Corresponding author. Mayfair Diagnostics, 6707 Elbow Drive Southwest 132, Calgary, Alberta T2V 0E3, Canada.
E-mail address: Peter.Salat@ucalgary.ca

Foot Ankle Clin N Am 23 (2018) 499–522
https://doi.org/10.1016/j.fcl.2018.07.011
1083-7515/18/© 2018 Elsevier Inc. All rights reserved.

foot.theclinics.com

Table 1 MRI features of normal lateral ligaments	
ATFL	13–25 mm long, 7–11 mm wide, and 2–3 mm thick[3,4] May have 1–3 distinct bands separated by fat tissue Closely associated with the fibular insertion of the anteroinferior tibiofibular ligament[5]
CFL	Average dimensions of 36 mm in length, 5 mm width, and thickness of 2 mm[3]
PTFL	Often has a striated appearance on MRI Closely associated with the posterior intermalleolar ligament[5]

and expertise. CT can be incorporated in the imaging algorithm if definition of fine bony anatomy is required.

DISCUSSION

MRI enables a comprehensive assessment of soft tissue and osseous structures and elegantly depicts the complex ligamentous structures of the foot and ankle. Cost, time, and availability are limiting factors of MRI as is a low predictive value for chronic sequela of acute injury.[6]

Typical MRI protocols of the foot and ankle include sequences in 3 orthogonal planes centered on the area of interest. Axial and coronal imaging with the foot in mild plantar flexion and slice thickness of 3 mm enables consistent visualization of the entire ligaments,[7,8] but various positions and sequences have been advocated in the literature (**Box 1**).[6,9]

On MRI, normal ligaments appear as low signal intensity structures often outlined by surrounding fat signal.[10] Some ligaments, such as the posterior talofibular ligament (PTFL), posterior tibiotalar component of the deltoid ligament, and the anterior inferior tibiofibular ligament, may normally contain internal striations, signal heterogeneity, and apparent areas of discontinuity, which are typically a reflection of interposed fat tissue.[7,8]

Box 1
Routine MRI protocol

Mild plantar flexion (~20°) decreases magic angle effect, accentuates the fat plane between the peroneal tendons, and allows better visualization of the CFL

An extremity surface coil enhances spatial resolution

A wrist coil or another small dedicated coil is often used to evaluate the forefoot.
- T1-WIs MRI:
    (repetition time/echo time 5–600/20 ms) 12-cm to 16-cm field of view
    256 × 192 to 512 acquisition matrix
    1 to 2 signals acquired
    3-mm to 5-mm section thickness, interleaved
- Marrow abnormalities are best evaluated with fat-suppressed fluid-weighted techniques, such as fat-suppressed proton density–weighted imaging or STIR sequences (1500/20; inversion time 5100–150 ms).
- STIR and Dixon sequences are superior to other fat suppression techniques, which are vulnerable to gradient inhomogeneity.
- Cartilage abnormalities are best visualized using high-resolution intermediate proton density or 3-D gradient-echo sequences.

Data from Rosenberg ZS, Beltran J, Bencardino JT. From the RSNA refresher courses. Radiological Society of North America. MR imaging of the ankle and foot. Radiographics 2000;20:S153–79.

Appearance of acute (<3 weeks) ligamentous injury on MRI:
- Discontinuity
- Detachment
- Contour irregularity
- Thinning
- Increased intraligamentous signal on T2-weighted images (WIs), indicating edema or hemorrhage

Secondary findings of acute ligamentous injury on T2-WI on MRI[9]:
- Extravasation of joint fluid or hemorrhage into the adjacent soft tissues
- Joint effusion
- Tenosynovial effusion
- Bone avulsion at ligamentous insertion
- Bone contusion

Subacute and chronic tears are mainly identified by morphologic changes on MRI:
- Heterogenous intrasubstance signal
- Wavy contour
- Thickening with low signal in chronic fibrosis
- Thinning
- Elongation
- Poor visualization or absence of ligament

Secondary findings of subacute and chronic tears on MRI:
- Decreased signal of periligamentous fat on T1-WI and T2-WI
  - Represents scarring or synovial proliferation

Ultrasound is also a valuable imaging modality especially for assessment of more superficial soft tissue structures, such as the ones relevant to ligamentous instability, and has the unique characteristic of dynamic imaging visualization of the ligament, tendon, or plantar plate with stress testing.[11]

Lateral Ankle Ligaments

Normal MRI appearances of the lateral ankle ligamentous complex and adjacent structures are depicted on images 1 to 28 in the axial plane and on images 37 to 53 in the coronal plane (Appendix 1). MRI features of normal lateral ligaments are summarized in **Table 1**.

Acute rupture of the anterior talofibular ligament (ATFL) may appear as a fluid signal defect in the expected location of the ligament with retracted wavy fibers and is often associated with a capsular rupture and leakage of joint fluid into the superficial soft tissues.[7] Ancillary abnormalities often seen with calcaneofibular ligament (CFL) injury include thickening of the superior peroneal retinaculum and peroneal tenosynovial effusion. Acute sprains of the PTFL manifesting as high intrasubstance T2 signal and a wavy contour.[12] Chronic tears manifest the appearances described above **(Fig. 1)**.

Defects within the substance of the ATFL can be detected on MRI within 2 weeks after injury. The defect closes by 7 weeks, resulting in a thin or thick ligament with possible additional morphologic changes, as described previously **(Fig. 2)**. The edema and hemorrhage associated with acute ATFL and CFL injury usually resolve by the fourth week, but periarticular edema is often present up to the seventh week postinjury. Injuries associated with or mimicking lateral instability, such as tenosynovitis, tendon tears, and osteochondral lesions, are concurrently demonstrated on MRI, which is an additional benefit of this modality.[13]

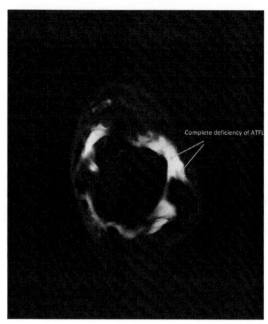

Complete deficiency of ATFL

Fig. 1. Fat-saturated T1-weighted axial MRI arthrogram of ankle: chronic full-thickness tear of ATFL.

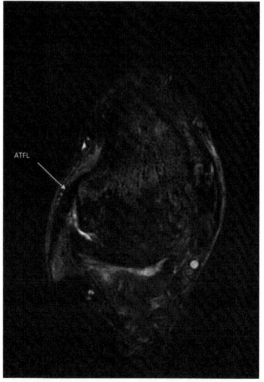

ATFL

Fig. 2. Axial fat-saturated T2-weighted MRI of ankle. Thickened ATFL representing chronic sprain.

Table 2 Imaging modalities in lateral ankle sprains	
Ultrasound	Accuracy for acute sprain of ATFL and CFL reported at 95% and 90%, respectively[14]
Radiography	Positive AP stress radiograph = 5° difference compared with normal ankle OR ≥ 10° absolute varus tilt[15]
CT scan	Accuracy for chronic ATFL sprain up to 94% using 3-D CT[2]
Arthrography	Sensitivity 96%, specificity 71% within 48 h of acute injury[16]
MRI arthrography	Accuracy of 100% for ATFL tear Accuracy of 82% for CFL tear[17]
MRI without contrast	Accuracy 94% for ATFL and CFL tears using 3D FISP sequence ATFL rupture sensitivity 100%, specificity 50% CFL rupture sensitivity 92% and specificity 100%[9]

Abbreviation: FISP, fast imaging with a steady-state precession.

Several imaging modalities are available for the assessment of lateral ankle sprain (**Table 2**). If a patient meets the Ottawa Ankle Rules,[18] the initial examination consists of routine 3 views of the ankle.

In the setting of chronic ankle pain of any origin, the best initial study is radiograph of the ankle. Radiographs may reveal clues to the presence of prior ligamentous injury, such as the presence of an effusion, which can be seen with an accuracy of 53% to 74%,[19] or ossific fragments, which may indicate ligamentous injury or retinacular avulsion.

With suspected ankle instability and normal or nonspecific ankle radiographs, the most appropriate tests are MRI of the ankle without contrast and MRI ankle arthrogram. Ultrasound of the ankle, radiograph stress view of the ankle, or CT ankle arthrography may be appropriate.

For assessment of prior ATFL injury, 1 study reported diagnostic accuracy relative to arthroscopy of 67% for stress radiography, 91% for US, and 97% for MRI with MRI identifying the location of the injury in 93% of cases compared with 63% with ultrasound.[20] In athletes with chronic ankle instability, ultrasound sensitivity for ATFL injury was reported at 61% compared with 71% for CT arthrography in 1 study.[21] For ATFL and CFL tears, MRI has reported accuracy relative to arthroscopy of 91.7% and 87.5%, respectively.

Medial Ankle Ligaments

Normal MRI appearances of the medial ankle ligamentous complex and adjacent structures are depicted on images 5 to 24 in the axial plane and on images 29 to 47 in the coronal plane. For a detailed discussion of the anatomy of the superficial and deep deltoid ligaments, refer to other publications. MRI features of normal deltoid ligament components are summarized in **Table 3**.[22]

If a patient meets the Ottawa Ankle Rules, the initial examination consists of the routine 3 views of the ankle. For suspected acute deltoid ligament injury in the setting of a supination-external rotation injury mechanism, a gravity stress view is reported to be a reliable alternative to the manual stress views.[23]

Deltoid ligament injuries manifest the features indicated previously (**Figs. 3** and **4**). On MRI, most of the deltoid ligament components are best seen in the coronal plane whereas the axial plane may best depict associated injuries of tendons and neurovascular structures. Syndesmotic injuries are associated with deltoid ligament sprains in up to 10% of cases. Ultrasound is reportedly highly accurate for assessing deltoid ligament injury after supination-external rotation fractures of the ankle.[24]

Table 3
MRI features of normal deltoid ligament components

Superficial components	
Tibionavicular ligament	Thickness of 1–2 mm, thicker in men
TSLs	Second thickest at 1–4 mm, thicker in men
Tibiocalcaneal ligament	May be difficult to distinguish from TSL on MRI
Deep components	
Anterior tibiotalar ligament	Best seen on coronal images, thin, multifascicular band seen in up to 84% of normal patients
Posterior tibiotalar ligament	Rectangular band, thickest component at 6–11 mm, commonly striated due to interposed fat
Pitfall on MRI of tibiotalar ligament, tibionavicular ligament, and tibiospring ligament	May show variable increased T2 signal in asymptomatic patients over age 45[22]

Distal Tibiofibular Syndesmosis Complex

Normal MRI appearances of the syndesmotic ligamentous complex and adjacent structures are depicted on images 1 to 12 in the axial plane and on images 37 to 48 in the coronal plane. MRI appearances of normal syndesmotic components are summarized in **Table 4**. Several imaging parameters are useful in the assessment of the normal syndesmosis, summarized in **Table 5**, and in the setting of acute or chronic injury (**Table 6**). Acute syndesmotic ligament sprain is illustrated in **Fig. 5**.

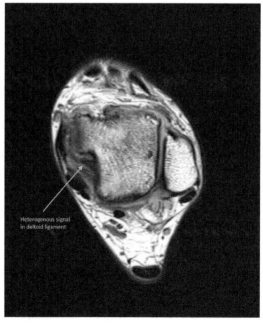

Heterogenous signal in deltoid ligament

Fig. 3. Axial proton density MRI ankle; deep deltoid ligament sprain.

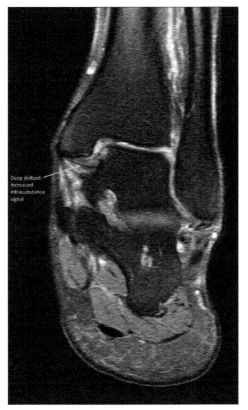

Deep deltoid:
Increased
intrasubstance
signal

Fig. 4. Coronal STIR MRI ankle. Deep deltoid ligament sprain.

Table 4	
MRI features of normal syndesmosis components	
AITFL	Trapezoidal, multiple fibers
	5 anatomic variations: number of fascicles, fascicle separations, attachment of inferior fascicle to main portion, presence of Bassett ligament[25]
Pitfall	Variable appearance of normal AITFL: thick or thin in normal patients[12]
PITFL	Triangular, broad tibial insertion[12]
Pitfall for AITFL and PITFL	Mimic intra-articular body on sagittal images[12]
IOL	Lowest thicker end of interosseous membrane[26]; multifascicular, broad, may be absent
ITL	Thick, deep labrum-like component of PITFL[26] overlaps with PTFL on coronal images
pIML	1–3 strips between ITL and PTFL on 19% of MRI[27,28]

Abbreviations: AITFL, anteroinferior tibiofibular ligament; IOL, interosseous ligament; ITL, inferior transverse ligament; pIML, posterior intermalleolar ligament; PITFL, posteroinferior tibiofibular ligament.

Table 5 Key imaging parameters of the syndesmosis	
Normal values AP radiographs	Talotibial angle 83° ± 4° Medial clear space <3 mm Talar tilt difference 2 mm[29]
Normal tibiofibular recess height on MRI	0.54 cm ± 0.68 cm[30]

Tears of the syndesmotic tibiofibular ligaments can be assessed with a reported perfect accuracy of 100% using MRI as can tears of the interosseous membrane based on one study. Tears of the interosseous membrane can also be detected using US, which has sensitivity of 89% and specificity of 94.5% compared with operative findings.

Spring Ligament Complex

The normal MRI appearance of the spring ligamentous complex is depicted on images 20 to 28 in the axial plane and on images 29 to 36 in the coronal plane.

The "spring" in spring ligament is a misnomer and arose from the mistaken belief that there were abundant elastin fibers in the ligament complex. Histologic assessment demonstrates the ligament to have normal collagen[31,32]

The anterior talus is contained by the cotyloid components of the navicular and calcaneus articular surfaces and the spring ligament complex (SLC), which form a talar acetabulum.[33] The first description of this anatomy was by Antonio Scarpa in 1803, who used the Italian term, *acetabolo*[34];more recently, this has been referred to as the "coxa pedis."[35]

The calcaneonavicular ligament acts to restrain the talar head and deepen the fossa, preventing medial and inferior displacement of the talar head, thus maintaining the medial longitudinal arch of the foot (**Fig. 6**).

Table 6 MRI features of syndesmosis injury	
Tibiofibular recess height	Acute injury: 1.2 cm ± 0.92 cm Chronic injury: 1.4 cm ± 0.57 cm[30]
Morphologic criteria of ligamentous injury	1. Discontinuity 2. Wavy/curved contour or nonvisualization
Associated findings	Ligament blurring Lateral fibular subluxation Fibular shortening Tibiofibular diastasis Fluid-like signal in the ligament ATFL injury (74%) Incongruous tibiofibular joint in chronic injury (33%) Bone bruise in acute injury (24%) Osteochondral lesion of talus in acute and chronic injury (28%)[30]
Features of interosseous membrane injury	1. Linear hyperintensity at distal tibia and fibula seen on: • Heavy T2-WI • Fat-suppressed proton density– weighted fast spin-echo • STIR 2. Low signal intensity foci: may reflect fibrosis, calcification, or hemosiderin

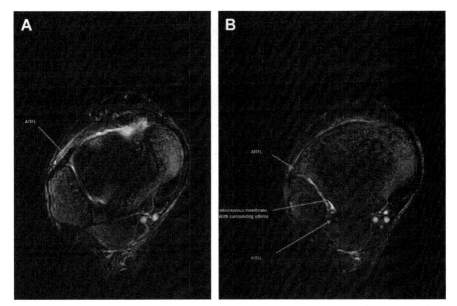

Fig. 5. (A) STIR MRI ankle. Acute low-grade AITFL sprain. (B) STIR MRI ankle. Edema along the interosseous membrane.

The tibialis posterior (TP) tendon is a dynamic stabilizer that locks the midfoot when contracted and has both medial and plantar distal attachments, resulting in a relatively elongated lever arm extending from the posterior calcaneus to the forefoot. Contraction of the calf muscles (gastrocnemius-soleus complex) result in elevation of the posterior calcaneus, with the fulcrum located at the metatarsal-phalangeal (MTP) joints. Failure of the TP tendon to stabilize the midfoot results in proximal positioning of the fulcrum at the midfoot and rotation of the diarthrodial talonavicular joint, with excessive strain at the plantar and medial aspect of the talar head constraining ligaments.[36] Kiter and colleagues[37] demonstrated that the presence of an accessory

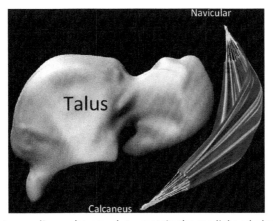

Fig. 6. The SLC acts as a sling or hammock to contain the medial and plantar aspect of the talar head articular surface.

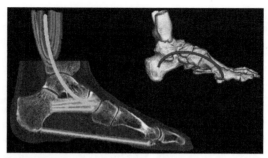

Fig. 7. Interplay of the dynamic (TP) and static stabilizers (SLC and plantar fascia) of the medial midfoot in maintaining the medial longitudinal arch.

navicular frequently resulted in an absent or non-functioning plantar component of the TP tendon (**Figs. 7** and **8**).[10]

The talus has no muscular nor tendon attachments[38] and acts as a bony meniscus, which is only stabilized by the surrounding ligaments, tendons and bones. If the surrounding constraints fail, it becomes inherently unstable.

The SLC is a group of ligaments connecting the medial and plantar aspect of the calcaneus to the plantar and medial aspect of the navicular, functioning as the static stabilizers of the medial midfoot. The complex consists of 3 components, the superomedial, medioplantar oblique, and inferoplantar (**Fig. 9**). The MRI features of these components are summarized in **Table 7**.

1. Superomedial calcaneonavicular ligament (SMCNL): the largest ligament, extending from the medial sustentaculum talus to the superomedial aspect of the navicular, forming a broad hammock shaped sling, which supports the medial talar head. The articular surface of the ligament is covered with fibrocartilage consistent with its role of withstanding load bearing forces generated by the talar head.[32] Superficial to the SMCNL is a gliding layer separating it from the TP tendon.[36]
2. Medioplantar oblique ligament (MPOCNL): the ligament extends from the coronoid fossa of the anterior calcaneus to the medioplantar navicular bone, located

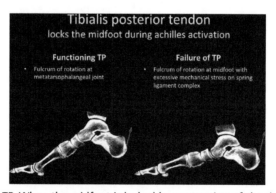

Fig. 8. Failure of TP. When the midfoot is locked by contraction of the dynamic stabilizers (primarily TP) the longitudinal integrity of the foot is maintained. The fulcrum of rotation is located at the MTP joints when the gastrocnemius-soleus complex contracts.

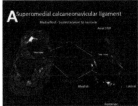 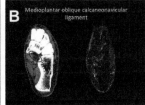 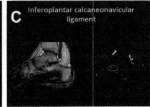

Fig. 9. (*A*) Coronal fat-saturated proton density MRI of the midfoot (*left*) demonstrating normal SMCNL of the midfoot, with low-signal gliding layer between SMCNL and TP tendon axial STIR MRI (*right*) demonstrating the relationship of TP tendon to spring ligament. (*B*) Coronal CT (*left*) and coronal fat-saturated proton density MRI of foot demonstrating normal MPOCNL. The circles identify the MPOCNL. (*C*) Sagittal proton density (*left*) and fat-saturated proton density demonstrating the normal IPCNL. The circles identify the IPCNL.

between the superomedial and the inferoplantar bands of the spring ligament, with sparse fibers fanning out and interposed by fat.[39] The adipose tissue deposits, particularly insertional angle fat, contain blood vessels and nerves and could play an important role in proprioception.[41]

3. Inferoplantar calcaneonavicular ligament (IPCNL) is a short fibrous band extending from the coronoid fossa of the calcaneus to the inferior beak of the navicular.[39] The spring ligament synovial recess of the talonavicular joint is located between the MPOCNL and IPCNL and can contain fluid, which can mimic a tear.

4. Included in the SCL is the tibiospring ligament (TSL), which is formed by the anterior superficial deltoid ligament.[36]

Integral to the functioning of the SLC are the dynamic stabilizers, most prominent of which is the TP, but including the flexor digitorum longus and flexor hallucis longus muscles.[34] Imaging assessment of the SLC includes careful assessment of the TP tendon, with failure of the TP a harbinger of SLC failure and acquired adult flat foot deformity[36] (**Figs. 10–13**). Isolated cases of SLC tears with intact TP tendon have been described.[42] The presence of an accessory navicular has been demonstrated to increase the probability of a central SMCNL tear.

Lisfranc Ligamentous Complex

Part of the soft tissue envelope of the Lisfranc joint, the Lisfranc ligament complex and the tarsometatarsal (TMT) ligaments are described in the literature as consisting of 3

Table 7 MRI features of the spring ligament components	
SMCNL	• Best seen on axial and coronal MRI (intermediate signal on T1 and low signal on proton density and T2 sequences).[39] • Normal thickness of 2 mm to 4 mm[40]
MPOCNL	• Best seen on axial and coronal MRI planes • Striated signal on T1, T2, and proton density sequences due to interposed fat[39]
IPCNL	• Intermediate to low signal on all MRI sequences • Best appreciated in the sagittal and axial planes and usually measures 4 mm in thickness[39]

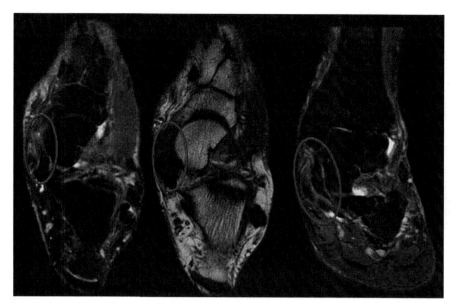

Fig. 10. Tear of the SMCNL and TP tendon. Axial proton density fat-saturated, T1, and coronal proton density fat-saturated weighted sequences through the midfoot demonstrating a tear of the SLC and tendon.

groups of ligaments—dorsal, interosseous, and plantar—and include intermetatarsal and intertarsal ligaments[43] (**Figs. 14** and **15**). The MRI features of the Lisfranc joint ligament components are summarized in **Table 8**.

Imaging findings of Lisfranc ligament injury are summarized in **Table 9**. For acute injury of the foot where physical examination is concerning for a Lisfranc injury, the

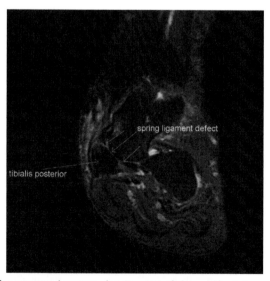

Fig. 11. Coronal fat-saturated proton density MRI of the midfoot demonstrating midsubstance tear of the SMCNL and thickened tendonopathic TP tendon.

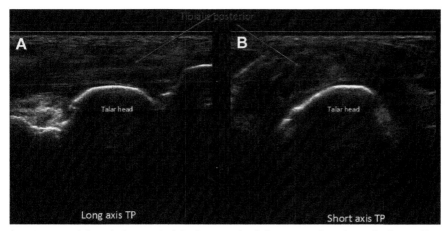

Fig. 12. Long (*A*) and short axis (*B*) ultrasound of the TP tendon through the midfoot demonstrating a tear of the SMCNL. The TP tendon rests directly on the talar head.

best first study is radiograph with weight bearing.[51] In addition to 3 views of the foot, weight-bearing anteroposterior (AP) foot with 20° craniocaudal angulation can be useful in the setting of suspected Lisfranc injury.

When a patient is unable to stand for weight-bearing radiographs but clinical examination is concerning for Lisfranc injury, MRI and CT are the next best test[44,52–55] (**Figs. 16–18**). Non–weight-bearing radiographs may miss Lisfranc injury in up to 10% of cases.[56] Superior sensitivity has been reported with 3-D volumetric acquisitions compared with orthogonal proton density fat-suppressed sequences.[57] With unstable Lisfranc injuries, MRI has high correlation with intraoperative findings,[58] with a reported sensitivity of 83% for traumatic injuries of the ligaments of the foot and ankle.[59] In the setting of significant Lisfranc injury, ultrasound may be another useful tool.[60]

Hallux Sesamoid Complex and Lesser Toe Plantar Plate

Suspected plantar plate injury at the first MTP joint is initially best assessed with weight-bearing AP, lateral, and axial sesamoid radiographs.[61] Including the contralateral side for comparison aids in assessment. Less subtle variations of these injuries include sesamoid fractures, which are readily visualized with plain radiographs (**Fig. 19**). Additionally, medial and lateral 40° oblique views offer better visualization

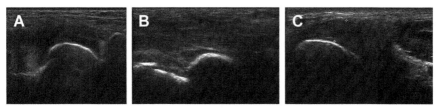

Fig. 13. (*A*) Expanded, hypoechoic partially torn spring ligament. (*B*) TP tendon applied directly to medial talar head articular cartilage consistent with complete tear of the spring ligament. (*C*) Chronic sprain with thickened SMCNL measuring up to 6.4 mm.

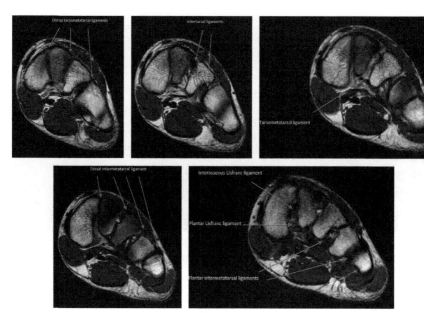

Fig. 14. Axial foot proton density–WI MRI. Lisfranc joint ligamentous complex.

of each sesamoid.[62] The axial sesamoid view illustrates the coronal positioning of the sesamoids relative to their sulci in the metatarsal head. In the case of capsular avulsions, a small fleck of bone can be observed adjacent to the proximal phalanx[63] (**Fig. 20**). CT scan can aid in delineating fractures of the sesamoid (**Fig. 21**) and can

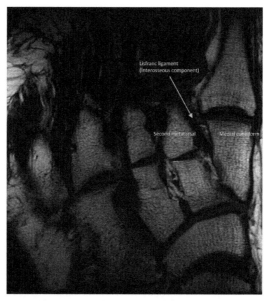

Fig. 15. Coronal proton density–weighted MRI of foot. Normal appearance of Lisfranc ligament.

Table 8 MRI feature of the Lisfranc ligament complex	
Dorsal TMT ligaments	Short, flat, homogenous best seen on sagittal and coronal images
Second plantar TMT (plantar Lisfranc) ligament	Best seen on axial and transverse oblique images Or short axis coronal plane
Lisfranc ligament	Length 7–11 mm Width 4–8 mm Thickness 5–9 mm[44] Oblique band Best seen on oblique axial long-axis images of foot[45]

better show erosions and sclerosis.[63] A CT arthrogram of the MTP joint can show tears of the capsuloligamentous complex; an example is shown in the second MTP joint (**Fig. 22**).

Under fluoroscopic assessment or on manual dorsiflexion lateral view of the MTP joint, the hallux sesamoids will not track distally when the plantar plate is disrupted.[61] A cadaveric biomechanical study demonstrated that 3 mm of increased sesamoid motion relative to the intact contralateral side is predictive of deficiency in 3 or more plantar ligaments.[64] This test can also enhance diastasis of bipartite or fractured sesamoids.[65]

Using high-resolution ultrasound, partial and complete tears of the plantar plate can also be detected and the soft tissue envelope at the first MTP joint can be assessed.[66,67] MRI, however, has been shown to be more accurate than ultrasound in diagnosing plantar plate tears.[68] MRI is the most robust modality to visualize soft tissues and cartilage around the MTP joint.

The non–fat-suppressed T1-weighted sequence or the proton density–weighted sequence should be used to visualize the anatomy.[69] Meanwhile, fluid and edema, suggestive of acute injury, is best visualized with fat-suppressed proton density–weighted sequences or short tau inversion recovery (STIR) sequences.[69]

The following structures are typically well seen on routine clinical MRI: sesamoid-phalangeal ligaments, metatarsal sesamoid ligaments, intersesamoid ligament (**Fig. 23**), MTP joint capsule, and collateral ligaments as well as the flexor and extensor tendons[69] (**Figs. 23** and **24**).

The plantar plate is best seen in the coronal and sagittal planes. A heterogeneous signal represents a plantar plate injury on a spectrum from partial to complete

Table 9 Imaging findings in Lisfranc injury	
Radiographs	• Malalignment of the TMT joints[46,47] • Gap between first and second metatarsals greater than 2 mm is suggestive of tear[48] • Complete tear = displacement of second metatarsal and medial cuneiform[48] • Bone avulsions: the fleck sign[49] • Associated fractures in 90% of cases[49]
MRI	Tear = complete absence or fragmentation of Lisfranc ligament[50]

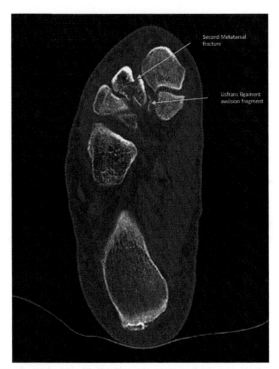

Fig. 16. Coronal CT foot. Acute Lisfranc fracture dislocation.

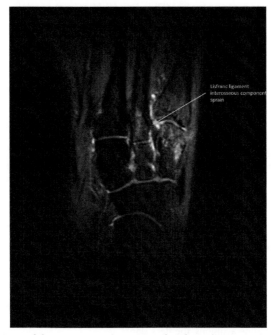

Fig. 17. Coronal STIR of foot. Low-grade sprain of Lisfranc ligament interosseous component: heterogenous signal within Lisfranc ligament surrounding soft tissue edema signal; bone marrow edema signal.

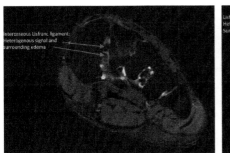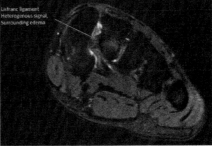

Fig. 18. Fat-saturated T2-WI MRI axial foot. Acute Lisfranc sprain.

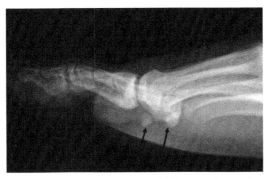

Fig. 19. Lateral radiograph demonstrating sesamoid fracture (*arrows*).

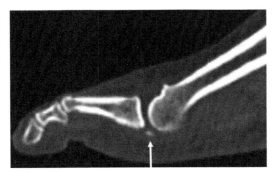

Fig. 20. Lateral CT foot demonstrating an avulsed fleck of bone (*arrow*) reflecting capsular avulsion at the second MTP joint.

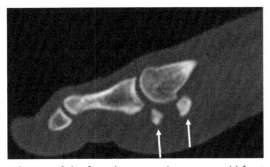

Fig. 21. Lateral CT reformat of the foot demonstrating a sesamoid fracture (*arrows*).

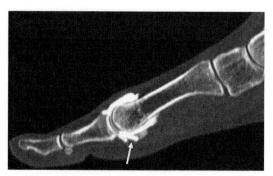

Fig. 22. CT arthrogram lateral reformat demonstrating contrast extensions (*arrow*) through tears in the plantar plate of the second MTP joint.

tear[70] (**Figs. 25** and **26**). The addition of MR arthrography has been shown to improve visualization of these structures.[71]

The lesser MTP joints are also subject to plantar plate injury. MRI is the modality of choice and injuries appear as described for the first MTP joint. A recent study described other morphologic findings on routine MRIs that suggest plantar plate injury, such as pericapsular fibrosis, plantar-plate-proximal phalanx distance, and thinning or nonvisualization of the plantar plate.[72]

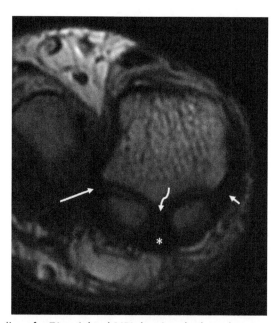

Fig. 23. Coronal slice of a T1-weighted MRI showing the lateral metatarsal sesamoid ligament (*long white arrow*), medial metatarsal sesamoid ligament (*short white arrow*), intersesamoid ligament with low signal intensity (*curved white arrow*), flexor hallucis longus tendon (*asterisk*) below.

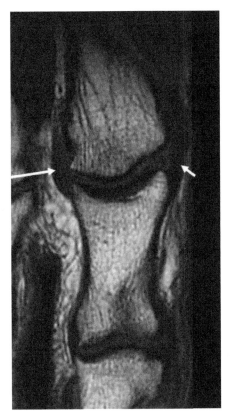

Fig. 24. Axial T1-weighted MRI slice showing the lateral collateral ligament (*long white arrow*) and medial collateral ligament (*short white arrow*) of the first MTP joint.

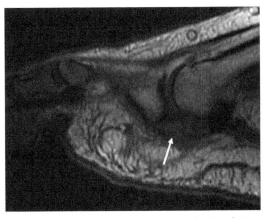

Fig. 25. Sagittal proton density–sequence demonstrating plantar plate partial tear with heterogeneous signal (*white arrow*).

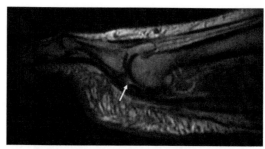

Fig. 26. Sagittal proton density–sequence demonstrating intermediate signal intensity region of plantar plate rupture (*white arrow*).

SUMMARY

The foot and ankle ligaments commonly contributing to clinical instability can be assessed in exquisite detail with MRI. Other imaging modalities have a role in the work-up of ligamentous instabilities; the first test is typically a routine radiographic series. This review has described the role of imaging and relevant findings in the work of instabilities of the foot and ankle.

ACKNOWLEDGMENTS

Mayfair Diagnostics for donating MRI time.

REFERENCES

1. Langner I, Frank M, Kuehn JP, et al. Acute inversion injury of the ankle without radiological abnormalities: assessment with high-field MR imaging and correlation of findings with clinical outcome. Skeletal Radiol 2011;40(4):423–30.
2. Nakasa T, Fukuhara K, Adachi N, et al. Evaluation of anterior talofibular ligament lesion using 3-dimensional computed tomography. J Comput Assist Tomogr 2006;30(3):543–7.
3. Dimmick S, Kennedy D, Daunt N. Evaluation of thickness and appearance of anterior talofibular and calcaneofibular ligaments in normal versus abnormal ankles with MRI. J Med Imaging Radiat Oncol 2008;52(6):559–63.
4. Milner CE, Soames RW. Anatomy of the collateral ligaments of the human ankle joint. Foot Ankle Int 1998;19(11):757–60.
5. Boonthathip M, Chen L, Trudell D, et al. Lateral ankle ligaments: MR arthrography with anatomic correlation in cadavers. Clin Imaging 2011;35(1):42–8.
6. Griffith JF, Brockwell J. Diagnosis and imaging of ankle instability. Foot Ankle Clin 2006;11(3):475–96.
7. Rosenberg ZS, Beltran J, Bencardino JT. From the RSNA refresher courses. Radiological Society of North America. MR imaging of the ankle and foot. Radiographics 2000;20(Spec No):S153–79.
8. Mesgarzadeh M, Schneck CD, Tehranzadeh J, et al. Magnetic resonance imaging of ankle ligaments. Emphasis on anatomy and injuries to lateral collateral ligaments. Magn Reson Imaging Clin N Am 1994;2(1):39–58.
9. Verhaven EF, Shahabpour M, Handelberg FW, et al. The accuracy of three-dimensional magnetic resonance imaging in the diagnosis of ruptures of the lateral ligaments of the ankle. Am J Sports Med 1991;19(6):583–7.

10. Muhle C, Frank LR, Rand T, et al. Collateral ligaments of the ankle: high-resolution MR imaging with a local gradient coil and anatomic correlation in cadavers. Radiographics 1999;19(3):673–83.

11. Sconfienza LM, Orlandi D, Lacelli F, et al. Dynamic high-resolution US of ankle and midfoot ligaments: normal anatomic structure and imaging technique. Radiographics 2015;35(1):164–78.

12. Gyftopoulos S, Bencardino JT. Normal variants and pitfalls in MR imaging of the ankle and foot. Magn Reson Imaging Clin N Am 2010;18(4):691–705.

13. DiGiovann BF, Fraga CJ, Cohen BE, et al. Associated injuries found in chronic lateral ankle instability. Foot Ankle Int 2000;21(10):809–15.

14. Peetrons P, Creteur V, Bacq C. Sonography of ankle ligaments. J Clin Ultrasound 2004;32(9):491–9.

15. Chan KW, Ding BC, Mroczek KJ. Acute and chronic lateral ankle instability in the athlete. Bull NYU Hosp Jt Dis 2011;69(1):17–26.

16. van Dijk CN, Molenaar AH, Cohen RH, et al. Value of arthrography after supination trauma of the ankle. Skeletal Radiol 1998;27(5):256–61.

17. Chandnani VP, Harper MT, Ficke JR, et al. Chronic ankle instability: evaluation with MR arthrography, MR imaging, and stress radiography. Radiology 1994;192(1):189–94.

18. Stiell IG, Greenberg GH, McKnight RD, et al. Decision rules for the use of radiography in acute ankle injuries. Refinement and prospective validation. JAMA 1993;269(9):1127–32.

19. Karchevsky M, Schweitzer ME. Accuracy of plain films, and the effect of experience, in the assessment of ankle effusions. Skeletal Radiol 2004;33(12):719–24.

20. Oae K, Takao M, Uchio Y, et al. Evaluation of anterior talofibular ligament injury with stress radiography, ultrasonography and MR imaging. Skeletal Radiol 2010;39(1):41–7.

21. Guillodo Y, Varache S, Saraux A. Value of ultrasonography for detecting ligament damage in athletes with chronic ankle instability compared to computed arthrotomography. Foot Ankle Spec 2010;3(6):331–4.

22. Mengiardi B, Pfirrmann CW, Vienne P, et al. Medial collateral ligament complex of the ankle: MR appearance in asymptomatic subjects. Radiology 2007;242(3):817–24.

23. Schock HJ, Pinzur M, Manion L, et al. The use of gravity or manual-stress radiographs in the assessment of supination-external rotation fractures of the ankle. J Bone Jt Surg Br 2007;89(8):1055–9.

24. Henari S, Banks LN, Radovanovic I, et al. Ultrasonography as a diagnostic tool in assessing deltoid ligament injury in supination external rotation fractures of the ankle. Orthopedics 2011;34(10):e639–43.

25. Ray RG, Kriz BM. Anterior inferior tibiofibular ligament. Variations and relationship to the talus. J Am Podiatr Med Assoc 1991;81(9):479–85.

26. Norkus SA, Floyd RT. The anatomy and mechanisms of syndesmotic ankle sprains. J Athl Train 2001;36(1):68–73.

27. Rosenberg ZS, Cheung YY, Beltran J, et al. Posterior intermalleolar ligament of the ankle: normal anatomy and MR imaging features. AJR Am J Roentgenol 1995;165(2):387–90.

28. Oh CS, Won HS, Hur MS, et al. Anatomic variations and MRI of the intermalleolar ligament. AJR Am J Roentgenol 2006;186(4):943–7.

29. Takao M, Ochi M, Naito K, et al. Arthroscopic diagnosis of tibiofibular syndesmosis disruption. Arthroscopy 2001;17(8):836–43.

30. Brown KW, Morrison WB, Schweitzer ME, et al. MRI findings associated with distal tibiofibular syndesmosis injury. AJR Am J Roentgenol 2004;182(1):131–6.

31. Hardy RH. Observations on the structure and properties of the plantar calcaneo-navicular ligament in man. J Anat 1951;85(2):135–9.

32. Davis WH, Sobel M, DiCarlo EF, et al. Gross, histological, and microvascular anatomy and biomechanical testing of the spring ligament complex. Foot Ankle Int 1996;17(2):95–102.

33. Smith EB. Astragalo-calcaneo-navicular joint. J Anat Physiol 1896;30(Pt 3):390–412.

34. Pisani G. "Coxa pedis" today. Foot Ankle Surg 2016;22(2):78–84.

35. Pisani G, Milano L. The ligamentous component in dysplasia of the "coxa pedis". Chir Organi Mov 1982;68(4–6):717–26 [in Italian].

36. Mengiardi B, Pinto C, Zanetti M. Spring ligament complex and posterior tibial tendon: MR anatomy and findings in acquired adult flatfoot deformity. Semin Musculoskelet Radiol 2016;20(1):104–15.

37. Kiter E, Gunal I, Karatosun V, et al. The relationship between the tibialis posterior tendon and the accessory navicular. Ann Anat 2000;182(1):65–8.

38. Pisani G. Peritalar destabilisation syndrome (adult flatfoot with degenerative glenopathy). Foot Ankle Surg 2010;16(4):183–8.

39. Omar H, Saini V, Wadhwa V, et al. Spring ligament complex: Illustrated normal anatomy and spectrum of pathologies on 3T MR imaging. Eur J Radiol 2016;85(11):2133–43.

40. Patil V, Ebraheim NA, Frogameni A, et al. Morphometric dimensions of the calcaneonavicular (spring) ligament. Foot Ankle Int 2007;28(8):927–32.

41. Benjamin M, Toumi H, Ralphs JR, et al. Where tendons and ligaments meet bone: attachment sites ('entheses') in relation to exercise and/or mechanical load. J Anat 2006;208(4):471–90.

42. Tryfonidis M, Jackson W, Mansour R, et al. Acquired adult flat foot due to isolated plantar calcaneonavicular (spring) ligament insufficiency with a normal tibialis posterior tendon. Foot Ankle Surg 2008;14(2):89–95.

43. Vogl TJ, Hochmuth K, Diebold T, et al. Magnetic resonance imaging in the diagnosis of acute injured distal tibiofibular syndesmosis. Invest Radiol 1997;32(7):401–9.

44. Castro M, Melao L, Canella C, et al. Lisfranc joint ligamentous complex: MRI with anatomic correlation in cadavers. AJR Am J Roentgenol 2010;195(6):W447–55.

45. Rosenberg ZS, Beltran J. Magnetic resonance imaging and computed tomography of the ankle and foot. In: Myerson MS, editor. Foot and ankle disorders, vol. 1. Philadelphia: Saunders; 1998. p. 123–56.

46. Rankine JJ, Nicholas CM, Wells G, et al. The diagnostic accuracy of radiographs in Lisfranc injury and the potential value of a craniocaudal projection. AJR Am J Roentgenol 2012;198(4):W365–9.

47. Shapiro MS, Wascher DC, Finerman GA. Rupture of Lisfranc's ligament in athletes. Am J Sports Med 1994;22(5):687–91.

48. Cheung Y, Rosenberg ZS. MR imaging of ligamentous abnormalities of the ankle and foot. Magn Reson Imaging Clin N Am 2001;9(3):507–31, x.

49. Myerson MS, Fisher RT, Burgess AR, et al. Fracture dislocations of the tarsometatarsal joints: end results correlated with pathology and treatment. Foot Ankle 1986;6(5):225–42.

50. Resnick D, Niwayama G. Osteonecrosis: diagnostic techniques, specific situations, and complications. In: Resnick D, Niwayama G, editors. Diagnosis of bone and joint disorders. Philadelphia: W, B. Saunders; 1995. p. 3495–558.

51. <ACR Appropriateness Criteria - Acute Trauma to the Foot.pdf>.

52. Melao L, Canella C, Weber M, et al. Ligaments of the transverse tarsal joint complex: MRI-anatomic correlation in cadavers. AJR Am J Roentgenol 2009;193(3): 662–71.

53. Preidler KW, Peicha G, Lajtai G, et al. Conventional radiography, CT, and MR imaging in patients with hyperflexion injuries of the foot: diagnostic accuracy in the detection of bony and ligamentous changes. AJR Am J Roentgenol 1999;173(6): 1673–7.

54. Haapamaki VV, Kiuru MJ, Koskinen SK. Ankle and foot injuries: analysis of MDCT findings. AJR Am J Roentgenol 2004;183(3):615–22.

55. Ting AY, Morrison WB, Kavanagh EC. MR imaging of midfoot injury. Magn Reson Imaging Clin N Am 2008;16(1):105–15, vi.

56. Arntz CT, Veith RG, Hansen ST Jr. Fractures and fracture-dislocations of the tarsometatarsal joint. J Bone Joint Surg Am 1988;70(2):173–81.

57. Ulbrich EJ, Zubler V, Sutter R, et al. Ligaments of the Lisfranc joint in MRI: 3D-SPACE (sampling perfection with application optimized contrasts using different flip-angle evolution) sequence compared to three orthogonal proton-density fat-saturated (PD fs) sequences. Skeletal Radiol 2013;42(3):399–409.

58. Raikin SM, Elias I, Dheer S, et al. Prediction of midfoot instability in the subtle Lisfranc injury. Comparison of magnetic resonance imaging with intraoperative findings. J Bone Joint Surg Am 2009;91(4):892–9.

59. Kuwada GT. Surgical correlation of preoperative MRI findings of trauma to tendons and ligaments of the foot and ankle. J Am Podiatr Med Assoc 2008;98(5): 370–3.

60. Woodward S, Jacobson JA, Femino JE, et al. Sonographic evaluation of Lisfranc ligament injuries. J Ultrasound Med 2009;28(3):351–7.

61. McCormick JJ, Anderson RB. Turf toe: anatomy, diagnosis, and treatment. Sports Health 2010;2(6):487–94.

62. York PJ, Wydra FB, Hunt KJ. Injuries to the great toe. Curr Rev Musculoskelet Med 2017;10(1):104–12.

63. Srinivasan R. The Hallucal-sesamoid complex: normal anatomy, imaging, and pathology. Semin Musculoskelet Radiol 2016;20(2):224–32.

64. Waldrop NE 3rd, Zirker CA, Wijdicks CA, et al. Radiographic evaluation of plantar plate injury: an in vitro biomechanical study. Foot Ankle Int 2013;34(3):403–8.

65. McCormick JJ, Anderson RB. The great toe: failed turf toe, chronic turf toe, and complicated sesamoid injuries. Foot Ankle Clin 2009;14(2):135–50.

66. Khoury V, Guillin R, Dhanju J, et al. Ultrasound of ankle and foot: overuse and sports injuries. Semin Musculoskelet Radiol 2007;11(2):149–61.

67. Nery C, Baumfeld D, Umans H, et al. MR imaging of the plantar plate: normal anatomy, turf toe, and other injuries. Magn Reson Imaging Clin N Am 2017; 25(1):127–44.

68. Duan X, Li L, Wei DQ, et al. Role of magnetic resonance imaging versus ultrasound for detection of plantar plate tear. J Orthop Surg Res 2017;12(1):14.

69. Crain JM, Phancao JP. Imaging of Turf Toe. Radiol Clin North Am 2016;54(5): 969–78.

70. Yao L, Do HM, Cracchiolo A, et al. Plantar plate of the foot: findings on conventional arthrography and MR imaging. AJR Am J Roentgenol 1994;163(3):641–4.

71. Theumann NH, Pfirrmann CW, Mohana Borges AV, et al. Metatarsophalangeal joint of the great toe: normal MR, MR arthrographic, and MR bursographic findings in cadavers. J Comput Assist Tomogr 2002;26(5):829–38.

72. Yamada AF, Crema MD, Nery C, et al. Second and third metatarsophalangeal plantar plate tears: diagnostic performance of direct and indirect MRI features using surgical findings as the reference standard. AJR Am J Roentgenol 2017; 209(2):W100–8.

Acute Lateral Ankle Instability

Kim Slater, MB BS, FRACS, FaORTHA*

KEYWORDS

- Acute • Lateral • Ankle • Ligament • Injury

KEY POINTS

- Acute injuries to the lateral ankle complex are common and in sports may result in significant player time lost.
- Grading of lateral ankle ligament injuries can still be classed I to III; however, it is more appropriate to determine if an ankle is mechanically stable or unstable.
- All grades of lateral ankle ligament injury can be successfully treated using rest, ice, compression, and elevation initially, followed by functional treatment in a semirigid brace with a low complication rate.
- Patients who develop chronic ankle instability can be successfully treated with delayed anatomic repair of the lateral ankle ligaments.
- Early surgical repair of the unstable ankle can be considered in elite athletes, with promising results and improved objective stability.

ANATOMY

The lateral ankle complex is composed of the anterior talofibular ligament (ATFL), the calcaneofibular ligament (CFL), and the posterior talofibular ligament. Other structures contributing to the stability of the lateral ankle include the distal tibiofibular syndesmosis, the peroneal tendons, and the lateral talocalcaneal ligaments.

MECHANISM OF INJURY

The majority of acute lateral ankle sprains occur with the ankle in a position of plantar flexion and inversion. With the foot plantar flexed, the ATFL acts as a virtual collateral ligament, which is why it is believed to rupture first and more commonly than the CFL (**Fig. 1**).[1]

INCIDENCE

The incidence of acute injury to the lateral ankle complex is estimated at approximately 1 per day for each 10,000 individuals[2]; however, it is considerably higher in the sporting population, in particular those involved in ball sports, such as soccer,

Disclosure: The author has nothing to disclose.
Mater Private Hospital, North Sydney, New South Wales, Australia
* Corresponding author. Mater Clinic, Wollstonecraft, New South Wales 2065, Australia.
E-mail address: hks1@optusnet.com.au

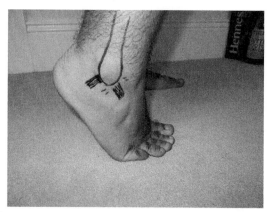

Fig. 1. In plantarflexion, the ATFL acts as a collateral ligament of the ankle, leading to a higher rate of injury than the CFL.

rugby, basketball, and volleyball, as well as in dance.[3] Approximately 20% to 25% of sports-related injuries are represented by lateral ankle complex injuries, resulting in the main contributor to player time lost. Similarly, the economic implications of time lost at work are significant after these injuries.[4]

CLINICAL PRESENTATION AND HISTORY

The patient with an acutely injured ankle presents with a history of the ankle giving way, or rolling, and there may be both intrinsic and extrinsic factors involved. The intrinsic factors include generalized ligamentous laxity, hindfoot varus, pes cavus, and, in the case of a previously injured ankle, any underlying mechanical instability that may predispose to a further acute injury. Extrinsic factors include the nature of the surface over which a patient or player is maneuvering as well as outside agencies that raise the center of gravity of the ankle and increase the likelihood of inversion, such as another player's foot, uneven surfaces, or shoe wear (ie, long cleats). A patient may describe a "pop" or a "crack", which raises the likelihood of a complete rupture of the ATFL and/or the CFL. A history of inability to bear weight after an injury raises the suspicion of an associated osteochondral lesion of the talar dome (OCD) or fracture (**Fig. 2**).

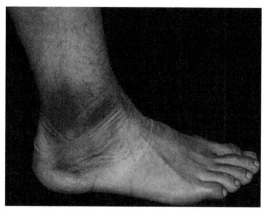

Fig. 2. The acutely sprained ankle shows features of swelling and bruising. Potential for damage to structures other than the ligaments should always be considered, especially with a history of inability to bear weight.

PHYSICAL EXAMINATION

After an acute lateral ankle ligament injury, a patient has swelling, bruising, and possibly a large hematoma in the perifibular region. The patient is generally limping but may present with an inability to weight bear due to a high severity of pain, in which case consideration needs to be given to the possibility of an underlying fracture or an intra-articular lesion, such as an osteochondral injury. Clinicians require an understanding of the potential for damage to associated structures, including the tibiofibular syndesmosis, and the medial complex, including the deltoid ligament, tibiotalar cartilage, peroneal tendons, and base of the fifth metatarsal, which are exposed to potential injury with an inversion mechanism (**Figs. 3** and **4**).

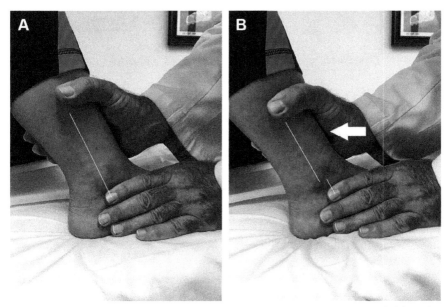

Fig. 3. Performing the anterior drawer test for ATFL integrity may be more reliable with a patient supine, with the hip and knee flexed. The foot is fixed (*A*), and firm pressure is applied to the distal tibia (*B*). This test can be performed reliably in the acute setting, and complements the same test performed with the patient sitting.

- Delayed physical examination shows a sensitivity of 96% in comparison with stress radiography, arthrography, and ultrasound in identifying ATFL rupture (level 2).[5]

INVESTIGATIONS

Studies have shown that many acute ankle sprain patients attend emergency departments or family practitioners and have radiographs, which may not be necessary.[1,5] The Ottawa ankle rules outline indications for radiological investigation, and these rules have been applied effectively to significantly reduce the unnecessary use of radiographs after these injuries.[5] The rules are outlined here:

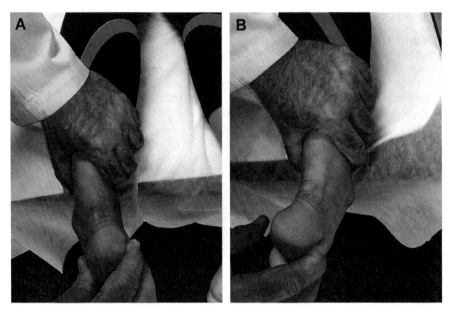

Fig. 4. The talar tilt test for CFL integrity can be performed with the patient prone. A firm endpoint is identified in a normal ankle (*A*), but increased laxity can be appreciated when the CFL has been damaged, as seen on the right (*B*). This test can be performed reliably in the acute setting.

Examination of bone tenderness over the posterior 6 cm of each malleolus, base of the fifth metatarsal, or medial tuberosity of the navicula raises suspicion for an underlying fracture and indicates the need for radiographs. Also, inability to weight bear at the time of injury or inability to take 4 steps at the time of examination satisfies the criteria for radiographic studies.[6]

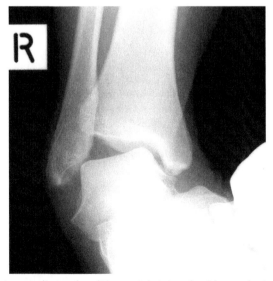

Fig. 5. Although stress radiographs of the acutely injured ankle may be impressive, they are considered unreliable in terms of planning treatment or in determining prognosis.

- The Ottawa ankle/foot rules have a sensitivity of 99% for the identification of fractures, when applied within 48 hours of injury.[6–8]

Stress radiographs are no longer commonly used in view of operator dependency and the minimal advantage over careful clinical examination, especially when physical examination is repeated at 4 days to 5 days postinjury (**Fig. 5**).[9,10]

Ultrasound

Oae and colleagues[11] noted 91% accuracy of ultrasound in detecting an acute ATFL tear compared with 97% for MRI. Due to operator dependency, ultrasound is not recommended as a first-line diagnostic tool.[2,12,13]

Arthrography has a similar sensitivity to delayed clinical examination; however, it is invasive and indirect and is rarely used in modern sports medicine.[14]

MRI

Radiologists may not have been able to discern the degree of ligament damage on MRI scans using a 1.5T magnet; however, the advent of 3T MRI scanners has resulted in far superior images, capable of fat suppression and excellent tissue imaging, to the extent that images now correlate closely with the clinical picture, and experienced MRI radiologists can grade the injury. In this way, the 3T MRI can be used as an independent predictor of clinical outcome and, therefore, may be beneficial in deciding treatment, especially in elite athletes (**Figs. 6–8**).[15,16]

In elite athletes, MRI is the preferred imaging modality, because it gives excellent detail regarding possible OCDs, the deltoid complex, the inferior tibiofibular syndesmosis, and the integrity of the peroneal tendons as well as imaging the lateral ankle ligament complex.

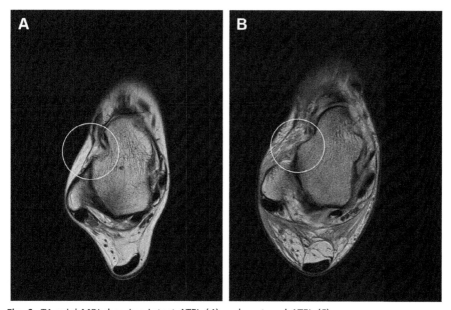

Fig. 6. T1 axial MRI showing intact ATFL (*A*) and ruptured ATFL (*B*).

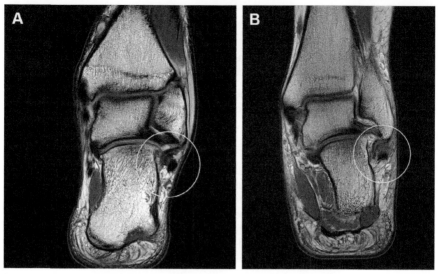

Fig. 7. Coronal T1 MRI showing intact CFL (*A*) and ruptured CFL (*B*).

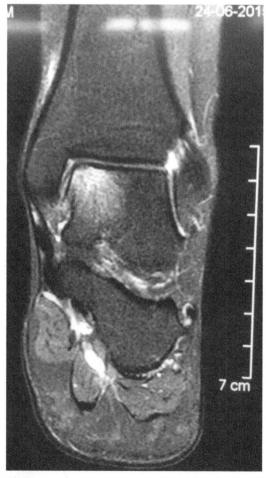

Fig. 8. Coronal MRI T2 image of an acute medial talar dome osteochondral lesion. Note the associated bone edema. These patients virtually always describe a period of inability to bear weight after their injury.

GRADING OF LATERAL ANKLE SPRAINS

Historically, lateral ankle sprains were graded I, II, or III based on a clinician's physical assessment of the ankle, where a grade I injury was considered a strain of the lateral ankle complex and grade III was a complete rupture of both the ATFL and CFL. In terms of functional grading, these injuries should be considered either stable or unstable.[5]

Therefore, a grade I injury involves a strain of the ATFL and/or the CFL without rupture, a grade II injury involves rupture of the ATFL but an intact CFL, and a grade III injury involves a complete rupture of both the ATFL and CFL. A grade III injury may involve rupture of the posterior talofibular "ligament;" however, this ligament is generally believed to rupture only in cases of ankle dislocation. Thus, the determination of whether an ankle is stable or unstable revolves around the differentiation between grade II and grade III injuries (**Table 1**).

Not all acute lateral ankle complex inversion injuries result in mechanical instability. Therefore, mechanical instability and functional instability need to be defined and how best to grade, assess, and treat these injuries considered.

- Mechanical instability is the objective finding of greater than normal (for a particular patient) laxity in the components of the lateral ankle complex, mainly the ATFL and CFL.
- Functional instability is the subjective patient experience of giving way or weakness during daily activities or sport.

This article does not address syndesmosis injuries, ankle fractures, and peroneal tendon injuries; however, those conditions may need to be considered in the differential of lateral ankle ligament injuries along with the possibility of subtalar joint instability, which may be difficult to assess even in the hands of experienced clinicians. The management of chronic lateral ankle instability of the ankle (CAI) is discussed in David A. Porter and Kreigh A. Kamman's article, "Chronic Lateral Ankle Instability: Open Surgical Management," in this issue.

PATHOLOGY OF LIGAMENT HEALING

The concern with inadequate ligament healing is that it may predispose to recurrent injury, CAI, and possibly posttraumatic osteoarthrosis (OA).[12] This sequence of events is seen more commonly in the knee, for example, after ACL injury, and there is debate about whether ACL reconstruction can prevent the onset or progression of posttraumatic OA.[12] It seems in the ankle that there is a less direct relationship between instability and the development of posttraumatic arthrosis than in the knee; however, OA remains an underlying concern for clinicians in the long-term management of these ankle injuries.

Table 1 Schematic of potential clinical instability			
Grade	Anterior Drawer (Anterior Talofibular Ligament)	Talar Tilt (Calcaneofibular Ligament)	Stability
I	Negative	Negative	Stable
II	Positive	Negative	+/− Stable
III	Positive	Positive	Unstable

The optimum result is ligamentous tissue healing as near to normal as possible, reducing the incidence of recurrent instability, and hopefully reducing the incidence of long-term OA.

- The normal ligament is composed predominantly of type 1 collagen with parallel bundles of collagen aligned with the lines of tensile stress. Microscopic studies have shown that with ligament strain there is a certain amount of elastic give, up to a point where the ligament may no longer withstand the force applied and in this situation it may rupture.
- Ligaments also have a proprioceptive function, and it is believed that mechano-receptors, such as Golgi organs, and specialized nerve endings, such as Pacinian corpuscles, provide feedback to fine tune muscular balance and control.[12] This in turn leads to dynamic stabilization of joints.
- When a ligament is injured, the inflammatory phase of healing begins immediately and continues for 48 hours to 72 hours. There is initial bleeding and clot formation, with release of healing growth factors from the platelets within the clot, and this is followed by activation of numerous growth factors, including neovascular factors and fibroblast growth factors. This histologic process aims to initiate the repair process after cellular damage.
- The proliferative or regenerative phase involves the influx of immune cells, further growth factors, and cytokines. There is fibroblast migration into the inflamed scar tissue, and these cells begin to lay down collagen and protein matrix; however, the collagen laid down is not type 1 collagen, although it does begin to align with lines of stress within the original ligament.
- Several weeks after the initial injury, the regenerative phase merges with the remodeling phase; this is the stage during which collagen maturation occurs and may last for months or up to a year after the original injury. Histologic studies during the remodeling phase show that this tissue is not the same as the original ligament biochemically, histologically, or biomechanically.
- Type 1 collagen confers stiffness, stability, and strength to a normal ligament; however, the type 3 collagen seen after injury is a result of fibroblast activity, which produces smaller-diameter collagen fibrils, less densely packed than in a normal ligament.
- In the months after the original injury, this remodeled collagenous scar tissue responds to extrinsic stressors and applied loads, and the ultimate functionality of that repair process depends largely on the quality of the tissue and the loads applied.[12]

TREATMENT

Advances in all fields of medicine in the twenty-first century have seen health professionals questioning treatment protocols and insurers and health departments demanding evidence-based support for patient treatment. This has resulted in systematic reviews of available literature as well as further research to answer the relevant questions about clinical interventions, including the management of lateral ankle ligament injuries. The Cochrane collaboration and the Kerkhoffs, van Dijk, et al have been at the forefront of examining the following questions with meta-analyses: What is the place of immobilization in the acutely injured ankle? What are the results of "functional treatment?" Is bracing preferable to taping? Is neuromuscular or proprioceptive training important? What is the place of surgical intervention in the acutely injured ankle?[17]

This article aims to address these questions and provide a reasonable contemporary approach to the management of these injuries.

WHAT IS KNOWN ABOUT TREATMENT OPTIONS FOR ACUTE LATERAL ANKLE SPRAINS?

- Stable lateral ankle complex injuries should be treated nonoperatively with ice, compression, and elevation (RICE), with the expectation of a good prognosis (level 1).[7]
- Numerous randomized controlled trials (RCTs) support functional treatment over immobilization, due to quicker recovery, greater patient satisfaction, and lower cost (level 1).[7]
- A semirigid ankle brace is more convenient and cost-effective than tape or an elastic bandage in the acute ankle sprain (level 2).[13]
- Unstable ankle sprains (grade II or III) should be treated nonoperatively with a semirigid ankle brace, early functional treatment, and supervised rehabilitation or physical therapy (level 2).[13]
- Cryotherapy is effective in reducing pain and swelling in acute ankle sprains when used in the first 3 days to 5 days (level 1).[7]
- Nonsteroidal anti-inflammatory drugs (NSAIDs) reduce pain and analgesic requirements when used in the first 3 days to 5 days postinjury (level 1). They should not be used, however, other than in the short term due to the adverse effects on cellular healing.[7]

Consideration should be given to patient factors when deciding on preferred treatment. Even the time-honored treatment of acute lateral ankle sprains with RICE has been questioned, and Kerkhoffs and colleagues[4] found "insufficient evidence from RCTs to determine the relative effectiveness of RICE therapy for acute sprains in adults." Despite this meta-analysis of 11 trials, including 868 patients, there was no clear evidence that RICE was deleterious; therefore, it remains a reasonable and widely used first line of treatment. Patients can expect good recovery in terms of mobility, function, pain, and swelling within 3 weeks of a grade I injury.

Van Rijn and colleagues[14] reported that after 1 year, 5% to 33% of patients after lateral ligament injury still had complaints of pain and instability (level 1).

There remains controversy about the management of grade II and grade III injuries. Factors to consider include the following: Is the ankle mechanically stable or unstable? What methods have been proved to optimize recovery and return to sport or return to work? Are there modalities available to reduce the rate of resprain over time?

Immobilization

Kerkhoffs and colleagues[4] examined 21 RCTs involving 2184 adult patients and concluded that functional treatment was superior to immobilization for 4 weeks to 6 weeks.

Petersen and colleagues'[13] review, however, recommended caution in interpretation of these results, because many were poorly reported, with variation in the functional treatments used.[13] Further RCTs found that a period of up to 10 days' immobilization for grade III injuries could be advantageous. RICE, despite lacking high-level evidence to support its use, remains the most common and practical method of initial treatment to reduce pain and swelling in the acutely injured ankle.[4]

Kerkhoffs' group[4] noted that several investigators recommended a short period of rest for 5 days to 7 days to reduce the pain and swelling of the inflammatory phase of soft tissue healing, followed by functional stress in the remodeling phase, allowing for improvement in the healing process.

The historical rationale for immobilization has been to reduce activity, thereby reducing pain and swelling, and thus minimizing further damage to the injured ligament and/or joint. Immobilization may be associated, however, with decreased collagen synthesis, formation of synovial adhesions, and the production of poorer quality replacement collagen.

Mobilization and Exercise

Kerkhoffs and colleagues'[4] study showed that functional treatment showed a statistically significant improvement for recovery of the affected joint when compared with immobilization. The patients treated with early active functional treatment were shown to return to work and sports activities sooner than the group who were treated with immobilization. They also had less objective instability (level 2). Other systematic reviews confirmed that early mobilization resulted in less pain, swelling, and stiffness and a quicker return to work.[18–20]

The beneficial effects of early mobilization, including repetitive loading of injured ligaments, have shown improved collagen proliferation and increased soft tissue mass and strength of healing tissue compared with those ligaments immobilized. These findings have been confirmed in animal studies, where it was shown that animals who were allowed to continue exercising had improved strength of repaired ligaments compared with those who were forced to rest.[21]

A functional controlled rehabilitation protocol seems to result in improved healing of ligament tissue as a result of microcellular changes and improved blood supply due to motion. At a cellular level, collagen quality and quantity are improved with motion, and the mobility of a functional rehabilitation program reduces the adverse effects of immobilization, including muscle wasting, stiffness, adhesions, and the formation of inadequate scar response.

Neuromuscular Training

Freeman and colleagues in 1965[22] first demonstrated the advantageous effects of proprioceptive training after a sprained ankle. They postulated that decreased coordination results from articular deafferentiation caused by afferent mechanoreceptor damage during injury.

Petersen and colleagues,[13] in a review article, identified evidence to support neuromuscular training after acute ankle sprains; however, Van Rijn and colleagues' article[23] concluded that "conventional treatment combined with supervised exercises compared to conventional treatment alone does not lead to differences in the occurrence of re-sprains or in subjective recovery, during the 1 year after an acute lateral ankle ligament sprain".

Nonsteroidal Anti-inflammatory Drugs

NSAIDs have been widely used in acute soft tissue injuries, such as ankle sprains; however, more recent research shows that there may be potential adverse effects in terms of soft tissue healing. This is because there may be inhibition of the normal prostaglandin response to injury, with less recruitment of healing cells in the postinjury matrix, and it is now believed that NSAIDs should be used sparingly if at all in the acute setting.[12]

Cortisone Injections

Steroid injections can be effective in terms of reducing immediate pain and swelling; however, they also have adverse effects in terms of preventing neutrophils and inflammatory cells from accumulating at the site of injury as well as disrupting inflammatory mediators and cytokines. Corticosteroid injections have been shown to inhibit fibroblast function and thus collagen synthesis at the site of injection. The quality of collagen tissue examined histologically after corticosteroid injection has been shown to be inferior[12]; therefore, particularly in athletes, these injections should be avoided.

Prolotherapy

Prolotherapy includes the injection of platelet-rich plasma (PRP), and there is some evidence that PRP injections have shown enhancement of the inflammatory healing response with respect to fibroblast activity and neovascular formation as well as growth factor stimulation. Whether this injection or enhancement of platelet activity provides any long-term benefit to the healing ligament remains to be proved.[24]

Paoloni and colleagues[25] in a review article found no scientific evidence in RCTs to support the use of PRP in acute ankle ligament injuries. They did note, however, significant commercial enthusiasm for this new technique.

THE ELITE ATHLETE

An elite athlete can be defined as an individual whose primary occupation relates to sporting endeavors. In most of these competitors, income depends on performance and participation. Given that up to 30% of patients after grade III lateral ankle ligament injury have residual symptoms of pain, swelling, or instability, surgeons have explored the potential for diminishing these residual symptoms by using early surgical repair. Discussion continues regarding the relative benefits and risks of this approach versus traditional nonoperative treatment.[1,10]

The place of Surgery in the Acutely Injured Ankle

Most clinicians and surgeons agree that nonoperative treatment is the preferred management of grade I and grade II lateral ankle ligament injuries.

- Nonoperative treatment of unstable acute lateral ankle ligament injuries, grade II or grade III, is preferred over surgical treatment due to lower complications, lower cost, and satisfactory results in a majority of patients (level 1).[5]
- The question of surgery arises in grade III lateral ankle injuries in the elite athlete. Surgical treatment may be a reasonable option in such an athlete with an unstable ankle, when considered on an individual basis.[1,2,10]

Identification of those patients who may not do well after a grade III injury is difficult. Experienced surgeons or clinicians may form a view at 7 days to 10 days postinjury that the normal healing response is inadequate and that acute repair is warranted. The rationale for recommending surgery at this point is that an elite athlete may be assessed as likely to have recurrent episodes of inversion instability (CAI) or symptoms secondary to postinjury synovitis and, therefore, may be considered candidates for acute repair.

- Due to their high athletic demands, the probability of a resprain in an elite athlete may be higher than in a nonathlete or social athlete.[26]

It is also possible that there is a higher incidence of peroneal tendinopathy and tears in this group, and surgical stabilization may reduce the incidence of these problems later (**Fig. 9**).

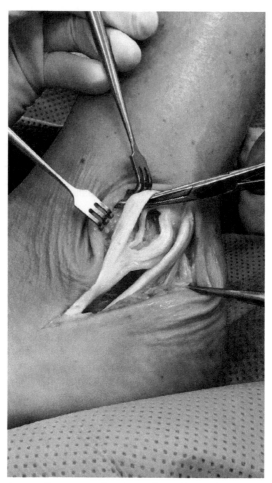

Fig. 9. Longitudinal tear of peroneus brevis tendon. The incidence of peroneal tendinopathy in CAI is another factor to consider when managing an elite athlete.

A surgeon who recommends early surgical stabilization can only justify this course of treatment if the surgeon forms the view that the assessed benefits of surgery outweigh the potential risks of surgery.[2] This is one of the basic principles of surgical intervention. The surgeon is obligated in this case (as in all cases) to explain to the patient the potential risks and benefits of surgical intervention.

There is little doubt that the risks of surgery can be avoided by avoiding surgery. If surgeon and patient agree that the risk of recurrent injury and time lost from sport outweighs the surgical risks, then it may be deemed reasonable to proceed with surgical repair. The particular risks associated with surgery include infection, venous thromboembolism (VTE), stiffness or loss of range, and residual pain due to scar tissue as well as the general risks associated with anesthesia and potential drug reactions (**Table 2**).

What is Known About Surgery in the Elite Athlete?

- Residual mechanical instability of the lateral ankle complex is a determinant of recurrent ankle sprains.[2]

Table 2		
Risks and benefits of surgery versus nonsurgery in acute lateral ankle instability		
	Nonsurgical	**Surgical**
Risks	• Neglect—"it's just a sprain" • Recurrent inversion episodes • Posttraumatic synovitis • CAI • Peroneal tendinopathy or tear • Missed talar dome lesions (OCDs)	• Infection • Thromboembolic disease (VTE) • Stiffness • Slower return to sports/work (historical)
Benefits	• Early functional treatment • Avoidance of surgical risks • More rapid return to sport/work when using semirigid brace	• Improved mechanical stability • Less recurrent instability • Ability to deal with intra-articular pathology, for example, talar dome lesions • Potential for reduced incidence of peroneal tendinopathy and OA

- Lateral ligament repair is a safe and effective treatment option for grade III lateral ankle ligament injury. It provides a stable ankle, with the expectation of return to sport at approximately 3 months (level 3).[2,10]
- Concomitant injuries, such as OCDs, deltoid complex injuries, and syndesmosis injuries, may be associated with residual symptoms and a delay in return to sport.[10]
- High-volume centers with surgeons experienced in lateral ankle ligament repair and reconstruction tend to have better results and lower complication rates than those with less experience.[10]
- Although there may be an appeal to elite athletes and surgeons for acute lateral ankle ligament repair, medically there is no urgency, because the results of later repair or reconstruction are comparable to nonoperative measures and are satisfactory.
- Elite athletes are more likely to be seen by an experienced surgeon as well as dedicated physical therapists, and the time available to these athletes for intensive and more frequent postoperative rehabilitation is often greater than for social athletes with work demands.[2,10] This may reduce the risk of stiffness, muscle wasting, and VTE.
- Over the past 2 decades, more aggressive rehabilitation protocols have been developed, with less postoperative time immobilized in plaster and earlier weight bearing, functional treatment, and mobility. This has significantly reduced recovery time for surgically treated elite athletes, with the result that return to sport is comparable with that seen in cases treated nonoperatively using traditional methods.[2,5,10,26]

SUMMARY

It is the responsibility of foot and ankle surgeons and specialized sports physicians to educate other medical and paramedical staff about the current evidence-based guidelines for the accurate assessment and treatment of acute lateral ankle ligament injuries.

Improvements in outcomes after acute lateral ankle ligament injuries will come more from improved and rigorous study design than from further poorly designed RCTs. This will allow clinicians to clarify the role of newer modalities, such as PRP, and those treatment methods that minimize the rate of resprain and to clearly identify the place of surgery.

Although encouraging results have been achieved with early surgical repair in the acute setting, the level of evidence is 3 to 4, and further RCTs are required to clarify the place of surgical intervention in elite athletes.

The aim of treatment is a stable ankle with less risk of recurrent instability, avoiding residual pain, swelling, peroneal tendinopathy, and long-term OA.

ACKNOWLEDGMENTS

Thank you to Dr James Linklater, Sydney, Australia, for the provision of MRIs.

REFERENCES

1. Kerkhoffs G, Van Dijk N. Acute lateral ankle ligament injuries in the athlete; the role of surgery. Foot Ankle Clin N Am 2013;18:215–8.
2. Van den Bekerom M, Kerkhoffs G, McCollum G, et al. Management of acute lateral ankle ligament injury in the athlete. Knee Surg Sports Traumatol Arthrosc 2013;21:1390–5.
3. Ekstrand J. The incidence of ankle sprains in football. Foot Ankle 1990;11:41–4.
4. Kerkhoffs G, van den Bekerom M, Elders L, et al. Diagnosis, treatment and prevention of ankle sprains: and evidence-based clinical guideline. Br J Sports Med 2012;46:854–60.
5. Van Dijk N, Lim L, Bossuyt P. Physical examination is sufficient for the diagnosis of sprained ankles. J Bone Joint Surg Br 1996;78:958–62.
6. Stiell I, McKnight R, Greenberg G, et al. Implementation of the Ottawa ankle rules. JAMA 1994;271:827–32.
7. Polzer H, Karz K, Prall W, et al. Diagnosis and treatment of acute ankle injuries: development of an evidence-based algorithm. Orthop Rev 2012;4:22–3.
8. Bachmann L, Kolb E, Koller M, et al. Accuracy of Ottawa Ankle Rules to exclude fractures of the ankle and midfoot: systematic review. BMJ 2003;326:417.
9. Frost SC, Amendola A. Is stress radiography necessary in the diagnosis of acute or chronic ankle instability? Clin J Sport Med 1999;9:40–5.
10. White WJ, McCollum GA, Calder JD. Return to sport following acute lateral ligament repair of the ankle in professional athletes. Knee Surg Sports Traumatol Arthrosc 2015;24(4):1124–9.
11. Oae K, Takao M, Uchio T, et al. Evaluation of anterior talofibular ligament injury with stress radiography, ultrasound and MR imaging. Skeletal Radiol 2010; 39(1):41–7.
12. Hauser R. Ligament injury and healing: a review of current clinical diagnostics and therapeutics. Open Rehabil J 2013;6:1–20.
13. Petersen W, Rembitzki I, Koppenberg A, et al. Treatment of acute ankle ligament injuries: a systematic review. Acta Orthop Trauma Surg 2013;133:1129–41.
14. Van Dijk CN, Molenaar AH, Cohen RH, et al. Value of arthrography after supination trauma of the ankle. Skeletal Radiol 1998;27:256–61.
15. Chhabra A, Soldatos T, Charlion M, et al. Current concepts review: 3T magnetic imaging of the ankle and foot. Foot Ankle Int 2012;33(2):164–71.
16. Van Rijn RM, van Os AG, Bernsen RM, et al. What is the clinical course of acute ankle sprains? A systematic literature review. Am J Med 2008;121:324–31.
17. Kerkhoffs G, Handoll H, de Bie R, et al. Surgical versus conservative treatment for acute injuries of the lateral ligament complex of the ankle in adults. Cochrane Database Syst Rev 2002;3:CD000380.

18. Kannus P, Renstrom P. Treatment for acute tears of the lateral ligaments of the ankle. Operation, cast, or early controlled mobilisation. J Bone Joint Surg Am 1991;73:305–12.

19. Tiling T, Bonk A, Hoher J, et al. Acute injury to the lateral ligament of the ankle joint in the athlete. Chirurg 1994;65:920–33.

20. Pijnenburg A, van Dijk CN, Bossuyt PM, et al. Treatment of ruptures of the lateral ankle ligaments: a meta-analysis. J Bone Joint Surg Am 2000;82:761–73.

21. Liu S, Yang R, al-Shaikh R, et al. Collagen in tendon, ligament, and bone healing: a current review. Clin Orthop Relat Res 1995;318:265–78.

22. Freeman M, Dean M, Hanham I. The aetiology and prevention of functional instability of the foot. J Bone Joint Surg Br 1965;47:678–85.

23. Van Rijn R, van Heest J, van der Weest P, et al. Some benefit from physiotherapy intervention in the subgroup of patients with severe ankle sprain as determined by the ankle function score: a randomised trial. Aust J Physiother 2009;55(2):107–13.

24. Moraes V, Lenza M, Falloppa F, et al. Platelet-rich therapies for musculoskeletal soft tissue injuries (review). Cochrane Database Syst Rev 2014;4:CD 010071.

25. Paoloni J, De Vos R, Hamilton B, et al. Platelet-rich plasma treatment for ligament and tendon injuries. Clin J Sport Med 2011;21(1):37–45.

26. Verhagen EA, van der Beek AJ, Bouter L, et al. A one season prospective cohort study of volleyball injuries. Br J Sports Med 2004;38(4):477–81.

Chronic Lateral Ankle Instability

Open Surgical Management

David A. Porter, MD, PhD[a],*, Kreigh A. Kamman, MD[b]

KEYWORDS

- Ankle instability • Modified Brostrom procedure • Lateral ankle ligament
- Open management • Bone tunneling • Video procedure

KEY POINTS

- Repeated ankle sprains with giving way leads to chronic lateral ankle Instability (CLAI).
- Numerous surgical reconstructions have been described for CLAI.
- The current recommendations are for anatomic repair/reconstructions.
- Rehabilitation is crucial to an optimal outcome; the authors' approach is listed, which involves early range-of-motion and intermittent immobilization.

 Video content accompanies this article at http://www.foot.theclinics.com.

INTRODUCTION

Ankle sprains are the most common lower limb musculoskeletal injury in physically active individuals[1]—occurring up to 30,000 times per day in the United States.[2] As one might expect, they are the most common athletic injury reported among collegiate NCAA student-athletes.[3,4] Among these ankle sprains, 85% involve the lateral ankle ligament complex,[5,6] of which the anterior talofibular ligament (ATFL, **Fig. 1**) is most vulnerable to injury, followed by a combined rupture of the ATFL and calcaneofibular ligament (CFL, **Fig. 2**).[7] Fortunately, most lateral ankle sprains (LAS) can be treated nonoperatively and recover uneventfully without long-term consequences (70%–95%).[8,9] Unfortunately, however, recurrence of LAS does occur: there is a 2-fold increased risk of reinjury within 1 year,[10] and up to 34% of patients will reinjure the lateral ankle ligaments within 3 years.[11] Recurrent sprains can lead to attenuation

Disclosure Statement: D.A. Porter is a consultant for Physician Rehab Consultants and a consultant for DJOrthopedics. K. Kamman has nothing to disclose.
[a] Methodist Sports Medicine, Volunteer Clinical Faculty, Department of Orthopedics, Indiana University, 201 Pennsylvania Parkway, Suite 100, Indianapolis, IN 46280, USA; [b] Department of Orthopedics, IU Health University Hospital, 550 N. University Boulevard, Suite 6201, Indianapolis, IN, USA
* Corresponding author.
E-mail address: dporter@methodistsports.com

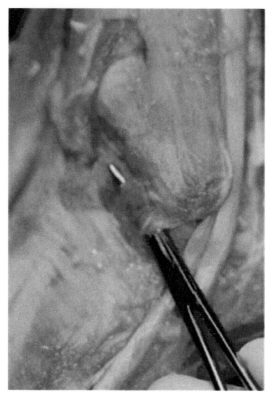

Fig. 1. Lateral view of cadaveric ankle showing ATFL with forceps underneath the ligament. The ATFL is seen originating off the anterior tip of the fibula and inserting on the lateral neck of the talus at the body/neck junction. Note the peroneal tendons posterior to the fibula and overlaying the calcaneal fibular ligament.

of the native lateral ligament complex, surreptitiously giving rise to chronic lateral ankle instability (CLAI), a feeling of giving way by the athlete and nonathlete. This feeling of giving way leads to a lack of confidence in the ankle and concern for recurrent and unexpected instability with sport and even activities of daily living (ADLs).

Up to 70% of patients with an initial LAS may develop secondary symptoms of chronic instability or pain.[6,12] In athletics, CLAI can be present in up to 25% of athletes[13] and even up to 59% of dancers.[14] Affected individuals may continue to experience pain with activity, giving way and recurrent sprains, difficulty walking on uneven ground, and feelings of instability in their ankle leading to persistent disability. These features of CLAI can result in significant time lost at work, in sport, or further disability in up to 60% of patients. Although deformities (ie, hindfoot varus [**Fig. 3A**], midfoot cavus, and so forth) and genetics (ie, ligamentous laxity [**Fig. 4**] and so forth) play a role in injury predisposition to the lateral ankle, the major factor in chronic ankle instability is the combination of mechanical and functional insufficiencies resulting from the initial and then recurrent ankle sprains. Functional insufficiencies alone, however, do not warrant surgery. It is, therefore, important to distinguish between *functional* and *mechanical* lateral ankle instability.

Patients with *functional* instability have subjective complaints about their ankle giving way; however, they can lack clinical and radiographic evidence of tibiotalar (ankle)

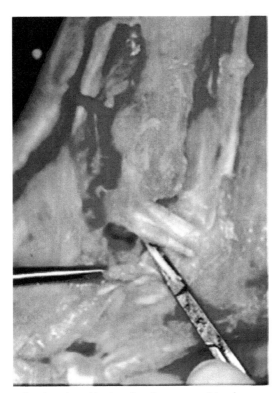

Fig. 2. Lateral view of cadaveric ankle showing the peroneal tendons removed with the CFL exposed and overlying the scissors. Note the CFL originating off the distal tip of the fibula just posterior to the ATFL. This relationship is critical to understand when doing an open Brostrom lateral ankle reconstruction (BLAR). The peroneal muscles will have to be retracted to access the CFL during BLAR.

instability (ie, no evidence of lateral ligament laxity). Factors leading to *functional* instability may include impaired proprioception, diminished neuromuscular control, compromised strength, tight Achilles and weak peroneal muscles, and/or decreased postural control and benefit from a structured rehabilitation program, not surgery. Conversely, patients with *mechanical* instability, exhibit clinical and radiographic evidence of excessive talar tilt within the ankle mortise and/or a significant difference from the contralateral ankle. Factors contributing to mechanical instability include pathologic ligamentous laxity, synovial changes, arthro-kinetic restriction, degenerative changes, and most commonly incompetent or stretched lateral ligaments (ATFL and CFL) due to repeated giving way.

Beyond functional or mechanical instability, the clinical diagnosis of CLAI has often been associated with other pathologic entities. These entities may include intraoperative findings of peroneal tendon pathological conditions (tear, dislocation, tenosynovitis, and so forth), ankle synovitis, anterolateral ankle impingement, talar dome osteochondral lesions (OCLs), intra-articular loose bodies, medial ankle tenosynovitis, and so forth.[15] Indeed, up to 93% of patients with CLAI may have associated intra-articular pathology of the ankle (ie, chondral or osteochondral fractures, synovitis, and so forth).[16] Varus (talar tilt) instability (**Fig. 5**) can shift contact pressures medially over the central medial talus region, potentially leading to OCLs.[17] Recurrent sprains

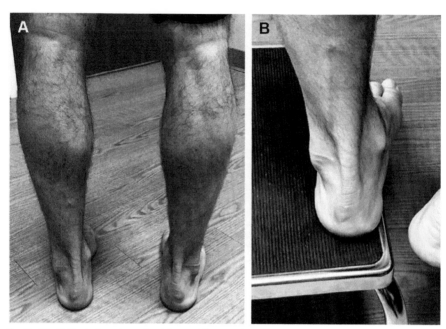

Fig. 3. (*A*, *B*) Posterior view of athlete with varus hindfoot, which leads to lateral foot overload and could require calcaneal and/or first metatarsal osteotomy to correct the varus alignment. (*A*) Hindfoot view showing the heel medially deviated resulting in lateral foot overload with weight bearing and leading to potential failure of a ligamentous lateral ankle reconstruction. (*B*) Coleman block test to evaluate if source of hindfoot varus is due to plantar flexed first ray (first metatarsal osteotomy to correct) or intrinsic varus in the calcaneus (calcaneal osteotomy to correct).

can alter ankle biomechanics, which over time can cause cartilage degeneration and/or spurring. Anterior drawer instability (**Fig. 6**) produces shear forces across the tibial and talar cartilage surfaces, which may lead to cartilage deterioration in chronic cases. Posttraumatic arthritis eventually develops in up to 78% of patients.[18] Therefore, in patients with long-standing CLAI, the need for an accurate diagnosis and appropriate treatment of other associated pathology is crucial. We, therefore, recommend an ankle arthroscopy in association with all open lateral ankle reconstructions if there is pain reported by athletes/patients. CLAI itself is not considered painful.

In general, an ankle instability episode (LAS) is treated with conservative, nonoperative treatment with a 90% success rate. The cornerstone of nonoperative treatment is early functional rehabilitation, including early aggressive range-of-motion (ROM) exercises (except plantar flexion (PF): we delay PF ROM until there is clinical stability up to 1–3 weeks), proprioception retraining, peroneal strengthening, aggressive Achilles tendon stretching, functional progression programs with progressive weight bearing, and intermittent bracing. Most grade II to III LAS can return to sport within 4 to 6 weeks. Some patients, however, fail these conservative measures and continue to experience symptomatic mechanical instability. These patients are candidates for lateral ligament reconstruction.

Although more than 50 operative techniques for ankle instability have been described, the short-term success rate is, fortunately, greater than 80% for all procedures.[19] Lateral ligament repair can broadly be divided into 3 categories: anatomic

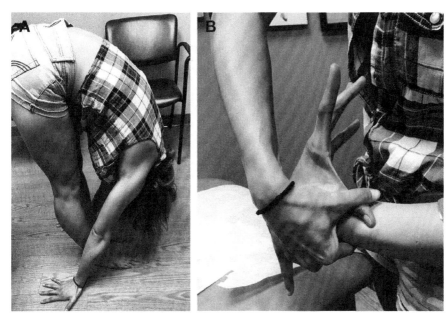

Fig. 4. (*A*, *B*) Clinical examination evidence for hyperlaxity. (*A*) Note the excess laxity of the back, hamstrings, and upper extremity allowing for the hypermobility. (*B*) Note the excess laxity of the wrist and thumb allowing hypermobility and ability to touch thumb to forearm.

repair/reconstruction, nonanatomic repair/reconstruction, and anatomic augmented tenodesis reconstructions. The goal of *anatomic repair/reconstruction* is to restore normal anatomy and joint biomechanics while maintaining tibiotalar and subtalar motion with stability. Originally described by Brostrom, anatomic repair is a division of

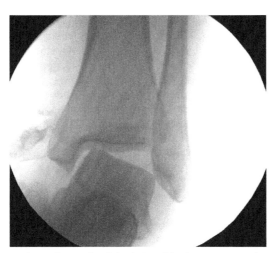

Fig. 5. Anterior-posterior radiograph of the left ankle demonstrating lateral ankle talar tilt instability due to CFL laxity. Note how the change in weight bearing of the talus is shifted medially and the amount of weight bearing surface significantly decreased. This varus instability must be corrected by CFL reconstruction in lateral ligament surgery.

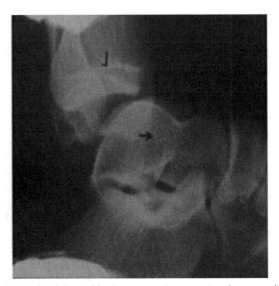

Fig. 6. Lateral radiograph of the ankle demonstrating anterior drawer ankle instability due to ATFL laxity. There are shear forces across the tibiotalar joint possibly leading to long-term cartilage damage and osteoarthritis if not corrected by ATFL reconstruction. *Arrow* demonstates direction of force to ankle during anterior draw test.

and imbrication of the ATFL; but various modifications have been described, including reinsertion into a bony trough, imbrication of the CFL, and reinforcement with the inferior extensor retinaculum (IER) creating a reconstruction of the native ligaments. *Nonanatomic reconstructions* do not recreate the native anatomy of the lateral collateral ligament complex. In these procedures, the peroneus brevis tendon is detached proximally, rerouted posterior to anterior through the fibula and secured to the talus ± calcaneus via variable techniques. Nonanatomic procedures are not discussed in this series, as they are known to alter subtalar joint mechanics, leading to hindfoot stiffness, eversion weakness, and, potentially, inferior outcomes.[20]

Although the Brostrom-Gould anatomic ligament repair/reconstruction (BLAR) largely remains the clinical gold standard, there are certain factors, such as severely attenuated tissue, history of prior repair, generalized ligamentous laxity (see **Fig. 4**), and cavovarus foot deformity (see **Fig. 3**), that may require alterations or augmentations to the basic BLAR. In these cases, some type of augmentation (revision surgery or ligamentous laxity) or realignment (cavovarus malalignment) should be considered. Clearly, a multitude of different techniques exists for CLAI. Therefore, this review explores open surgical techniques for CLAI, with particular focus on the well-studied and validated modified Brostrom technique with our personal application and modification as well as reported outcomes of open surgical management.

ANATOMY AND BIOMECHANICS

Understanding the normal anatomy of the lateral ligamentous complex (LLC) and biomechanics of the ankle is essential to the diagnosis and surgical treatment of chronic ankle instability. The LLC comprises 3 main structures: the ATFL, CFL, and posterior talofibular ligament (PTFL). Tearing, stretching, and recurring sprains of these ligaments can result in chronic lateral ankle instability. These ligaments are extra-articular and heal with scar tissue initially, but repeated giving way episodes ultimately compromise ankle stability because of stretching out of the ligaments despite healing. The ATFL is involved in 90% of all lateral sprains, whereas the CFL is involved in 50% to 75% of these sprains and the PTFL less than 10%.[7]

Lateral Ankle Anatomy

The ATFL is essentially a capsular thickening that consists of 1 to 2 bands that run anteromedially, originating from the anterior aspect of the distal fibula and inserting on the talar body/neck junction just anterior to the articular dome margin (see **Fig. 1**). This anatomy is critical to understanding the open BLAR. The ATFL is the weakest of all 3 ligaments with an ultimate failure load of 138 to 160 N, as such, the ATFL is most susceptible to injury during inversion sprain of the ankle with concomitant plantar flexion.[21]

Crossing both tibiotalar and subtalar joints, the CFL acts as the primary restraint to varus stress during ankle dorsiflexion and is also thought to play a role in subtalar stability. Originating on the anterior border of the fibula, confluent with the ATFL, the CFL courses deep to the peroneal tendons and inserts obliquely and posteriorly along the calcaneal tubercle (see **Fig. 2**). Isolated injuries to the CFL are rare[22]; a CFL rupture typically occurs only in conjunction with an ATFL rupture, in approximately 20% of cases, and rarely needs to be repaired.[23] An isolated CFL sprain most commonly occurs with the ankle dorsiflexed with inversion, such as with landing short in gymnastics/tumbling or in football pileups. Landing with the ankle dorsiflexed with inversion results in an isolated lateral subtalar sprain without anterior drawer instability.

Unlike the ATFL or CFL, the PTFL does not greatly contribute to ankle stability in the typical inversion ankle sprain. This point is true largely because the ligament is relaxed in plantarflexion.

Subtalar joint ligaments, such as the IER, may also play a role in ankle stability by contributing to subtalar joint stability.[24] These ligaments may very well be injured in conjunction with the LLC, but the patho-mechanics are poorly understood. Many surgeons use the IER during their repair/reconstruction, asserting that the calcaneal attachments of the IER provide further stability to the repair.[25] The IER anatomy can be variable (ie, the superolateral band is present in only 25% of cases); therefore, some surgeons think the sural fascia is more likely incorporated rather than the true IER, which is only used as the Gould modification in cases with such an anatomic variant.[26] This IER incorporation into an open reconstruction is crucial to reinforcing the CFL reconstruction and is thought to aid subtalar and varus stability.

Several comparison studies have been published examining the biomechanical outcomes following different operative techniques: the Brostrom procedure, modified Brostrom procedure, tendon transfer/allograft techniques, arthroscopic ligament repairs, and so forth. Despite efforts to restore normal anatomy, these procedures, including both open and arthroscopic techniques, continue to remain inferior to native, healthy ATFL tissue.[21,22,27] We do think, however, that the open BLAR with our described modification and bony reinsertion reliably recreates as functional as possible these native, uninjured ligaments.

OPERATIVE MANAGEMENT
Evolution of the Open Surgical Technique

Open surgical treatment of CLAI dates back to 1932 when a nonanatomic peroneus brevis tendon transfer was used in attempt to restore ankle stability. Over the ensuing years, a variety of procedures were developed in order to better restore ankle biomechanics—the Watson-Jones, Evans, and Chrisman-Snook to name a few—yet most of them continued to sacrifice the peroneal tendon. The results were largely suboptimal with continued pain, stiffness, subtalar arthritis, and/or recurrent instability. In 1966, however, a technique emerged that actually preserved the peroneal tendons: the direct, open, anatomic ligament repair that later became known as the Brostrom procedure, after its creator, Dr Lennart Brostrom (source).[7] Then came a myriad of modifications, such as the Gould modification of incorporating the IER into the repair. The Gould modification has been shown to improve biomechanical strength of the repair by 60%[28] as well as more closely restore ankle joint contact pressures.[29] This procedure, called the modified Brostrom, became popularized over the years; the open approach is currently considered the gold standard for surgical treatment of CLAI. In recent years, surgeons are performing concurrent diagnostic arthroscopy immediately preceding open ligament repair. With the advent of newer, improved technology and fixation devices, some surgeons now favor performing all-arthroscopic ligament repair as opposed to the traditional open repair. We still favor the open approach because of the anatomic reproducibility and ease of direct reattachment to the distal fibular, bony reattachment, and ease of adding the IER to the reconstruction.

Types of Operative Techniques

Surgical options are broadly divided into 2 categories: anatomic (repair or reconstruction) versus nonanatomic reconstruction. The latter procedure follows a nonanatomic course, as the name might suggest; there have been several techniques described. The most well-known nonanatomic reconstruction involves passing the peroneal brevis tendon through a predrilled tunnel in the fibular malleolus and suturing it to itself near the insertion on the fifth metatarsal base. This procedure alters subtalar joint biomechanics by creating a tenodesis effect, leading to stiffness[30,31] (similar to a subtalar coalition) and inferior outcomes.[32] For these reasons, nonanatomic reconstruction is rarely ever used anymore in the setting of a primary lateral ankle ligament surgery. Therefore, our focus is on anatomic techniques, which can be performed as a repair or a reconstruction.

Anatomic ligament repair/reconstruction

With patient satisfaction rates more than 90%,[33] the most popularized technique, the modified Brostrom is routinely considered the first-line treatment of CLAI. We prefer the open approach with the use of bone tunnels with an absorbable suture (BT) rather than suture anchors (SAs). A recent level II prospective cohort study comparing BT and SA techniques in 81 patients undergoing the modified Brostrom procedure demonstrated similar outcomes.[34] The mean Karlsson scores, American Orthopedic Foot and Ankle Society scores, anterior talar translation, and talar tilt (see **Fig. 5**) improved significantly with both procedures after intervention. There were no significant differences between the two cohorts, yet there was a clear trend in preoperative scores favoring the SA group over the BT group, suggesting the BT patients had more attenuated ligaments preoperatively. Associated pathology (defined as synovitis, OCL of talus, anterior bony impingement, loose body, and ossicles at the lateral malleolus) occurred in 53% of BT patients and 63% of SA patients. SA displacement, breakage, and pullout have all been reported in the literature[35]; but these complications that are unique to the SA technique were not investigated in this study. Indeed, one disadvantage of SAs is the unique complications that are inherent to its use. For these reasons, as well as the cost of SA and the ease of using BT, we advocate the use of bone tunnels for our open approach BLAR.

Role of Arthroscopy in Open Anatomic Ligament Repair

Arthroscopy is routinely performed concomitantly before open ligament repair in order to evaluate for intra-articular lesions and determine potential sources for pain (as mentioned, CLAI itself is not painful). Studies have shown that more than 90% of patients undergoing lateral ligament surgery have intra-articular lesions,[36–38] such as impingement lesions, ankle synovitis, intra-articular loose bodies, talar OCLs, and medial ankle tenosynovitis; extra-articular peroneal tendon pathology has also been reported. Yasui and colleagues[39] recommended performing concomitant ankle arthroscopy after retrospectively analyzing 16,069 patients undergoing a lateral ankle ligament procedure. Therefore, we too advocate the use of routine, concurrent ankle arthroscopy preceding open ligament reconstruction (BLAR) if there is any report of patient pain.

In overview, the BLAR operative technique begins with diagnostic arthroscopy using anterolateral and anteromedial portals (and other auxiliary portals as needed) and, after appropriately evaluating for and treating intra-articular pathology, finishes with an open modified Brostrom ligament reconstruction using bone tunnels. Arthroscopy time should be minimized to limit soft tissue edema and induration.

We describe this surgical technique, as well as the postoperative rehabilitation, in further detail next.

Modification of the Modified Brostrom Lateral Ankle Reconstruction

Technique (see Video 1 of open BLAR of left ankle).

Setup

Patients are placed in the supine position with a bump under the involved hip. A sequential compression device is placed on the uninvolved extremity throughout the procedure. The involved extremity is placed in a unilateral leg holder for the duration of the arthroscopy. An ankle block anesthetic is performed, and a well-padded tourniquet is applied in the supramalleolar region. We often do not use the tourniquet at the beginning of the arthroscopy and sometimes do not elevate the tourniquet until we start the Brostrom procedure. During draping, we exclude the toes from the operative field with the use of an inexpensive Coban wrap (3M, Saint Paul, MN). We then elevate the leg for exsanguination rather than using an Esmarch.

Arthroscopy

Two arthroscopic portals are always used: a standard anterolateral arthroscopy portal just lateral to peroneus tertius and an anteromedial portal at the soft spot between the tibialis anterior tendon, anterior medial malleolus, and dorsal medial neck of the talus. A diagnostic and therapeutic arthroscopy is then performed, taking care to address any additional intra-articular pathologic condition (eg, soft tissue impingement, bony impingement, OCLs, synovitis) that exists before proceeding with the modified Brostrom ligament procedure. An accessory inferior medial portal is occasionally added if inferior medial malleolar and/or medial talar neck pathology cannot be addressed through traditional portals. Posterior portals are not typically required unless further posterior ankle pain and pathology is suspected preoperatively.

The anterior inferior tibiofibular ligament (AITLF) can sometimes be hypertrophied with CLAI, causing anterolateral soft tissue ankle impingement.[40] We debride the AITFL back to the origin (fibula) and insertion (tibia) to alleviate this impingement. Also frequently encountered is anteromedial spurring that results from repeated medial bony impingement. We debride any excessive spurring that has accumulated on the anterior and inferior medial malleolus through the anteromedial portal using a

4.0-mm acromionizer. Using this same portal and arthroscopic burr, we also debride and remove any dorsal medial talar neck kissing spurs. We have the surgical assistant dorsiflex the ankle, which improves access and visualization of the spurs.

We also attempt to remove hypertrophied synovium and debride, microfracture, and sometimes even bone graft OCLs of the talar dome. In general, debridement alone is performed for cartilage with a rough surface or fibrillation; microfracture is performed for small cartilage defects that exhibit poor healing potential; and osteochondral autografting is performed only for patients with large cartilage talar dome defects (>1.0 cm diameter).

Open brostrom

After arthroscopy is completed, we remove the leg holder, paint the ankle with povidone-iodine (Betadine), flatten the operative table, and place a small bump underneath the distal tibia to allow the talus to sit more for ATFL reconstruction.

The anterolateral arthroscopy portal is incorporated into the anterolateral reconstruction incision (**Figs. 7** and **8**A) along Langerhans lines, and a blunt dissection is carried down to the peroneal tendons inferiorly. The superficial peroneal nerve is identified first and retracted dorsally and medially while the peroneal tendons are retracted inferiorly out of harm's way. Once both of these structures are identified, there are no other critical structures at risk during the procedure. We keep our retractors positioned to protect these structures throughout the remaining procedure. Dissection is carried down through subcutaneous tissue in order to easily visualize the ATFL (see **Fig. 1**) and CFL (see **Fig. 2**).

After subcutaneous dissection, the ATFL and CFL must be detached at their origin off the fibula (see **Fig. 8**B). First, however, the IER, running parallel to the CFL, is identified, preserved, and mobilized for later reattachment. A small Freer elevator is then placed under each individual ligament, which are then sharply dissected down to bone and shaved off the distal fibula. Both the ATFL and CFL ligamentous origins are then subperiosteally dissected off their respective origins to create a subperiosteal flap (see **Fig. 8**C) that is later imbricated to the distal stump of each respective reattached ligament (see **Fig. 8**D).

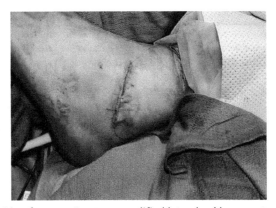

Fig. 7. Lateral incision for open Brostrom modified lateral ankle reconstruction (BLAR). The anterolateral arthroscopy portal is incorporated into the anterolateral reconstruction incision along Langerhans lines. Closure uses a subcuticular nonabsorbable suture for anatomic, cosmetic closure.

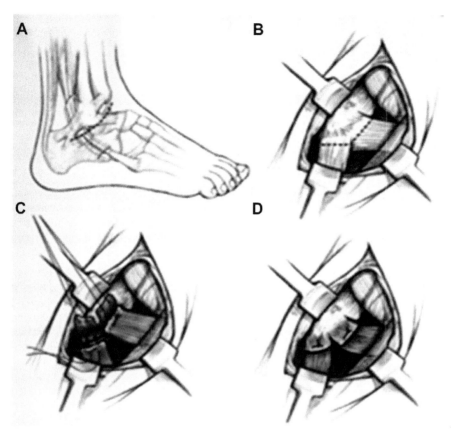

Fig. 8. (*A–D*) Lateral view of right ankle for open Brostrom lateral ankle reconstruction. (*A*) Lateral incision in Langerhans line incorporating anterolateral scope portal. (*B*) Location of release of lateral ankle ligaments off distal fibula. (*C*) Subperiosteal dissection of origin of lateral ankle ligaments with reattachment of native ligament into bony trough with suture through drill holes in distal fibula. (*D*) Imbrication of origin of lateral ankle ligaments down to distal stump of native ligaments to give soft tissue imbrication of ligaments. IER augmentation is included in our open procedure but is not demonstrated in this diagram.

Bone tunneling

A small egg burr (4.0 mm) is used to create a small trough at the ligaments' origin in the distal fibula. It is important to localize the anatomic footprints of the ligaments within the trough to ensure reestablishment of normal ankle biomechanics. Aware of these footprints, 1.5-mm drill holes are placed from the lateral fibula into the trough. The distal stump of the ATFL and CFL are then reattached through the drills holes using size 1 Vicryl (Ethicon Inc, Somerville, NJ) sutures via a horizontal mattress technique, so that the ATFL and CFL fit into the trough (see **Fig. 8**C). The foot/ankle is placed in maximal *plantar flexion* and *eversion* for all the CFL sutures applied. Then, the foot/ankle is placed in maximal *dorsiflexion* and *eversion*, for securing all the ATFL sutures.

Augmentation/Gould

The repair is augmented via vest-over-pants fashion, imbricating the origin of the ATFL and CFL into the distal stump of each ligament with a size 1 Vicryl horizontal mattress suture (see **Fig. 8**D). The Gould modification is then added to provide additional stability and protection as well as some proprioceptive feedback bringing the IER into the lateral fibular periosteum using a size 0 Vicryl suture in a figure-of-eight fashion. Before closure, stability is always checked.

Closure

Subcutaneous tissues are then reapproximated, and cosmetic skin closure is performed with 3-0 Monocryl (Ethicon, Inc) dermal sutures and 3-0 Prolene (Ethicon, Inc) subcuticular sutures (see **Fig. 8**A). A low-profile compressive dressing is applied. A thromboembolic device hose, ankle cold-compression device, and a long plastic walking boot are placed on the operative extremity in the operating room to give stability and cold compression therapy.

Postoperative care/rehabilitation

Postoperative rehabilitation occurs over 4 distinct phases with emphasis on early weight bearing and the goal of returning to sports or work-related activity in a brace by 3 to 4 months and, ultimately, return to full unrestricted activity as early as 4 to 6 months.

- Phase I (0–4 weeks) focuses on restoring full passive eversion and dorsiflexion ROM, controlling edema, weaning off crutches to full weight bearing in an Aircast walking boot (DJO Global Vista, CA), desensitization massaging, and improving Achilles flexibility while restricting strengthening exercises to only *light* eversion and dorsiflexion strengthening. We do allow stationary biking with the boot on at 1 week. We have the athlete sleep in the boot during the first 4 weeks to position the ankle in dorsiflexion.[41]
- Phase II (4–8 weeks) focuses on restoring full passive/active ROM and strength in all 4 directions (dorsiflexion, plantar flexion, inversion, eversion) as compared with the contralateral, unaffected limb, restoring complete Achilles flexibility, weaning out of the Aircast boot into an a stiff-up style brace, beginning proprioceptive retraining in the brace, and progressing to aerobic exercise, such as a bike and StairMaster/elliptical with the brace.
- Phase III (8–12 weeks) focuses on implementing a sport-specific functional progression program while continuing to restore/maintain full ankle ROM, strength, flexibility, and proprioception, such that patients can return to sport or work-related activity by the end of phase III or the beginning of phase IV.
- Phase IV (3–12 months) focuses on progressing to return to full, unrestricted sports or work-related activity with Cybex testing (60°/s, 120°/s, 180°/s) at 6 months and 1 year.

Clinical outcomes

The modified Brostrom technique described earlier, along with the postoperative rehab protocol, have been performed in more than 300 lateral ankle reconstructions by the senior author at our affiliated institution (Methodist Sports Medicine Center, Indianapolis, IN) over a 20-year period (1996–2016). To date, only 3 patients greater than 2 years out from surgery have required revisions (3 of 250 revision rate, 1.2%), of which 2 patients required suture removal. Unfortunately, during the initial phase of this study, we used a synthetic absorbable suture that we no longer use (since March 2006) because of its known postoperative complications, including spitting sutures, which likely accounted for the 2 suture removals in the study. Nevertheless, the BLAR technique described yielded a revision rate substantially lower than those generally reported in the literature (1.2% vs 5.9%–20.0%).[39] Our reported revision rate of 1.2% is validated by a level III systematic review on intermediate- to long-term longevity and incidence of revision following the modified-Gould procedure. Also, 11 studies involving 669 Brostrom-Gould–specific procedures (ie, procedures excluded were those that used industry SAs, tendon autograft or allograft, nonanatomic repairs, and/or an arthroscopic approach; those with a follow-up period of <5 years; or those that included patients with generalized hypermobility) also reported a revision rate of 1.2% at a weighted mean follow-up of 8.4 years.[42]

Special Considerations

Varus malalignment

We use the Dwyer lateral closing wedge osteotomy when the lateral foot overload is due to intrinsic heel varus (see **Fig. 3**). When the lateral overload is due to a plantar flexed first ray (see **Fig. 3**B), we use a dorsal first metatarsal closing wedge osteotomy with a 3-hole T plate for fixation. Rarely, we implement both osteotomies. With a Dwyer calcaneal osteotomy, weight bearing is delayed 2 to 4 weeks.

Ligamentous hyperlaxity

Historically, ankle ligament laxity in patients with generalized joint hypermobility (GJH) has resulted in suboptimal outcomes (see **Fig. 4**). However, this has recently been called into question. A case series of 32 patients with GJH, who underwent the modified Brostrom procedure for CLAI and had normal stress radiographs of the uninvolved ankle, demonstrated excellent postoperative functional Karlsson-Peterson ankle scores.[43] Although 9 patients reinjured their ankle and 3 ankles were unstable on stress radiographs, all patients were satisfied and none required reoperation at a mean follow-up of 27.4 months. We augment our open BLAR with a gracilis allograft via drill holes in the talus and calcaneus to provide more normal collagen in cases of pathologic hyperlaxity.

Revisions

We approach the revision cases the same as the hyperlaxity cases. We use the same incision (if no peroneal pathology), perform our traditional modified BLAR, and then augment with gracilis allograft with SAs and a trough in the talus and calcaneus. We have found this to provide significant improvement in stability as well as maintaining full ROM without sacrificing any otherwise normal peroneal tendons. We keep our revision and hyperlaxity patients in a boot for sleep and ADLs until the 6-week timeframe.

Future considerations

Recently, an augmented Brostrom repair technique using tape augmentation has been studied for primary lateral ankle ligament surgery in order to enhance stability and accelerate recovery. One such example, called the InternalBrace (Arthrex, Naples, FL), uses a suture tape and interference screw construct to augment the repair. Use of this construct in human cadaveric models increases mean ultimate load to failure as compared with the traditional Brostrom with suture or SAs,[44,45] but it is unclear how it compares with the modified Brostrom because the Gould modification was not performed. In a case series, the InternalBrace used in patients resulted in return to running within 12 weeks.[46] However, most rehab protocols following the normal modified Brostrom procedure allow patients to return to running within that same time frame. Additionally, the InternalBrace did not improve proprioception in a similar manner as imbricating the ligaments. We have considered using this augmentation in hyperlaxity. We have also considered using this technique for revision cases. Recently, a prospective case series on 30 patients undergoing a revision surgery using the modified Brostrom procedure augmented with suture tape, after a failed primary modified Brostrom procedure, demonstrated satisfactory clinical outcomes for revision cases at the intermediate-term follow-up.[47]

SUMMARY

We have been pleased with our open BLAR for chronic lateral ankle instability. We find the technique easily reproducible, reliable if there is no pathologic hyperlaxity, and relatively simple in approach and execution. We favor an aggressive early weight bearing and early limited ROM. We use intermittent immobilization with cold compression for pain control and edema management. Biking in a boot can begin as early as 1 week if protected by boot wear. Return to sports can begin as early as 3 months after reconstruction. Hyperlaxity requires augmentation with the open approach, and lateral overload from a cavovarus hindfoot requires realignment osteotomies. Revision surgery requires augmentation.

SUPPLEMENTARY DATA

Supplementary data related to this article can be found online at https://doi.org/10.1016/j.fcl.2018.07.002.

REFERENCES

1. Waterman B, Owens B, Davey S, et al. The epidemiology of ankle sprains in the United States. J Bone Joint Surg Am 2010;92:2279–84.
2. DiGiovanni BF, Partal G, Baumhauer JF. Acute ankle injury and chronic lateral instability in the athlete. Clin Sports Med 2004;23(1):1–19.
3. Roos KG, Kerr ZY, Mauntel TC, et al. The epidemiology of lateral ligament complex ankle sprains in National Collegiate Athletic Association Sports. Am J Sports Med 2017;45(1):201–9.
4. Hootman JM, Dick R, Agel J. Epidemiology of collegiate injuries for 15 sports: summary and recommendations for injury prevention initiatives. J Athl Train 2007;42:311–9.
5. Maffulli N, Ferran NA. Management of acute and chronic ankle instability. J Am Acad Orthop Surg 2008;16:608–15.
6. Gribble PA, Bleakley CM, Caulfield BM, et al. Evidence review for the 2016 international ankle consortium consensus statement on the prevalence, impact, and long-term consequences of lateral ankle sprains. Br J Sports Med 2016;50:1496–505.
7. Brostrom L. Sprained ankles: a pathologic, arthrographic, and clinical study, dissertation. Stockholm (Swedan): Karolinksa Institute; 1966.
8. Medina McKeon JM, Bush HM, Reed A, et al. Return-to-play probabilities following new versus recurrent ankle sprains in high school athletes. J Sci Med Sport 2014;17(1):23–8.
9. Gerber JP, Williams GN, Scoville CN, et al. Persistent disability associated with ankle sprains: a prospective examination of an athletic population. Foot Ankle Int 1998;19:653–60.
10. Beynnon BD, Murphy DF, Alosa DM. Predictive factors for lateral ankle sprains: a literature review. J Athl Train 2002;37:376–80.
11. Van Rijn RM, Van Os AG, Bernsen RM, et al. What is the clinical course of acute ankle sprains? A systematic literature review. Am J Med 2008;121(4):324–31.
12. Hiller CE, Nightingale EJ, Raymond J, et al. Prevalence and impact of chronic musculoskeletal ankle disorders in the community. Arch Phys Med Rehabil 2012;93:1801–7.

13. Attenborough AS, Hiller CE, Smith RM, et al. Chronic ankle instability in sporting populations. Sports Med 2014;44:1545–56.
14. Simon J, Hall E, Docherty C. Prevalence of chronic ankle instability and associated symptoms in university dance majors: an exploratory study. J Dance Med Sci 2014;18(4):178–84.
15. DiGiovanni BF, Fraga CJ, Cohen BE, et al. Associated injuries found in chronic lateral ankle instability. Foot Ankle Int 2000;21(10):809–15.
16. Komenda GA, Ferkel RD. Arthroscopic findings associated with the unstable ankle. Foot Ankle Int 1999;20(11):708–13.
17. Sugimoto K, Takakura Y, Okahashi K, et al. Chondral injuries of the ankle with recurrent lateral instability: an arthroscopic study. J Bone Joint Surg Am 2009; 91(1):99–106.
18. Lofvenberg R, Karrholm J, Lund B. The outcome of nonoperated patients with chronic lateral instability of the ankle: a 20-year follow-up study. Foot Ankle Int 1994;15(4):165–9.
19. Clanton TO. Athletic injuries to the soft tissues of the foot and ankle. In: Coughlin MJ, Mann RA, editors. Surgery of the foot and ankle. 7th edition. St Louis (MO): Mosby; 1999. p. 1153–65.
20. DiGiovanni CW, Brodsky A. Current concepts: lateral ankle instability. Foot Ankle Int 2006;27(10):854–66.
21. Viens NA, Wijdicks CA, Campbell KJ, et al. Anterior taolofibular ligament ruptures, part 1: biomechanical comparison of augmented Brostrom repair techniques with the intact anterior talofibular ligament. Am J Sports Med 2014; 42(2):405–11.
22. Rigby R, Cottom JM, Rozin R. Isolated calcaneofibular ligament injury: a report of two cases. J Foot Ankle Surg 2015;54(3):487–9.
23. Lee KT, Park YU, Kim JS, et al. Long-term results after modified Brostrom procedure without calcaneofibular ligament reconstruction. Foot Ankle Int 2011;32(2): 153–7.
24. Neuschwander TB, Indresano AA, Hughes TH, et al. Footprint of the lateral ligament complex of the ankle. Foot Ankle Int 2013;34(4):582–6.
25. Acevedo JI, Mangone PG. Arthroscopic lateral ankle ligament reconstruction. Tech Foot Ankle Surg 2011;10(3):111–6.
26. Dalmau-Pastor M, Yasui Y, Calder JD, et al. Anatomy of the inferior extensor retinaculum and its role in lateral ankle ligament reconstruction: a pictorial essay. Knee Surg Sports Traumatol Arthrosc 2016;24(4):957–62.
27. Waldrop NE, Wijdicks CA, Jansson KS, et al. Anatomic suture anchor versus Brostrom technique for anterior talofibular ligament repair: a biomechanical comparison. Am J Sports Med 2012;40(11):2590–6.
28. Aydogan U, Glisson RR, Nunley JA, et al. Extensor retinaculum augmentation reinforces anterior talofibular ligament repair. Clin Orthop Relat Res 2006;442: 210–5.
29. Prisk VR, Imhauser CW, O'Laughlin PF, et al. Lateral ligament repair and reconstruction restore neither contact mechanics of the ankle joint nor motion patters of the hindfoot. J Bone Joint Surg Am 2010;92(14):2375–86.
30. Sugimoto K, Takakura Y, Akiyama K, et al. Long-term results of Watson-Jones tenodesis of the ankle. Clinical and radiographic findings after ten to eighteen years of follow-up. J Bone Joint Surg Am 1998;80(11):1587–96.
31. Krips R, van Dijk CN, Halasi T, et al. Long-term outcome of anatomical reconstruction versus tenodesis for the treatment of chronic anterolateral instability of the ankle joint: a multicenter study. Foot Ankle Int 2001;22:415–21.

32. Hennrikus WL, Mapes RC, Lyons PM, et al. Outcomes of the Chrisman-Snook and modified-Brostrom procedures for chronic lateral ankle instability. A prospective, randomized comparison. Am J Sports Med 1996;24(4):400–4.

33. Bell SJ, Mologne TS, Sitler DF, et al. Twenty-six year results after Brostrom procedure for chronic lateral ankle instability. Am J Sports Med 2006;34(6):975–8.

34. Hu CY, Lee KB, Song EK, et al. Comparison of bone tunnel and suture anchor techniques in the modified Brostrom procedure for chronic lateral ankle instability. Am J Sports Med 2013;41(8):1877–84.

35. Messer TM, Cummins CA, Ahn J, et al. Outcome of modified Brostrom procedure for chronic lateral ankle instability using suture anchors. Foot Ankle Int 2000; 21(12):996–1003.

36. Ferkel RD, Chams RN. Chronic lateral instability: arthroscopic findings and long-term results. Foot Ankle Int 2007;28:24–31.

37. Hua Y, Chen S, Li Y, et al. Combination of modified Brostrom procedure with ankle arthroscopy for chronic ankle instability accompanied by intra-articular symptoms. Arthroscopy 2010;26:524–52.

38. Taga I, Shino K, Inoue M, et al. Articular cartilage lesions in ankles with lateral ligament injury. An arthroscopic study. Am J Sports Med 1993;21:120–6.

39. Yasui Y, Murawski CD, Wollstein A, et al. Reoperation rates following ankle ligament procedures performed with and without concomitant arthroscopic procedures. Knee Surg Sports Traumatol Arthrosc 2017;25(6):1908–15.

40. McCarroll JR, Schrader JW, Shelbourne KD, et al. Meniscoid lesions of the ankle in soccer players. Am J Sports Med 1987;15(3):255–7.

41. Smith R, Reischl S. The Influence of Dorsiflexion in the Treatment of Severe Ankle Sprains: An Anatomical Study Foot & Ankle International 1988;9(1):28–33.

42. So E, Preston N, Holmes T. Intermediate- to long-term longevity and incidence of revision of the modified Brostrom-Gould procedure for lateral ankle ligament repair: a systematic review. J Foot Ankle Surg 2017;56(5):1076–80.

43. Huang B, Kim YT, Kim JU, et al. Modified Brostrom procedure for chronic ankle instability with generalized joint hypermobility. Am J Sports Med 2016;44(4): 1011–6.

44. Schuh R, Benca E, Willegger M, et al. Comparison of Brostrom technique, suture anchor repair, and tape augmentation for reconstruction of the anterior talofibular ligament. Knee Surg Sports Traumatol Arthrosc 2016;24(4):1101–7.

45. Willegger M, Benca E, Hirtler L, et al. Biomechanical stability of tape augmentation for anterior talofibular ligament (ATFL) repair compared to the native ATFL. Knee Surg Sports Traumatol Arthrosc 2016;24(4):1015–21.

46. Mackay GM, Ribbans WJ. The addition of an "internal brace" to augment the Brostrom technique for lateral ankle ligament instability. Tech Foot Ankle Surg 2016;15(1):47–56.

47. Cho BK, Kim YM, Choi SM, et al. Revision anatomical reconstruction of the lateral ligaments of the ankle augmented with suture tape for patients with a failed Brostrom procedure. Bone Joint J 2017;99-B(9):1183–9.

Arthroscopic Treatment of Ankle Instability: Brostrom

Jorge I. Acevedo, MD[a],*, Robert C. Palmer, MD[b],
Peter G. Mangone, MD[c]

KEYWORDS

- Ankle instability • Arthroscopy • Brostrom • Ankle sprain • Lateral ligament repair

KEY POINTS

- Over the last 10 years, significant advances have been made and successful techniques have now been developed that effectively treat ankle instability via the arthroscope.
- Currently arthroscopic lateral ligament repair techniques can be grouped into "arthroscopic-assisted techniques," "all-arthroscopic techniques," and "all-inside techniques."
- Recent studies have proven these arthroscopic techniques to be a simple, safe, and biomechanically equivalent, stable alternative to open Brostrom Gould lateral ligament reconstruction.

EPIDEMIOLOGY

An ankle sprain refers to an injury of the ankle ligaments and is the most common injury in physically active patients.[1] This injury occurs approximately 30,000 times per day with an estimated annual incidence of 2 per 1000 people in the United States.[2] Eighty-five percent of ankle sprains involve the lateral ankle ligaments.[3] An MRI study of ankle inversion injuries showed that the anterior talofibular ligament (ATFL) was involved in 75% of the injuries, the calcaneofibular ligament (CFL) in 41%, and 5% were combined.[4] Chronic ankle instability (CAI) develops in 20% to 40% of patients with a history of lateral ankle sprains and is prevalent among basketball, soccer, and volleyball players as well as ballet dancers.[1,2] Odak[5] discovered a high incidence of synovitis (63%) associated with chronic lateral ankle instability as well as osteochondral lesions (17%) and signs of anterior impingement (12%). Several arthroscopic studies

Disclosure Statement: Drs J.I. Acevedo and P.G. Mangone are consultants and speakers for Arthrex, Inc and they receive royalties from the company as well. Also, speakers for Wright Medical. Dr R.C. Palmer has nothing to disclose.
[a] Department of Orthopedics, Southeast Orthopedic Specialists, 6500 Bowden Road, Suite 103, Jacksonville, FL 32216, USA; [b] Department of Orthopedics, University of Florida, 2nd Floor ACC Ortho Department, 655 W 8th Street, Jacksonville, FL 32209, USA; [c] Department of Orthopedics, Blue Ridge Division of Emergeortho, Foot and Ankle Center, 2585 Hendersonville Road, Arden, NC 28704, USA
* Corresponding author.
E-mail address: Ace4foot@gmail.com

have shown a high rate of chondral lesions in chronic lateral ankle instability with some reporting upwards of 90% of patients with intra-articular problems with a mean time from initial injury of 2 years and mean patient age in the third decade of life.[6–9]

MECHANISM OF INJURY

The mechanism of injury of lateral ankle ligament tears are commonly caused by an inverted and plantar flexed foot with a rotational force component that typically involves sequential rupture of the ATFL, CFL, and less frequently, the posterior talofibular ligament (PTFL).[3] As proposed by Hertel,[10] the cause of chronic lateral ankle instability is divided into 2 broad categories of mechanical instability and functional instability.[11] Mechanical instability refers to abnormal movement of the talus within the ankle joint complex and is historically referred to as pathologic ligamentous laxity, and was subsequently expanded to include abnormal bony anatomy of the talocrural joint (ie, wider talar dome or reduced talar coverage by the tibial plafond). Conversely, functional instability as introduced by Freeman refers to instability that is due to proprioceptive or neuromuscular deficits (ie, slower peroneal tendon responsiveness to inversion/supination stimuli).[2] Others have described this definition of functional instability as motion beyond voluntary control but not exceeding physiologic range of motion.[12] This homogeneous model has been questioned and revised by Hiller and colleagues[1] in order to incorporate the perceived multifactorial nature of CAI development.

RISK FACTORS

CAI may alter the ankle joint biomechanics causing degenerative changes. It has been shown in some studies that upwards of 90% of CAI patients have intra-articular pathologic condition, such as osteochondral lesions.[11] One theory suggests that varus instability shifts contact pressure medially leading to articular damage of the central and medial talar regions. This shift of contact pressure may be observed in patients with cavovarus foot deformity, tibia vara, peroneal tendon injuries, tight Achilles tendon, and hyperligamentous laxity syndrome who are at increased risk of CAI.[13] In a normal ankle, the center of pressure during heel strike lies lateral to the subtalar joint axis, which produces a pronation torque, whereas in a varus hindfoot, the center of pressure is placed medially, producing a supinating torque and stressing the lateral ankle ligamentous complex. Likewise, a tightened Achilles tendon produces prolonged periods of plantar flexion during the gait cycle and consequently increased stress upon the ATFL.[14] Furthermore, White and colleagues[15] demonstrated significantly longer (116 days vs 72 days) to return to play in a cohort of professional athletes with concomitant ankle injuries (ie, osteochondral lesion, deltoid tear). Improved outcomes have been shown by simultaneously addressing associated pathologic condition (ie, cavovarus deformity) during the treatment of lateral ligamentous laxity.[16]

CLASSIFICATION AND NONOPERATIVE MANAGEMENT

Lateral ankle ligament injuries are graded from I to III. Grade I indicates ligament stretching; grade II is classified as a partial tear of one or several ligaments, and grade III translates to complete rupture of the lateral ligament complex.[3] The normal treatment of a patient with CAI focuses on a combination of peroneal muscle strengthening, balance reflex training, and external bracing to prevent recurrent injury.[13] Better outcomes have been demonstrated with initial immobilization and functional rehabilitation compared with 6 weeks of cast immobilization for acute ankle sprains. Although most patients will recover with conservative management, those who fail conservative measures, typically after 6 months, are considered candidates for lateral ankle ligament repair or reconstruction.[4,13]

LATERAL LIGAMENTOUS COMPLEX AND BIOMECHANICS OF THE NORMAL LATERAL ANKLE

The lateral ligamentous support of the ankle comprises 3 main structures: the ATFL, the CFL, and the PTFL. The ATFL is the weakest (ultimate failure, load 138N-160N) of the 3 ligaments and is most commonly injured in lateral ankle sprains.[13,14] Traditionally, the ATFL has been described as a flat, quadrilateral ligament. Later, Sarrafian described the ligament as having 2 distinct bands. A recent systematic review by Matsui and colleagues[17] revealed the distribution of bundle anatomic variability across 10 studies of 263 specimens was found to be single bundle in 61.6%, double bundle in 35.7%, and triple bundle in 2.7%. The origin of the ATFL has been reported approximately 10 to 14 mm from the tip of the distal fibula and inserts on the lateral portion of the talar neck with a mean length of 11.8 mm to 24.8 mm.[17,18]

The origin of the CFL is 5 to 8 mm from the tip of the lateral malleolus. It courses deep to the peroneal tendons to insert on a tubercle on the lateral wall of the calcaneus. This footprint lays approximately 3 cm posterior and superior to the peroneal tubercle. The CFL serves a role in providing subtalar stability extending across the tibiotalar and subtalar joints. However, clinical and biomechanical studies have not demonstrated direct repair of this ligament to be essential for good outcomes.[3,18–20] The PTFL originates on the medial surface of the lateral malleolus and in a multifascicular fashion inserts along the posterolateral talus. Because this ligament is relaxed in plantarflexion, it is unlikely to be a major contributor to stability in the typical inversion sprain but may be involved in posterior ankle impingement syndromes.[13]

The inferior extensor retinaculum (IER) is typically described as a thickening of the crural fascia and is a Y-shaped structure formed by the stem ligament, an oblique superomedial band, and an oblique inferomedial band. In up to 64% of cases, an additional superolateral band is formed giving the IER an X-shaped morphology.[21] Because of the calcaneal attachments of the IER, the investigators believe this ligament imparts further stability to the modified Brostrom repair. Given the variable anatomy, some investigators have questioned the validity of IER incorporation into the repair, and to the contrary, have postulated that it is the sural fascia.[22]

The superficial peroneal nerve has been found to run a mean distance of 32 mm (24–48 mm) at 90° from the center of the ATFL origin. As the nerve courses distally, it runs more anterior, thus placing an accessory incision more distal may serve to decrease the risk of iatrogenic injury.[18] Matsui and colleagues[23] have shown that the fibular obscure tubercle (FOT) is a reliable landmark in 100% of cases by using a combination of palpation and fluoroscopy and may serve as a clinically relevant landmark for locating the ATFL for percutaneous MIS procedures aimed at treating CLAI. The FOT is located on the anterior border of the fibula between the inferior tip and anterior tubercle of the distal fibula. The ATFL origin had a mean measurement of 3.7 mm (range 0–6.7 mm) proximal to the FOT, and the CFL origin had a mean measurement of 4.9 mm (range 1.1–10.9 mm) distal to the FOT. Alternatively, Clanton and colleagues[24] suggested that the origin of the ATFL could be placed at 50% of the distance along the anterior fibular border in order to account for the measurement variability in patients who deviate from the mean.

EVOLUTION OF SURGICAL TECHNIQUE

Gallie's work[25] treating paralytic clubfoot in 1913 is credited as inspiring the first surgical procedure targeted at lateral ligament instability using a nonanatomic peroneus brevis transfer.[26] Throughout the ensuing decades, many evolutions of the nonanatomic procedures occurred (ie, Watson-Jones, Evans, Chrisman-Snook), but patient outcomes were underscored by persistent pain, hindfoot stiffness, resultant subtalar arthritis, and recurrent instability.[3] The Broström technique was first described in 1964 and involved direct repair of the ATFL and CFL or transosseous fixation.[27] Later, the Gould modification was popularized in 1993 by Hamilton and colleagues[28] after successful outcomes in professional ballet dancers. Subsequent studies have shown that the incorporation of the IER can improve biomechanical strength of the repair by 60%.[29]

Despite failures for the treatment of shoulder and knee instability, thermal shrinkage was thought to be more effective in the chronically unstable ankle due to the intrinsic stability of the ankle mortise. Initial series implemented this technique for mild or functional ankle instability with 80% to 86% good to excellent results.[30,31] A recent case series by Vuurberg and colleagues[32] demonstrated a high rate of recurrent instability and residual symptoms following arthroscopic thermal capsular shrinkage and thus did not recommend this procedure for joint stabilization in patients with chronic lateral ankle instability.

Arthroscopic ankle stabilization was first reported in 1987 by Hawkins[33] using a staple technique for plication of the lateral ankle ligaments. Although they had promising results with only one recurrence and the remaining complications were attributed to staple prominence, the study lacked adequate follow-up of outcomes. Subsequently, Kashuk and colleagues[34] produced an iteration to this technique, which was the first arthroscopic technique to use suture anchors for lateral ligamentous complex repair. These arthroscopic stabilization techniques potentially offer the benefit of quicker recovery and decreased morbidity in addition to offering a single approach to address intra-articular pathologic condition and faster surgical time.[3] Touted as a safe procedure early on, it is important to draw attention to the wide variation in reported complication rates (0% to 29%), which includes delayed wound healing, nerve pain, and deep vein thrombosis (**Table 1**). A systematic review found the overall complication rate of open ligament repair to be 8% versus 15% for those performed arthroscopically.[16] Analysis of this systematic review reveals inclusion of arthroscopic techniques that used accessory incisions[46] and others[37] with heterogeneity in considering complications, such as asymptomatic suture knots and transient skin irritation as significantly reportable. If these variances are eliminated, the effective complication rate for both open and arthroscopic ligament repair would be similar (8%). Compared with open repair, arthroscopic repair has shown similar functional scores, talar tilt, and return to play.[47]

ARTHROSCOPIC LIGAMENT REPAIR ANATOMY

Both anatomic and biomechanical investigations have demonstrated that the IER can function in stabilization of the subtalar joint similar to the CFL.[21] The Gould modification, which involves the incorporation of the IER, has been supported by functional outcomes data.[28] Recently, the utility of the IER for arthroscopic ligament repair has been questioned. In a recent anatomic study, it was purported that the variable structure of the IER, specifically Y-shaped variations, may lead to incorporation of the sural fascia, which is not thought to confer the same biomechanical stability.[22] Moreover, it has been suggested that overtightening of the IER may promote stiffness in the

Table 1
Arthroscopic lateral ankle ligament repair peer reviewed publications

Author, Year	Level of Evidence	Repair Type	No. of Ankles	Follow-up (mo or y)	Time from Injury to Surgery (mo or y)	Preoperative AOFAS/Karlsson	Postoperative AOFAS/Karlsson	Satisfaction Rate (%)
Acevedo & Mangone,[35] 2011	IV, retrospective case series	Arthroscopic	24	10.9 mo	NA	NA	NA	95.8
Acevedo & Mangone,[13] 2015	IV, retrospective case series	Arthroscopic	73	28 mo	NA	NA/28.3	NA/90.2	94.5
Corte-Real,[54] 2009	IV, retrospective case series	Arthroscopic	28	27.5 mo (6–48 mo)	7 mo (2–30 mo)	—	85.3 (65–100)	NA
Cottom & Rigby,[36] 2013	IV case series	Arthroscopic	40	12.13 mo (6–21 mo)	NA	41.2 (23–64)	95.4 (84–100)/93.6	NA
Kim,[37] 2011	IV, retrospective case series	Arthroscopic	28	15.9 mo (13–25 mo)	—	60.78	92.48	—
Labib & Slone,[38] 2015	IV, retrospective case series	Arthroscopic	14	3 mo (6–54 wk)	NA	NA	92.8 (80–100)	86
Li et al,[39] 2017	III, retrospective cohort	— Arthroscopic Open	60 23 37	— 39.7 35.5	16 mo (3–60) 39 mo (3–120)	69.3/61.8 69.2/59.7	93.3/90.3 92.4/89.4	— — —
Nery et al,[40] 2011	IV, retrospective case series	Arthroscopic	38	9.8 y (5–14 y)	9 mo (6–19 mo)	NA	90 (44–100)	94.7
Nery et al,[41] 2017	II, prospective cohort	Arthroscopic	26	27 mo (21–36 mo)	NA	58	90	NA

(continued on next page)

Table 1
(continued)

Author, Year	Level of Evidence	Repair Type	No. of Ankles	Follow-up (mo or y)	Time from Injury to Surgery (mo or y)	Preoperative AOFAS/Karlsson	Postoperative AOFAS/Karlsson	Satisfaction Rate (%)
Song et al,[42] 2017	III, retrospective cohort	—	28	—	—	—	@ 12 mo	—
		Arthroscopic	16	16.3	—	59.3	93	—
		Reconstruction	12	19.3	—	61.3	94.4	—
Vega et al,[43] 2013	IV, retrospective case series	Arthroscopic	16	22.3 mo (12–35 mo)	NA	67 (59–77)	97 (95–100)	NA
Yeo et al,[44] 2016	I, randomized control trial	—	48	NA	NA	—	@ 12 mo	—
		Arthroscopic	25	NA	NA	67.5/45.0	90.3/76.2	—
		Open	23	NA	NA	69.9/48.6	89.2/73.5	—
Yoo & Yang,[45] 2016	III, retrospective cohort	—	85	—	—	—	@ 24 wk	—
		W/internal brace	22	—	—	65.8	98	—
		W/o internal brace	63	—	—	66.7	96.5	—

posterior subtalar joint.[48] Jorge and colleagues[18] advised that an anteriorly placed accessory portal improves the odds of incorporating the IER rather than the sural fascia, noting that the distance should be less than 22 mm from the lateral malleolus to decrease risk of injury to the superficial peroneal nerve (SPN). Based on this information, some investigators have debated the utility of incorporating the IER in the arthroscopic lateral ankle ligament repair. In 2015, Acevedo and colleagues[49] reported the internervous safe zone between the intermediate branch of the SPN and sural nerve was a mean of 51 mm (range, 39–64 mm) and the intertendonous safe zone between the peroneus tertius and peroneus brevis was a mean of 43 mm (range, 37–49 mm). The investigators stressed the importance of passing sutures at least 15 mm anterior to the distal fibula with the ankle held in neutral position in order to incorporate a sufficient portion of the IER. Based on this study and their clinical results, the senior authors maintain the importance of the IER to the lateral ligament complex repair.

BIOMECHANICS OF ARTHROSCOPIC LATERAL ANKLE LIGAMENT RECONSTRUCTION

Both Drakos and colleagues[50] and Giza and colleagues[51] in 2013 published data revealing biomechanically equivalent results of arthroscopic versus open techniques when using matched cadaver pairs. Drakos's technique used 2 anchors with one anchor inserted in the inferior fibula through an accessory portal. Giza's research used the ArthroBrostrom "all-arthroscopic" technique using the typical standard anteromedial and anterolateral arthroscopic portals. In a recent cadaveric biomechanical study, Lee and colleagues[52] found no significant difference between torque to failure in open modified Brostrom technique (MBO) (19.9 Nm) and arthroscopic MBO (23.3 Nm). Yoshimura and colleagues[53] investigated optimal suture anchor placement and recommend the suture anchor should be placed at an angle of less than 45° to the longitudinal axis of the fibula to avoid complications with anchors penetrating posteriorly.

ARTHROBROSTROM INTRAOPERATIVE TECHNIQUE

Although there are several different published arthroscopic techniques for lateral ankle ligament reconstruction, in this review, the authors discuss the technique the senior authors (J.I.A., P.G.M.) developed, which currently is the only technique with published data supporting biomechanical equivalency to the standard open Brostrom Gould procedure.

- Anesthesia: Most patients can have a regional popliteal block plus monitored anesthesia care (MAC). Some patients may require a general anesthesia. If a regional popliteal is performed, the surgeon or anesthesiologist usually must perform a separate local block for the saphenous nerve to cover the anteromedial portal.
- Distraction versus no distraction: The arthroscopy and arthroscopic lateral ligament reconstruction can be performed with either method. The surgeon should use his or her preference. It is important to remember that if distraction is used, the distraction is removed before tying the sutures to tighten the lateral ankle ligament complex.
- Preoperative drawing of anatomic landmarks: This is critical for success and involves marking the "safe zone" in the lateral ankle region. The peroneal tendons, distal fibula, and intermediate branch of the superficial peroneal nerve are identified and outlined on the skin. The location of the IER is estimated and drawn using the lateral calcaneal tubercle to help identify the margin of this tissue (**Fig. 1**).
- Use standard anteromedial and anterolateral arthroscopy portals.

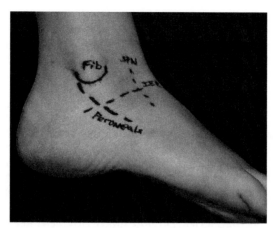

Fig. 1. Anatomic landmarks.

- Perform normal diagnostic arthroscopy and address any additional intra-articular pathologic condition that exists before the ligament procedure. The surgeon must perform a more extensive debridement of the lateral gutter for 2 purposes: to reduce impingement and clean out the pathologic fibrotic tissue that usually fills the lateral gutter; and to allow for adequate visualization of the anterior distal face of the fibula.
- The inferior tip of the fibula is identified with a probe.
- Using the standard anterolateral portal, the first bone anchor is then placed 1 cm superior to the tip of the fibula with the sutures being brought out of the standard anterolateral portal. Anchor placement at an angle of less than 45° to the longitudinal axis of the fibula is recommended. This first set of sutures is then passed one at a time using a sharp-tipped suture passer. This can be performed with either an "inside-out" technique or an "outside-in" technique. Care is taken to make sure the exit point is at least 1.5 cm distal to the anterior face of the fibula to ensure capture of the IER. This is performed while visualizing it from the anteromedial portal.
  - First set of sutures: The first suture is passed just superior to the peroneal tendons, and the second suture is passed 1 cm dorsal/anterior to the first suture along the arc of the IER (**Fig. 2**).
- The second anchor is then placed 1 cm superior to the first anchor in the anterior face of the fibula. This should still be located inferior to the level of the talar dome as the ATFL anatomic origin is inferior to the talar dome. The second set of sutures is then passed with a sharp-tipped suture passer while visualized through the anteromedial portal.
  - Second set of sutures: The first suture is passed about 1 cm dorsal/anterior to the last suture from the first anchor along the arc of the IER. The second suture from the second anchor is then passed through the tissue 1 cm dorsal/anterior from the first suture. Care is taken to make sure the surgeon stays inferior to the intermediate branch of the superficial peroneal nerve within the safe zone (**Fig. 3**).
- A small incision (4 mm) is then made between the 2 sets of sutures, and using a small arthroscopic hook, the suture sets are then passed through this central incision (**Fig. 4**). If the surgeon is concerned about the intermediate branch of

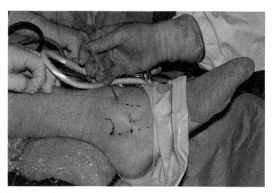

Fig. 2. Passage of first set of sutures using a sharp-tipped suture passer. First suture limb is shown already passed through lateral ligament complex and exiting skin.

the superficial peroneal nerve, he or she can simply retract the tissue anteriorly through the incision to make sure the more superior set of sutures has been passed deep to the nerve to prevent entrapment.

- The ankle is then held in neutral to slight eversion at 90° with a slight posterior drawer pressure. The sutures are tied down over the capsule and IER allowing these to imbricate and pull up to the face of the anterior fibula when viewed through the arthroscope.
- The construct is tested for stability. If the surgeon prefers, supplemental suture techniques, such as a suture bridge or internal brace, can be added to the construct. Should the surgeon decide that the arthroscopic technique has not adequately stabilized the lateral ligaments, the procedure can easily be converted to an open technique at any point.
- If the surgeon is concerned about a possible peroneal tendon tear, a small incision can be made directly over the peroneal tendons to examine and perform a repair as necessary. The senior authors prefer to perform a peroneal tendonoscopy to examine the anatomy and debride through the scope unless a tear is present.

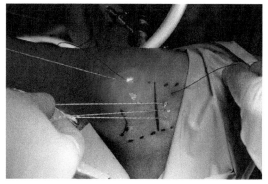

Fig. 3. Passage of second set of sutures after passage of first suture set and first limb of second set. The looped wire is shown in proper position to shuttle last suture limb after sharp-tipped suture passer is removed.

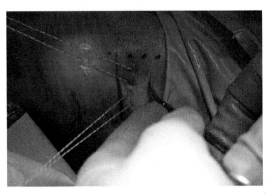

Fig. 4. Small (4-mm) incision is shown before subcutaneous passage and tying of suture.

- The arthroscopic portals and the small incision for suture tying are then closed with a small nylon mattress suture. With the smaller incisions and less soft tissue dissection, immediate postoperative swelling is far less than normal, and the long-term cosmetic appearance is excellent (**Fig. 5**).

CLINICAL RESULTS OF ARTHROSCOPIC LATERAL LIGAMENT REPAIR

Arthroscopic lateral ligament repair techniques have been continuously refined over the past 10 years (**Table 2**). Among the more modern techniques, there are 3 relatively distinct methods, which should be differentiated to better analyze study results. For discussion purposes, these can be grouped into "arthroscopic assisted techniques," "all-arthroscopic techniques," and "all-inside techniques." Arthroscopic-assisted repairs use either an accessory portal or an accessory incision for suture passage through the lateral ligamentous complex and sutures are tied extracapsular. In

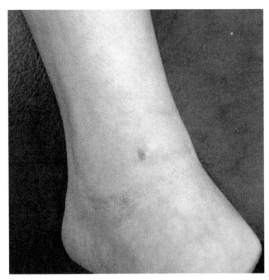

Fig. 5. Six weeks postoperatively from all-arthroscopic ligament repair. Note minimal swelling and cosmesis.

Table 2		
Complications with arthroscopic lateral ankle ligament repair		
Author, Year	**Number of Complications (%)**	**Type of Complications**
Acevedo & Mangone,[13] 2015	9 (12.32)	1 residual instability 3 persistent lateral pain 5 neuritis
Corte-Real & Moreira,[46] 2015	9 (29)	3 delayed wound healing 3 neuritis SPN 2 acute ankle sprains
Cottom & Rigby,[36] 2013	3 (7.5)	1 deep vein thrombosis 1 neuritis dorsal cutanoeus nerve 1 distal fibular fracture
Li et al,[39] 2017	1 (4.3)	1 persistent pain
Nery et al,[40] 2011	0	—
Nery et al,[41] 2017	1 (3.8)	1 neuritis SPN
Song et al,[42] 2017		
Reconstruction	1 (8.3)	1 neuritis sural nerve
Repair	2 (12.5)	2 neuritis SPN
Vega et al,[43] 2013	2 (12.5)	1 superficial infection 1 delayed wound healing
Yeo et al,[44] 2016	5 (20)	2 neuritis SPN 1 neuritis sural nerve 2 knot pain
Yoo & Yang,[45] 2016		
Internal brace	0	—
w/o internal brace	2 (3.2)	2 neuritis DCN

contrast, all-arthroscopic repairs, such as the Arthrobrostrom, involve suture passage under direct arthroscopic visualization using a sharp-tipped suture passer. Additional portals are not necessary for this technique, and sutures are also tied extracapsularly. All-inside techniques also involve suture passage under direct visualization with the arthroscope, but suture knots are tied within the joint.

Arthroscopic-Assisted Techniques

Arthroscopic-assisted techniques involve the use of one or more accessory portals to pass either bone anchors or sutures through the joint and the ligament. Multiple clinical studies have reported favorable outcomes for patients treated with the arthroscopic-assisted repairs. In 2009, Corte-Real and Moreira[46] reported the first European study on 28 of their 31 patients using an arthroscopic-assisted technique. The investigators used one double-loaded suture anchor as well as an accessory anterolateral portal. At 24.5-months average follow-up, American Orthopaedic Foot and Ankle Society (AOFAS) scores averaged 85.3, and only 2 patients, demonstrated recurrent instability. Although their complication rate was relatively high (29%), their technique contributed positively to the early development of arthroscopic ligament repair and marks the beginning of modern techniques. Kim[37] subsequently published the results on 28 ankles also using one double-loaded suture anchor. Unlike the prior technique, these investigators used a soft tissue penetrator to pass sutures and an accessory anteroinferior portal. At a 15.9-month average follow-up, 3 patients had laxity with stress radiographs, but all were able to return to their preinjury level. In

2012, Nery and colleagues[40] reported on their first cohort of 38 patients with an average 9.8-year follow-up. Their technique also used one double-loaded anchor into the anterior fibula and an accessory portal to lasso the lateral ligamentous complex. The mean AOFAS score was 90%, and 87% of active patients continued to practice sport at the same preoperative level 10 years after the repair. All of these techniques used either an accessory portal or an accessory incision for suture passage through the lateral ligamentous complex.

All-Arthroscopic Techniques

All-arthroscopic techniques use only the 2 traditional ankle arthroscopy portals for passage of the bone anchors and/or sutures through the joint and ligaments, but still use a small incision to tie the sutures. In 2011, the senior authors[35] published the first fully arthroscopic technique that did not rely on accessory portals or incisions for anchor placement or suture passage. This study included 24 ankles with a 95.8% satisfaction rate at a 10.9-month follow-up. Several subsequent studies using the same techniques have reported comparable results.[13,36,38,41,45] The largest study to date included 73 patients evaluated retrospectively at an average 28 months with a 94.5% satisfaction rate. The mean Karlsson score improved from a preoperative score of 28.3 to a postoperative score of 90.2.[13] Despite 4 of 73 patients who were dissatisfied, only one patient had recurrent instability. In 2016, Nery and colleagues[41] published a prospective cohort study that included 26 patients who underwent inside-out technique for arthroscopic repair. The postoperative AOFAS score improved to a mean of 90 from 58 preoperatively with an average of 27 months of follow-up. Regular-poor scores were present in 4 (15.4%) patients.

All-Inside Techniques

All-inside techniques use only the 2 traditional and accessory ankle arthroscopy portals for passage of the bone anchors and/or sutures through the joint and ligaments but either tie the knot with arthroscopic techniques or use a knotless technique to secure the repair. These techniques have been developed more recently with promising results. Vega and colleagues[43] investigated using a knotless suture anchor as a means to prevent complications related to suture prominence (ie, neuritis, suture pain). A total of 16 patients were included and followed for an average of 22.3 months (12–35). Patient AOFAS scores improved from a mean of 67 (59–77) to 97 (95–100) using an all-inside technique. One patient had a superficial infection of the distal portal site that resolved with conservative management, and another patient had delayed wound healing of the anterolateral portal, which also resolved. No major or neurologic complications were reported. Li and colleagues[39] reported on 23 patients who underwent arthroscopic repair and compared these with a subgroup of 37 open MBOs. Postoperative AOFAS scores for the arthroscopic procedure was 93.3, Karlsson score 90.3, and Tegner score 5, which showed equivalence to the open technique scores of 92.4, 89.4, and 5, respectively. One (4.3%) patient in the arthroscopic group reported persistent pain following the procedure; otherwise, no additional complications were reported in this group. Yeo and colleagues[44] performed the only published randomized control trial comparing open modified Brostrom operation with an all-inside arthroscopic technique for ankle instability. There were 25 patients in the arthroscopic group and 23 patients in the open group. The arthroscopic group's mean Karlsson and AOFAS improved from 45 and 76.2 to 67.5 and 90.3, respectively. Similarly, in the open group the scores improved from 48.6 and 73.5 to 69.9 and 89.2. There were 5 (20%) complications in the arthroscopic group, which included SPN neuritis (2), sural neuritis (1), and knot pain (2).

Arthroscopic Versus Augmented Repair

Several studies have compared arthroscopic lateral ligament repair techniques to augmented repairs with tendon grafts or internal brace. Yoo and Yang[45] performed a retrospective cohort study that compared the arthroscopic modified Brostrom operation with and without the use of an internal brace. Twenty-two patients underwent the procedure with the internal brace and 63 patients underwent the procedure without the internal brace. The AOFAS scores of the patients with the brace improved from 65.8 to 98 and those without the brace improved from 66.7 to 96.5. There were no complications in the internal brace group, and there were 2 (3.2%) cases of dorsal cutaneous neuritis in the group without an internal brace. Although there was no statistical difference between the groups in terms of outcomes scores, the internal brace group was able to return to activity and sports more quickly. Song and colleagues[42] compared arthroscopic MBO repair (16 patients) versus reconstruction (12 patients) of the ATFL with a semitendinosus autograft. The arthroscopic repair group AOFAS score improved to 93 from 59.3, and the reconstruction group improved to 94.4 from 61.3 at the 12-month follow-up visit. Similarly, there was no statistically significant difference in outcome scores at 12 months, although early results at 6 months favored the tendon reconstruction group.

SUMMARY

Since the mid 1980s, significant advances have been made using arthroscopic techniques for stabilizing major joints, such as the shoulder and the knee. Ankle arthroscopy, on the other hand, has been a relative novelty with its main use being inspection of the joint and treating associated intra-articular pathologic condition, such as removal of loose bodies, impingement debridement, and microfracture. Ankle arthroscopy in combination with open lateral ligament reconstruction is now performed more frequently due to a better understanding of the importance of defining intra-articular pathologic condition secondary to ankle instability. Similar to the knee and shoulder, this combination has prompted multiple surgeons from across the globe to investigate the use of arthroscopic techniques to stabilize the ankle. Over the last 10 years, significant advances have been made, and successful techniques have now been developed that effectively treat ankle instability via the arthroscope. In particular, the 2-anchor ArthroBrostrom technique detailed in this article has been the most rigorously studied and proven to be a simple, safe, and biomechanically equivalent, stable alternative to open Brostrom Gould lateral ligament reconstruction. Reviewing the history of shoulder and knee arthroscopy, significant further advances will continue to occur in the next 20 years. Techniques and instruments will evolve to undoubtedly make arthroscopic lateral ankle ligament reconstruction the standard of care in the world of foot and ankle orthopedics.

REFERENCES

1. Gribble PA, Bleakley CM, Caulfield BM, et al. 2016 consensus statement of the International Ankle Consortium: prevalence, impact and long-term consequences of lateral ankle sprains. Br J Sports Med 2016;50(24):1493–5.

2. Freeman MA, Dean MR, Hanham IW. The etiology and prevention of functional instability of the foot. J Bone Joint Surg Br 1965;47:678–85.

3. Shakked RJ, Karnovsky S, Drakos MC. Operative treatment of lateral ligament instability. Curr Rev Musculoskelet Med 2017;10(1):113–21.

4. Ballal MS, Pearce CJ, Calder JD. Management of sports injuries of the foot and ankle: an update. Bone Joint J 2016;98-B(7):874–83.

5. Odak S. Arthroscopic evaluation of impingement and osteochondral lesions in chronic lateral ankle instability. Foot Ankle Int 2015;36(9):1045–9.

6. Cannon LB, Slater HK. The role of ankle arthroscopy and surgical approach in lateral ankle ligament repair. 2005;11(1):1–4.

7. Hintermann B, Boss A, Schäfer D. Arthroscopic findings in patients with chronic ankle instability. Am J Sports Med 2002;30(3):402–9.

8. Hua Y, Chen S, Li Y, et al. Combination of modified Broström procedure with ankle arthroscopy for chronic ankle instability accompanied by intra-articular symptoms. Arthroscopy 2010;26(4):524–8.

9. Komenda GA, Ferkel RD. Arthroscopic findings associated with the unstable ankle. Foot Ankle Int 1999;20(11):708–13.

10. Hertel J. Functional anatomy, pathomechanics and pathophysiology of lateralankle instability. J Athl Train 2002;37(4):364.

11. Tourné Y, Mabit C. Lateral ligament reconstruction procedures for the ankle. Orthop Traumatol Surg Res 2017;103(1S):S171–81.

12. Tropp H. Commentary: functional ankle instability revisited. J Athl Train 2002;37(4):512–5.

13. Acevedo JI, Mangone P. Ankle instability and arthroscopic lateral ligament repair. Foot Ankle Clin 2015;20(1):59–69.

14. Hossain M, Thomas R. Ankle instability: presentation and management. Orthopaedics and Trauma 2015;29(2):145–51.

15. White WJ, McCollum G, Calder JD. Return to sport following acute lateral ligament repair of the ankle in professional athletes. Knee Surg Sports Traumatol Arthrosc 2016;24(4):1124–9.

16. Vega J, Dalmau-Pastor M, Malagelada F, et al. Ankle arthroscopy: an update. J Bone Joint Surg Am 2017;99(16):1395–407.

17. Matsui K, Takao M, Tochigi Y, et al. Anatomy of anterior talofibular ligament and calcaneofibular ligament for minimally invasive surgery: a systematic review. Knee Surg Sports Traumatol Arthrosc 2017;25(6):1892–902.

18. Jorge JT, Gomes TM, Oliva XM. An anatomical study about the arthroscopic repair of the lateral ligament of the ankle. Foot Ankle Surg 2018;24(2):143–8.

19. Lee KT, Lee JI, Sung KS, et al. Biomechanical evaluation against calcaneofibular ligament repair in the Brostrom procedure: a cadaveric study. Knee Surg Sports Traumatol Arthrosc 2008;16(8):781–6.

20. Lee KT, Park YU, Kim JS, et al. Long-term results after modified Brostrom procedure without calcaneofibular ligament reconstruction. Foot Ankle Int 2011;32(2):153–7.

21. Dalmau-Pastor M, Yasui Y, Calder JD, et al. Anatomy of the inferior extensor retinaculum and its role in lateral ankle ligament reconstruction: a pictorial essay. Knee Surg Sports Traumatol Arthrosc 2016;24(4):957–62.

22. Dalmau-Pastor M. X-shaped inferior extensor retinaculum and its doubtful use in the Bröstrom-Gould procedure. Knee Surg Sports Traumatol Arthrosc 2017. https://doi.org/10.1007/s00167-017-4647-y.

23. Matsui K, Oliva XM, Takao M, et al. Bony landmarks available for minimally invasive lateral ankle stabilization surgery: a cadaveric anatomical study. Knee Surg Sports Traumatol Arthrosc 2017;25(6):1916–24.

24. Clanton TO, Campbell KJ, Wilson KJ, et al. Qualitative and quantitative anatomic investigation of the lateral ankle ligaments for surgical reconstruction procedures. J Bone Joint Surg Am 2014;96(12):e98.

25. Gallie WE. VIII. Tendon fixation: a preliminary report of a simple operation for the prevention of deformity in paralytic Talipes. Ann Surg 1913;57(3):427–9.
26. Nilsonne H. Making a new ligament in ankle sprain. J Bone Joint Surg Am 1932; 14(2):380–1.
27. Broström L. Sprained ankles. VI. Surgical treatment of "chronic" ligament ruptures. Acta Chir Scand 1966;132(5):551–65.
28. Hamilton WG, Thompson FM, Snow SW. The modified Brostrom procedure for lateral ankle instability. Foot Ankle 1993;14(1):1–7.
29. Aydogan U, Glisson RR, Nunley JA. Extensor retinaculum augmentation reinforces anterior talofibular ligament repair. Clin Orthop Relat Res 2006;442:210–5.
30. Berlet GC, Saar WE, Ryan A, et al. Thermal-assisted capsular modification for functional ankle instability. Foot Ankle Clin 2002;7(3):567–76.
31. Maiotti M, Massoni C, Tarantino U. The use of arthroscopic thermal shrinkage to treat chronic lateral ankle instability in young athletes. Arthroscopy 2005;21(6): 751–7.
32. Vuurberg G, de Vries JS, Krips R, et al. Arthroscopic capsular shrinkage for treatment of chronic lateral ankle instability. Foot Ankle Int 2017;38(10):1078–84.
33. Hawkins RB. Arthroscopic stapling repair for chronic lateral instability. Clin Podiatr Med Surg 1987;4(4):875–83.
34. Kashuk KB, Landsman AS, Werd MB, et al. Arthroscopic lateral ankle stabilization. Clin Podiatr Med Surg 1994;11(3):407–23.
35. Acevedo JI, Mangone PG. Arthroscopic lateral ankle ligament reconstruction. Tech Foot Ankle Surg 2011;10(3):111–6.
36. Cottom JM, Rigby RB. The "all inside" arthroscopic Brostrom procedure: a prospective study of 40 consecutive patients. J Foot Ankle Surg 2013;52(5):568–74.
37. Kim ES. Arthroscopic anterior talofibular ligament repair for chronic ankle instability with a suture anchor technique. Orthopedics 2011;34(4). https://doi.org/ 10.3928/01477447-20110228-03.
38. Labib SA, Slone HS. Ankle arthroscopy for lateral ankle instability. Tech Foot Ankle Surg 2015;14(1):25–7.
39. Li H, Hua Y, Li H, et al. Activity level and function 2 years after anterior talofibular ligament repair: a comparison between arthroscopic repair and open repair procedures. Am J Sports Med 2017;45(9):2044–52.
40. Nery C, Raduan F, Del Buono A, et al. Arthroscopic-assisted Broström-Gould for chronic ankle instability: a long-term follow-up. Am J Sports Med 2011;39(11): 2381–8.
41. Nery C, Fonseca L, Raduan F, et al. Prospective study of the "inside-out" arthroscopic ankle ligament technique: preliminary result. Foot Ankle Surg 2017. https://doi.org/10.1016/j.fas.2017.03.002.
42. Song B, Li C, Chen N, et al. All-arthroscopic anatomical reconstruction of anterior talofibular ligament using semitendinosus autografts. Int Orthop 2017;41(5): 975–82.
43. Vega J, Golanó P, Pellegrino A, et al. All-inside arthroscopic lateral collateral ligament repair for ankle instability with a knotless suture anchor technique. Foot Ankle Int 2013;34(12):1701–9.
44. Yeo ED, Lee KT, Sung IH, et al. Comparison of all-inside arthroscopic and open techniques for the modified brostöm procedure for ankle instability. Foot Ankle Int 2016;37(10):1037–45.
45. Yoo JS, Yang EA. Clinical results of an arthroscopic modified Brostrom operation with and without an internal brace. J Orthop Traumatol 2016;17(4):353–60.

46. Corte-Real NM, Moreira RM. Arthroscopic repair of chronic lateral ankle instability. Foot Ankle Int 2015;5:213–7.
47. Matsui K, Takao M, Miyamoto W, et al. Early recovery after arthroscopic repair compared to open repair of the anterior talofibular ligament for lateral instability of the ankle. Arch Orthop Trauma Surg 2016;136(1):93–100.
48. Prisk VR, Imhauser CW, O'Loughlin PF, et al. Lateral ligament repair and reconstruction restore neither contact mechanics of the ankle joint nor motion patterns of the hindfoot. J Bone Joint Surg Am 2010;92(14):2375–86.
49. Acevedo JI, Ortiz C, Golano P, et al. ArthroBroström lateral ankle stabilization technique: an anatomic study. Am J Sports Med 2015;43(10):2564–71.
50. Drakos M, Behrens S, Hoffman E, et al. A biomechanical comparison of an open vs. arthroscopic approach for the treatment of lateral ankle instability (SS-57). Arthroscopy 2011;27(5):809–15.
51. Giza E, Shin EC, Wong SE, et al. Arthroscopic suture anchor repair of the lateral ligament ankle complex: a cadaveric study. Am J Sports Med 2013;41(11): 2567–72.
52. Lee KT, Kim ES, Kim YH, et al. All-inside arthroscopic modified Broström operation for chronic ankle instability: a biomechanical study. Knee Surg Sports Traumatol Arthrosc 2016;24(4):1096–100.
53. Yoshimura I, Hagio T, Noda M, et al. Optimal suture anchor direction in arthroscopic lateral ankle ligament repair. Knee Surg Sports Traumatol Arthrosc 2017. https://doi.org/10.1007/s00167-017-4587-6.
54. Corte-Real NM, Moreira RM. Arthroscopic repair of chronic lateral ankle instability. Foot Ankle Int 2009;30(3):213–7.

Arthroscopic Treatment of Ankle Instability - Allograft/ Autograft Reconstruction

João Teixeira, MD[a], Stephane Guillo, MD[b],*

KEYWORDS

- Ankle instability • Ankle arthroscopy • Ankle endoscopy
- Lateral ligament reconstruction • Gracilis autograft

KEY POINTS

- Arthroscopic techniques used to repair or reconstruct lateral ankle ligaments in patients with chronic ankle instability are a theme of increasing interest.
- Reconstruction procedures should be reserved for cases of failed previous ligament repair, insufficient remaining tissue, general laxity, excessive body mass index, and in those who are heavy laborers or participate in aggressive sports.
- Arthroscopic reconstruction of lateral ankle ligaments using autologous gracilis autograft is a technically challenging but reproducible and safe procedure.

INTRODUCTION

Inversion ankle sprains represent one of the most common traumatic injuries in the active sports population. It is globally accepted that most of these lesions can be managed conservatively. However, recent scientific trends in the foot and ankle community note the prevalence of hidden lesions associated with these apparently simple ankle sprains.[1] In fact, up to 30% of the patients do not respond to conservative treatment, developing chronic ankle instability (CAI).[2,3]

The group of patients that develop CAI is not homogeneous, so its etiology is thought to be multifactorial versus caused by individual predisposing factors.[2]

When left untreated, CAI is thought to be responsible for multiple repetitive trauma events to the cartilage, leading to the predisposition of osteochondral lesions with possible evolution to ankle arthrosis.[1,2] It is therefore important to look for reparable ligamentous structures in order to avoid or potentially delay the natural evolution to ankle arthritis.

Disclosure: Dr Teixeira is nothing to disclose and Dr Guillo is arthrex consultant.
a Departament of Orthopaedics and Traumatology, Centro Hospitalar de Entre o Douro e Vouga, rua Dr. Cândido de Pinho, Santa Maria da Feira 4520-211, Portugal; b Clinique du Sport, 2 rue Negrevergne, Bordeuax-Mérignac 33700, France
* Corresponding author.
E-mail address: steguillo@gmail.com

Foot Ankle Clin N Am 23 (2018) 571–579
https://doi.org/10.1016/j.fcl.2018.07.004
1083-7515/18/© 2018 Elsevier Inc. All rights reserved.

foot.theclinics.com

Lateral ankle ligament injuries occur in more than 80% of all ankle sprains, and the anterior talo-fibular ligament (ATFL) is the primary ligament involved, followed by the calcaneo-fibular ligament (CFL). The posterior talo-fibular ligament (PTFL) is rarely injured.[4]

Whenever conservative treatment fails, CAI patients should be considered for ligament repair/reconstruction surgery. The main surgical goal is to restore the normal ankle anatomy, ligamentous balance, and function of the ankle.

Ligament repair, most notably the Brostrom procedure associated with Gould augmentation, has become the gold-standard procedure to deal with CAI in the past decade, with the widest and most reproducible use.[2,5] However, it assumes the existence of viable remnant ligamentous tissue suitable for repair and a favorable environment for biologic healing.

Actually, the repair procedures showed substandard results in overweight patients, those with generalized ligamentous laxity, bad remnant ligament quality, presence of ossicles greater than 1 cm, and revision procedures. In these cases, reconstructive procedures, where the native ligaments are replaced instead of being repaired, are preferable.[4]

NONANATOMIC VERSUS ANATOMIC RECONSTRUCTION SURGERY

The first reconstruction procedures, such as Chrisman- Snook, Evans, and Watson-Jones, advocate ankle stabilization through a nonanatomic tenodesis or graft interposition. Besides showing promising results in the first studies, the following studies showed progressive range of motion loss, with consequent evolution to early arthrosis.[6] It is thought this arthrosis was a result of the rigidity produced by overconstraining the talo-crural and subtalar joints.[7] Besides that, normal ankle kinematics and biomechanics are altered, as most of these nonanatomical reconstructions utilize/sacrifice the peroneal tendons, which are important dynamic hindfoot stabilizers, thus leading to stabilization failure.[2,6]

In 2013, a consensus in CAI agreed that nonanatomic procedures should be avoided, as they did not achieve reconstruction surgery goals.[2]

The objective of anatomic reconstruction is to achieve ankle stability without overconstraining the talo-crural or subtalar joints. There are several anatomic reconstructions described in the literature,[8] with the common goal of recreating the native anatomy by positioning the graft closest to the anatomic landmarks of the native ATFL and CFL origin and insertion sites.

Anatomic ligament reconstruction has been proven to effectively stabilize a chronically unstable ankle without compromising articular range of motion.[2,9] As such, this is considered the preferred option in lateral ligament reconstructive procedures.[2,9]

MINIMALLY INVASIVE AND ENDOSCOPIC ANATOMIC RECONSTRUCTION TECHNIQUES

The natural evolution in every successful surgical technique is to reduce morbidity while being as minimally invasive as possible. Considering that more than 90% of CAI patients have intra-articular lesions found in anterior ankle arthroscopy, it is logical to associate both procedures.[10]

In the last years, several endoscopic-assisted and mini-invasive procedures emerged.[7,11-13] In 2005, Takao[7] described a mini-invasive technique assisted by arthroscopy where the ATFL and CFL graft limbs were fixed to a common fibular origin by interference screws. Later, in 2016, the ankle instability group[14] presented a revised totally arthroscopic lateral ligament reconstruction based on a new technique presented 2 years before by Guillo and colleagues.[11]The technique has been simplified subsequent to the article due to the fact that peroneal tendoscopy is not required each time. The reliability of this technique was tested in a cadaveric study that proved its safety and reproducibility.[15]

Matsui and colleagues[3] recently reviewed all minimally invasive surgical treatment for CAI. They only found 6 studies (1 level IV study and 5 level V studies) regarding arthroscopic reconstruction procedures. Besides the good results reported in these initial descriptions, the grade of recommendation was only grade C.[3] There is also insufficient evidence to state the superiority of one technique against another.[3,4]

The endoscopic lateral ankle ligament reconstruction procedures represent natural progress in ankle surgery, similar to what happened in shoulder and knee in the past decade. However, there is still a long way to go to prove these techniques are efficient in CAI treatment. It is therefore necessary to perform more quality studies to reach better grades of recommendations.

SURGICAL TECHNIQUE

Surgical indications include chronic ankle instability associated with[2]:
- Overweight patients (BMI >25)
- Heavy labor occupation or sports requirement
- Congenital ligament laxity (Beighton scale >8)
- Nonviable remnant ligament tissue
- Previously failed repair procedure
- Lateral ossicle >1 cm

The Graft

Contrary to other common ligament reconstruction surgeries, the graft needed to replace the lateral ankle ligaments does not have to be particularly thick or long. In fact, the ideal graft can be less than 12 cm long and must be thin enough to avoid impingement with the surrounding structures. The tensile strength also is not a problem, because the maximum failure of the ATFL is around 350N, which is less than a half of the maximum failure load of commonly used tendons (eg, Gracilis 838N).[6]

There are several different graft options described in the literature; however there is still no consensus about the best graft option to use in ankle lateral ligament reconstruction.[4] Among them, the autologous gracilis tendon was proved to be adequate for lateral ankle ligament reconstruction.[6]

As in other articulations, such as the knee, the debate between autografts and allografts is still inconclusive. A recent meta-analysis about hamstring grafts used in anterior cruciate knee reconstruction showed no statistically significant differences between autografts and allografts.[16]

In the ankle, Xu and colleagues[17] did a retrospective review comparing semitendinosus autograft and allograft, and concluded that both grafts were effective. They only found a slightly faster healing time in the autograft group without any significant additional donor site morbidity.

Considering the costs and limited availability of the allografts, and assuming the safety and mini-invasiveness of the new hamstring harvest techniques, the authors prefer the use of gracilis autograft.

Equipment

A standard 4 mm 30° arthroscope and 4.5 mm bone/soft tissue shaver blade are used. Irrigation is provided by gravity pressure with hanging saline 3 L bag.

The main surgical goal is to make 3 bone tunnels (fibular, talar, and calcaneal) corresponding to the lateral ligament attachments, and then secure the graft with the best devices available.

Currently the authors use several graft fixation devices (but others are available with similar efficacy):

1. Fibular fixation: Toggle Lock (Biomet) or ACL TightRope (Arthrex). According to the authors' experience, it is preferable to have a fixation device that pushes the graft when the shuttle suture is tensioned in the opposite direction of the graft movement.
2. Talar tunnel: Considering a 6 × 20 mm tunnel, a BioTenodesis (Arthrex) 5.5 × 15 mm screw is used. It is important to downsize the screw diameter because of the hardness of talar bone.
3. Calcaneal tunnel: Considering a 6 × 30 mm tunnel, a 7 × 25 mm full-thread interference screw is used. Contrary to the talus, the calcaneus mostly consists of soft cancellous bone, so it is important to upsize the screw size to improve fixation.

Patient positioning

The patient is in lateral decubitus position with the pelvis rotated 30° posterior to ensure the ability to perform the 3 positions needed for the surgery (**Fig. 1**).

Position 1 (graft harvest): externally rotated hip and flexed knee (see **Fig. 1**A)
Position 2 (anterior arthroscopy): externally rotated hip and extended knee (see **Fig. 1**B)
Position 3 (lateral endoscopy): neutral hip and extended knee (see **Fig. 1**C)

Graft harvest

With the patient in position 1, the gracilis tendon is harvested by a minimally invasive antero-medial incision as previously described by other authors.[18]

Step 1

The first portal to be made is the antero-medial one. It is important to place this portal just medial to the tibialis anterior tendon, with the ankle in dorsiflexion, in order to have clear access to the lateral gutter. Transillumination is used to create the second portal. This second portal is placed in the talus tunnel direction, so it will be slightly more distal and lateral than the regular anterolateral portal. Complete lateral gutter debridement is performed, essentially next to the fibular ATFL attachment to facilitate the next step.

Step 2

The arthroscope is now moved to portal 2, and medial intra-articular inspection is completed with management of existent lesions.

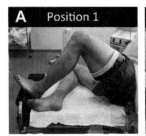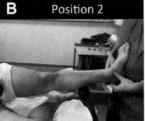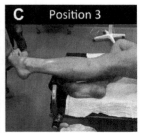

Fig. 1. Patient positioning.

The portal 3 is then created in the intersection between a line that follows the superior border of the peroneus brevis and a second line that follows the direction of the fibular tunnel (**Fig. 2**). A mosquito clamp is introduced through this portal in the direction of lateral malleolus, creating the working space through this portal.

Calcaneal tunnel With the arthroscope in portal 2, the subtalar joint and the lateral calcaneal wall is exposed to find the CFL footprint. It is usually located 17 mm inferior to the lateral midpoint of the posterior subtalar calcaneal facet.[19]

Correct debridement of the surrounding area is performed. A guidewire is then introduced through the CFL footprint. It is directed distal, posterior, and medial, exiting in the postero-medial calcaneal border in order to make the maximal possible tunnel length. A 6 mm tunnel is then overdrilled through both cortices.

With the aid of eyelet pin, another lead suture (n° 1) is passed through the calcaneal tunnel and retrieved medially.

Fibular tunnel The obscure tubercle is the first landmark to search for. It is found in the transition between the 2 different bone plane directions (**Fig. 3**) and corresponds to the common anatomic ATFL and CFL origin.[19,20]

With the 4.0 mm bone cutter, a small hole is made in this spot in order to transform this convex slippery surface into a concave one, avoiding guidewire slide. The guidewire is then introduced immediately lateral to the lateral malleolar cartilage and advanced in a postero-superior direction through both lateral malleolar cortices. The peroneal tendons should always be protected when the pin passes the posterior fibular cortex. A 4.5 mm drill is then passed through both fibular cortices, and a 10 mm tunnel is then made with a 6 mm drill. An eyelet guidewire is then retrieved from the posterior-superior position, passing a strong suture through the tunnel that will be used to pull the graft into the tunnel in a subsequent step (lead suture n° 2).

Step 3: talar tunnel
The arthroscope is now moved to portal 3, and the talus ATFL footprint is debrided through portal 2. The footprint's main landmark is the bottom of the triangular talar surface without cartilage. The tunnel insertion point should be located halfway between the superior and inferior talus lateral surface (usually coincident with the deepest point of its lateral surface). In the horizontal plane, it should be aligned with the bottom end of the peroneal tunnel.

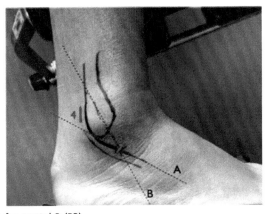

Fig. 2. Landmarks for portal 3 (P3).

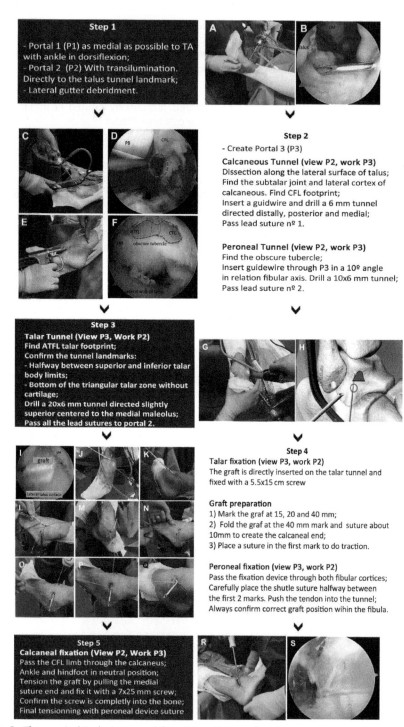

Step 1
- Portal 1 (P1) as medial as possible to TA with ankle in dorsiflexion;
- Portal 2 (P2) With transillumination. Directly to the talus tunnel landmark;
- Lateral gutter debridment.

Step 2
- Create Portal 3 (P3)

Calcaneous Tunnel (view P2, work P3)
Dissection along the lateral surface of talus;
Find the subtalar joint and lateral cortex of calcaneous. Find CFL footprint;
Insert a guidewire and drill a 6 mm tunnel directed distally, posterior and medial;
Pass lead suture nº 1.

Peroneal Tunnel (view P2, work P3)
Find the obscure tubercle;
Insert guidewire through P3 in a 10º angle in relation fibular axis. Drill a 10x6 mm tunnel;
Pass lead suture nº 2.

Step 3
Talar Tunnel (View P3, Work P2)
Find ATFL talar footprint;
Confirm the tunnel landmarks:
- Halfway between superior and inferior talar body limits;
- Bottom of the triangular talar zone without cartilage;
Drill a 20x6 mm tunnel directed slightly superior centered to the medial maleolus;
Pass all the lead sutures to portal 2.

Step 4
Talar fixation (view P3, work P2)
The graft is directly inserted on the talar tunnel and fixed with a 5.5x15 cm screw

Graft preparation
1) Mark the graf at 15, 20 and 40 mm;
2) Fold the graf at the 40 mm mark and suture about 10mm to create the calcaneal end;
3) Place a suture in the first mark to do traction.

Peroneal fixation (view P3, work P2)
Pass the fixation device through both fibular cortices;
Carefully place the shuttle suture halfway between the first 2 marks. Push the tendon into the tunnel;
Always confirm correct graft position wihin the fibula.

Step 5
Calcaneal fixation (View P2, Work P3)
Pass the CFL limb through the calcaneus;
Ankle and hindfoot in neutral position;
Tension the graft by pulling the medial suture end and fix it with a 7x25 mm screw;
Confirm the screw is completely into the bone;
Final tensionning with peroneal device suture

Fig. 3. The surgical technique used for allograft reconstruction.

The guidewire is then inserted through portal 2, aiming to medial malleolus in a slightly superior direction. With this orientation, a completely safe 20 × 6 mm tunnel can be drilled as shown by Michels.[15] At this point, all the lead sutures are passed to portal 2.

Step 4: talar fixation and graft preparation

The graft is introduced in the talar tunnel through portal 2 under direct visualization from portal 3. A bioabsorbable 5.5 × 15 mm screw is used for fixation.

The graft is then prepared:

1. 3 marks are made on the graft: at 15 mm from the talus, 20 mm from the first mark, and 40 mm from the second mark (see **Fig. 3**).
2. The graft is folded in the distal mark (40 mm from the second mark), and about 10 mm are sutured to create the calcaneal end of the graft (see **Fig. 3**). The remaining free portion of the graft distal to the calacaneal portion is rejected.
3. A suture is placed in the first mark for traction.

Fibular fixation

The lateral malleolar fixation device is introduced in the fibular tunnel through portal 2 by pulling the lead suture n° 1. After confirming proper device fixation to the postero-lateral fibular cortex, the shuttle suture is carefully placed halfway between the first 2 marks (see **Fig. 3**). This ensures the creation of a folded 10 mm graft that will be pushed inside the peroneal tunnel. It is important to always confirm the graft position inside the fibula through direct vision.

The ATFL limb tension is achieved by pulling on the loop of the fibular fixation device with the ankle in neutral position.

Step 5: calcaneal tunnel fixation The CFL limb is passed into to the respective calcaneal tunnel with aid of lead suture n° 1, and is then tensioned by pulling on the medial calcaneal side maintaining the ankle and hindfoot in neutral position. The graft is then secured with a 7 × 25 mm bioabsorbable screw. It is important to always ensure the correct positioning of the screw inside the calcaneal tunnel to avoid impingement on the peroneal tendons.

POSTOPERATIVE CARE

The passive and active dorsi and plantar flexion range of motion are allowed immediately after surgery. Inversion and eversion movements are protected during the first 6 weeks by an ankle splint. At 6 weeks postoperative, the patients start walking without crutches and are allowed to full athletic activity at 6 months after surgery.

SUMMARY

Symptomatic patients with mechanical CAI are often forced to reduce or abandon sports activities because of repetitive sprain episodes. In addition, they are at risk of developing osteochondral lesions with possible evolution to osteoarthritis.[1,7] It is therefore important to deal with CAI in order to re-establish normal ankle kinematics and biomechanics.

As in every surgical procedure, the first key for success is a good surgical indication. Thus, the reconstruction procedures should be reserved for cases of failed previous ligament repair, insufficient remaining ligamentous tissue, general laxity, excessive body mass index, and those individuals with heavy labor occupations or aggressive sports requirement.

Arthroscopic lateral ankle ligament reconstruction is a challenging new procedure described to treat CAI. Although technically demanding, it is a reproducible and safe technique.[15] The arthroscopic approach, in addition to minimizing soft tissue damage, enables to one to treat coexistent intra-articular lesions that have been noted to be present in more than 90% of the cases.[10]

Despite being a promising solution, the level of evidence is still low, and further investigation is needed to prove the value of this procedure.

REFERENCES

1. Kerkhoffs GM, Kennedy JG, Calder JD, et al. There is no simple lateral ankle sprain. In: Knee Surgery Sports Traumatology Arthroscopy. Springer; 2016.
2. Guillo S, Bauer T, Lee JW, et al. Consensus in chronic ankle instability: aetiology, assessment, surgical indications and place for arthroscopy. Orthop Traumatol Surg Res 2013;99(8 Suppl):S411-9.
3. Matsui K, Burgesson B, Takao M, et al. Minimally invasive surgical treatment for chronic ankle instability: a systematic review. Knee Surg Sports Traumatol Arthrosc 2016;24(4):1040-8.
4. Shakked RJ, Karnovsky S, Drakos MC. Operative treatment of lateral ligament instability. Curr Rev Musculoskelet Med 2017;10(1):113-21.
5. Acevedo JI, Mangone P. Ankle instability and arthroscopic lateral ligament repair. Foot Ankle Clin 2015;20(1):59-69.
6. Coughlin MJ, Schenck RC Jr, Grebing BR, et al. Comprehensive reconstruction of the lateral ankle for chronic instability using a free gracilis graft. Foot Ankle Int 2004;25(4):231-41.
7. Takao M, Oae K, Uchio Y, et al. Anatomical reconstruction of the lateral ligaments of the ankle with a gracilis autograft: a new technique using an interference fit anchoring system. Am J Sports Med 2005;33(6):814-23.
8. Karlsson J, Eriksson BI, Bergsten T, et al. Comparison of two anatomic reconstructions for chronic lateral instability of the ankle joint. Am J Sports Med 1997;25(1):48-53.
9. Schmidt R, Cordier E, Bertsch C, et al. Reconstruction of the lateral ligaments: do the anatomical procedures restore physiologic ankle kinematics? Foot Ankle Int 2004;25(1):31-6.
10. Choi WJ, Lee JW, Han SH, et al. Chronic lateral ankle instability: the effect of intra-articular lesions on clinical outcome. Am J Sports Med 2008;36(11):2167-72.
11. Guillo S, Archbold P, Perera A, et al. Arthroscopic anatomic reconstruction of the lateral ligaments of the ankle with gracilis autograft. Arthrosc Tech 2014;3(5):e593-8.
12. Lopes R, Decante C, Geffroy L, et al. Arthroscopic anatomical reconstruction of the lateral ankle ligaments: a technical simplification. Orthop Traumatol Surg Res 2016;102(8S):S317-22.
13. Michels F, Cordier G, Guillo S, et al, ESKKA-AFAS Ankle Instability Group. Endoscopic ankle lateral ligament graft anatomic reconstruction. Foot Ankle Clin 2016; 21(3):665-80.
14. Guillo S, Takao M, Calder J, et al. Arthroscopic anatomical reconstruction of the lateral ankle ligaments. Knee Surg Sports Traumatol Arthrosc 2016;24(4):998-1002.
15. Michels F, Cordier G, Burssens A, et al. Endoscopic reconstruction of CFL and the ATFL with a gracilis graft: a cadaveric study. Knee Surg Sports Traumatol Arthrosc 2016;24(4):1007-14.

16. Cvetanovich GL, Mascarenhas R, Saccomanno MF, et al. Hamstring autograft versus soft-tissue allograft in anterior cruciate ligament reconstruction: a systematic review and meta-analysis of randomized controlled trials. Arthroscopy 2014; 30(12):1616–24.
17. Xu X, Hu M, Liu J, et al. Minimally invasive reconstruction of the lateral ankle ligaments using semitendinosus autograft or tendon allograft. Foot Ankle Int 2014; 35(10):1015–21.
18. Lanternier H, de Cussac JB, Collet T. Short medial approach harvesting of hamstring tendons. Orthop Traumatol Surg Res 2016;102(2):269–72.
19. Matsui K, Oliva XM, Takao M, et al. Bony landmarks available for minimally invasive lateral ankle stabilization surgery: a cadaveric anatomical study. Knee Surg Sports Traumatol Arthrosc 2017;25(6):1916–24.
20. Thes A, Klouche S, Ferrand M, et al. Assessment of the feasibility of arthroscopic visualization of the lateral ligament of the ankle: a cadaveric study. Knee Surg Sports Traumatol Arthrosc 2016;24(4):985–90.

Percutaneous Ankle Reconstruction of Lateral Ligaments

Mark Glazebrook, MSc, MD, PhD, FRCSC[a],*,
Mohammad Eid, MSc, MD, MRCS[a], Meshal Alhadhoud, MD[a],
James Stone, MD[b], Kentaro Matsui, MD, PhD[c],
Masato Takao, MD, PhD[d,e]

KEYWORDS

- Ankle instability • Ligament • P-anti RoLL • Pathology • Y-graft

KEY POINTS

- The Percutaneous Ankle Reconstruction of the Lateral Ligaments (Anti RoLL) provide a near anatomic reconstruction of the anterior talo fibular ligament and the calcaneal fibular ligament to treat chronic ankle instability This Surgery can also be done as a Arthroscopic Anti RoLL and an Open Anti RoLL technique.
- The Ankle Reconstruction of the Lateral Ligaments (Anti RoLL) Is a minimally invasive surgical reconstruction technique that is indicated when a surgical repair is not possible due to deficient remanent native ligaments Or when the patient or surgeon desires a more robust surgical solution to chronic ankle instability.
- The Ankle Reconstruction of the Lateral Ligaments (Anti RoLL) may be done with an autograft or allograft to construct the near anatomic "Y" reconstruction graft.

INTRODUCTION

Chronic ankle instability following ankle sprains causes pain and functional problems such as recurrent giving way. Within the 3 ligaments of the lateral ligament complex, 80% of patients tear the anterior talofibular ligament (ATFL), whereas the other 20% of patients tear the ATFL and calcaneofibular ligament (CFL). Rarely, the posterior talofibular ligament is involved.[1] An incidence of 10% to 30% of patients will fail conservative treatment and result in chronic ankle instability (CAI) that may require surgical

Disclosure Statement: The authors have nothing to disclose.
[a] Division of Orthopedic Surgery, Department of Surgery, Dalhousie University, Queen Elizabeth II Health Sciences Center, Room 4867, Halifax Infirmary, 1796 Summer Street, B3H3A7, Halifax, Nova Scotia B3H 3A6, Canada; [b] Orthopedic Surgery, Medical College of Wisconsin, Milwaukee, WI, USA; [c] Department of Orthopedic surgery, Teikyo University School of Medicine, 2-11-1 Kaga, Itabashi, Tokyo 173-8605, Japan; [d] Department of Orthopaedic Surgery, Teikyo Institute of Sports Science & Medicine, Tokyo, Japan; [e] Department of Sport and Medical Science, Teikyo Institute of Sports Science & Medicine, Tokyo, Japan
* Corresponding author.
E-mail address: markglazebr@hotmail.com

Foot Ankle Clin N Am 23 (2018) 581–592
https://doi.org/10.1016/j.fcl.2018.07.013
1083-7515/18/© 2018 Elsevier Inc. All rights reserved.

treatment.[2–5] To date, numerous open surgical procedures for anatomic repair or reconstruction of ATFL and/or CFL provide good clinical results.[5–7]

If nonoperative treatments fail, operative ankle stabilization may be required to improve pain and function.[3,8] Operative options include both anatomic repair and reconstruction techniques.[7] Anatomic repair techniques use preexisting ligament remnants that are either reattached or tightened to improve stability of the ankle.[1] If preexisting ligament structures have been damaged beyond repair or are insufficient to allow repair, then it is appropriate to choose an anatomic reconstructive technique.[7,9] These procedures have traditionally been performed using open techniques and have been successful in restoring function and decreasing pain.[7,10] In this article, the authors describe a Percutaneous Ankle Reconstruction of the Lateral Ligaments (P-Anti RoLL), which is a new minimally invasive surgical technique for anatomic reconstruction of the lateral ligaments of the ankle that uses the anatomic Y-graft and inside-out technique.[10] The P-Anti RoLL technique can be performed percutaneously using fluoroscopic guidance.

Recently, there have been advances in arthroscopic[11] and minimally invasive[12–16] ankle stabilization techniques that may allow faster recovery compared with open techniques.[17] The arthroscopic procedure allows one to assess and treat intraarticular pathology of the ankle concurrently with stabilization[9,18] but may be more technically demanding.[12] In contrast, the advantage of the percutaneous technique is its generally simple concept that does not require the skill of an experienced arthroscopist.[12] In addition, the use of fluoroscopic guidance allows more reliable and anatomic positioning of the graft to the ATFL and CFL insertion sites.[19]

Operative Technique

General preoperative technique considerations

- Standard ankle arthroscopy is recommended before the percutaneous stabilization procedure if there is any associated ankle pathology.
- The P-Anti RoLL technique does not require arthroscopy to reconstruct the lateral ligaments of the ankle and may be performed in isolation if there is no associated ankle pathology present.[20]

Landmark drawing and patient positioning

- The patient is positioned lateral with a support under the leg to allow access to the medial side of the ankle on an operating table that will allow perfect anterior-posterior and lateral fluoroscopic examinations throughout the procedure to enable accurate anatomic landmark identification.
- Anatomic landmarks should be drawn on the patient's skin before starting surgery (**Fig. 1**).[20]
- The P-Anti RoLL anatomic landmarks include the distal edge of the tibial plafond, the lateral and medial malleoli, the extensor digitorum tendon, and the peroneal tendon.
- The bony landmarks for the origin and insertion sites of the ATFL and CFL should be drawn under fluoroscopic view.

Landmark of the fibular bone tunnel

- The landmark for the fibular origin of the ATFL and CFL when using an anatomic Y-graft should be between the ATFL and CFL origin sites on the fibula.
- This ATFL and CFL origin site can be localized at the fibular obscure tubercle (FOT) on the anterior-inferior border of the fibula (**Figs. 2** and **3**).

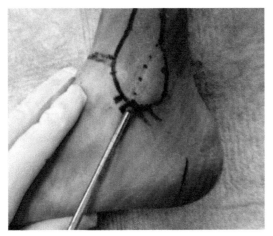

Fig. 1. Anatomic landmark drawn on the patient's skin.

- In case the FOT is not detectable with fluoroscopic view or palpation, the inferior one-third point between the inferior tip and anterior tubercle of the fibula on its anterior border would be the alternative (see **Figs. 2** and **3**).

Landmark of the talar bone tunnel

- The landmark for the talar insertion of the ATFL should be the talar obscure tubercle (TOT) on the anterolateral border of the talar body (**Figs. 4** and **5**).[21]
- If the TOT is not detectable with fluoroscopy or palpation, the point just proximal to the midpoint between the superior corner and inferior corner of the talar body would be the alternative (see **Figs. 4** and **5**).[20,22,23]

Landmark of the calcaneal bone tunnel

- The landmark for the calcaneal insertion of the CFL should be the tuberculum ligamenti calcaneofibularis (TLC) on the lateral wall of the calcaneus (**Figs. 6** and **7**).[21]
- If the TLC is not detectable with fluoroscopy or palpation, the point at 13 mm distal and on the vertical line down from the center of the subtalar joint would be the alternative (see **Figs. 6** and **7**).[19,20]

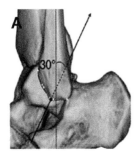
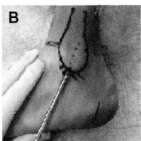
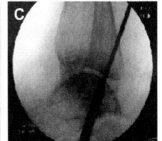

Fig. 2. Landmark (*black dot*) and direction (*arrow lines and broken lines*) of each guide pin for fibular bone tunnel, lateral view. (*A*) Diagram, (*B*) cadaveric model, (*C*) fluoroscopic view (lateral view).

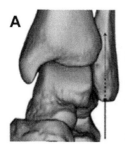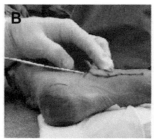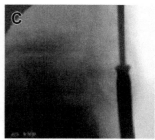

Fig. 3. Landmark (*black dot*) and direction (*arrow lines and broken lines*) of each guide pin for fibular bone tunnel, lateral view. (*A*) Diagram, (*B*) cadaveric model, (*C*) fluoroscopic view (anterior posterior view).

Constructing the anatomic Y-graft for anti-RoLL

- The surgeon and patient may choose an autograft (eg, gracilis tendon) harvested from the ipsilateral knee using a tendon harvester or an allograft of sufficient size (at least 135 mm length, 15-mm × 9 components, and ~5 mm diameter) and strength for the reconstruction of the ATFL and CFL.
- The graft is prepared in the anatomic "Y" configuration with 3 (fibular, talar, and calcaneal) looped stems by doubling the graft to a length of 15 mm at all 3 ends of the "Y" configuration to facilitate attachment of a "tensioning thread" for graft delivery and tensioning (**Fig. 8**).
- The looped stems will be anchored in a bone tunnel and single 15- and 30-mm parts between the stems to the ATFL and CFL, respectively.[20]

Incisions and guide pin insertion

- Three 1-cm incisions are made in sequence using a "nick and spread" technique (cut the skin only and then bluntly spread the subcutaneous tissue) for preparation of the 3 bone tunnels (fibula, talus, and calcaneus) and insertion of a passing thread in each bone tunnel, which is required to accept the Y-graft insertion and interference screw fixation.
- The first incision is used to construct the common ATFL and CFL origin site and designate the Y-graft delivery site (see **Fig. 2**B).
- A guide pin is introduced at the common ATFL and CFL origin site using the anatomic and fluoroscopic landmarks on the fibula described earlier and passed through the far cortex of the bone and the skin (**Fig. 9**A) using fluoroscopic guidance.
- The fibular guide pin is inserted from the FOT or the alternative landmark mentioned earlier on the lateral ankle fluoroscopic view (see **Fig. 2**C).

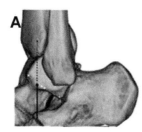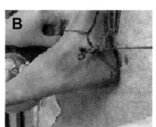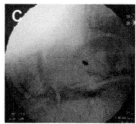

Fig. 4. Landmark (*black dot*) and direction (*arrow lines and broken lines*) of each guide pin for talar bone tunnel. (*A*) Diagram, (*B*) cadaveric model, (*C*) fluoroscopic view (lateral view).

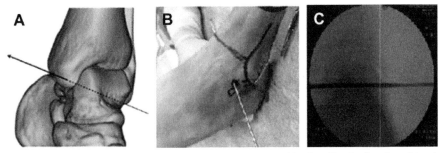

Fig. 5. Landmark (*black dot*) and direction (*arrow lines and broken lines*) of each guide pin for talar bone tunnel. (*A*) Diagram, (*B*) cadaveric model, (*C*) fluoroscopic view (anterior posterior view).

- The guide pin is directed to the posterior cortex of the fibula approximately 30° to the long axis of the fibula on the lateral view (see **Figs. 2**C and **9A**).
- Fluoroscopic anterior-posterior views are taken to ensure that the guide pin is passed through the central portion of the fibula to assure accurate placement and prevent fracture (see **Fig. 3**C; **Fig. 9**B).
- The talar guide pin is inserted from the TOT or the alternative landmark mentioned earlier on the anterolateral border of the talar body using the lateral ankle fluoroscopic view (see **Fig. 4**C).
- The guide pin should be directed slightly proximal and posterior toward a point just proximal of the medial malleolus (see **Fig. 4**B; **Fig. 10**A).
- This pin direction allows the guide pin to run through the talar body to place the interference screw in dense cancellous bone and prevents talar neck fracture, misdirection through the talus or sinus tarsi, and damage to the posterior tibial neurovascular bundle.
- The calcaneal guide pin is inserted from the TLC or the alternative landmark on the lateral wall of the calcaneus (see **Fig. 6**C).
- The guide pin should be directed toward the inferior, medial, and posterior area of the calcaneus without damaging the medial calcaneal branch of the tibial nerve (see **Fig. 6**B; **Fig. 10**B).

Construction of the bone tunnels and insertion of passing threads

- A cannulated drill is then used to overdrill the guide pins, constructing a bone tunnel to diameter of 6 mm and a depth of 20 mm in the fibula and talus and 30 mm in the calcaneus (see **Fig. 9**B).

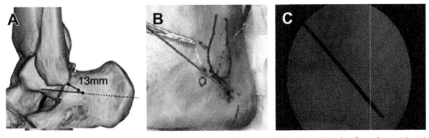

Fig. 6. Landmark (*black dot*) and direction (*arrow lines and broken lines*) of each guide pin for calcaneal bone tunnel, lateral view. (*A*) Diagram, (*B*) cadaveric model, (*C*) fluoroscopic view (lateral view).

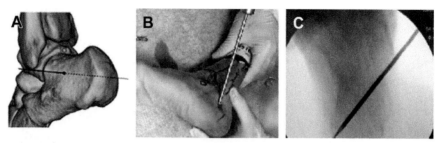

Fig. 7. Landmark (*black dot*) and direction (*arrow lines and broken lines*) of each guide pin for calcaneal bone tunnel. (*A*) Diagram, (*B*) cadaveric model, (*C*) fluoroscopic view (axial view).

- A passing thread is attached to the hole at the end of the guide pin (**Fig. 9**C) and introduced through the bone tunnel by antegrade pulling of the guide pin (**Fig. 9**D).
- Leave one end (closed loop) of the passing thread exiting from the pin entry site incision (**Fig. 9**E) and the other end (the second limb of the thread) exiting from the skin at the guide pin exit site.
- These 2 ends are clamped (see **Fig. 9**E; **Fig. 10**C).
- It is essential that local neurovascular structures and tendons be protected when using these techniques to avoid complications using "nick and spread" technique and a drill guide and targeting guide system to allow more precision when passing the guide pin and drill through the bone to protect the surrounding soft tissues.[20]

Delivery and fixation of each looped stem of the Y-graft to the corresponding bone tunnels with inside-out technique

- All 3 looped stems of the Y-graft are delivered through the Y-graft delivery site using an inside-out technique by pulling each passing thread (**Fig. 11**B).

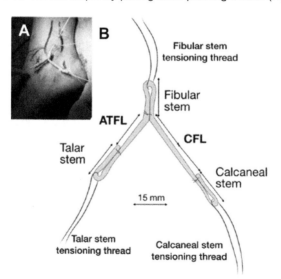

Fig. 8. Construction of the anatomic Y-graft. (*A*) Intraoperative photograph shows the configuration of the Y-graft and skin incisions. (*B*) Y-graft showing its 15-mm × 9 components and construction of each looped stem, the ligament parts (anterior talofibular ligament [ATFL] and calcaneofibular ligament [CFL]), and each tensioning thread (*gray line*).

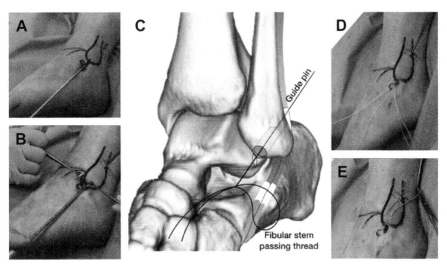

Fig. 9. Construction of the fibular bone tunnel. (*A*) Inserting a guide pin under fluoroscopy. (*B*) Overdrilling with cannulated drill. (*C*) Changing the guide pin to the fibular passing thread. (*D*) Introducing the passing thread by pulling the guide pin. (*E*) Holding the passing thread with a clamp.

- First, a tensioning thread is passed through the fibular looped stem of the Y-graft into the fibula passing suture loop that exits in the fibular site skin incision (**Fig. 11**A).
- Then the other end of the passing thread that comes out from the posterior aspect of the fibula is pulled through.

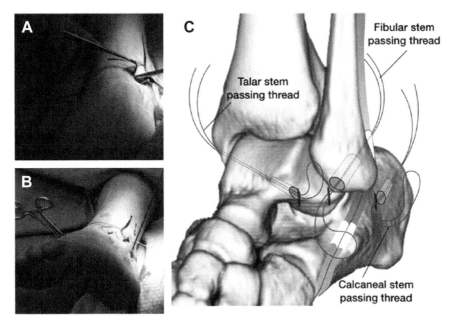

Fig. 10. Construction of the talar and calcaneal bone tunnel. (*A*) Drilling the talar bone tunnel. (*B*) Inserting the guide pin for the calcaneal bone tunnel. (*C*) Three bone tunnels and passing thread out from each skin incision.

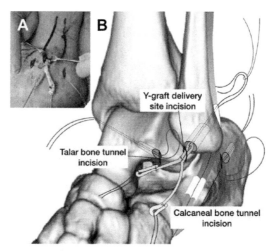

Fig. 11. Inside-out passage of the anatomic Y-graft stem into the fibular bone tunnel. (*A*) Intraoperative photograph of inserting the Y-graft into fibular bone tunnel. (*B*) Inserting the Y-graft into fibular bone tunnel.

- This series of inside-out technique allows the fibular stem of the Y-graft to be delivered into the fibular bone tunnel, with the tensioning thread exiting the posterior aspect of the fibula (see **Fig. 11**B).
- An interference screw guide pin is inserted into the fibular bone tunnel, and the looped fibular stem of the Y-graft in the bone tunnel is fixed using a 6 × 15 mm interference screw (**Fig. 12**B).
- Next, the talar and calcaneal stems are introduced into each bone tunnel using the same inside-out technique.
- To deliver the talar stem, a mosquito forceps is passed through the Y-graft delivery incision site and along the lateral wall of the talus exiting at the talus

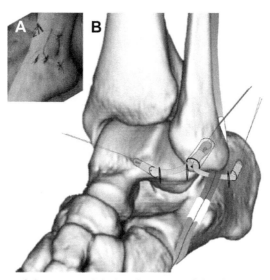

Fig. 12. Final image of the surgery. (*A*) The placement of the skin incisions. (*B*) The placement and the fixation of the Y-graft with tensioning the tension threads.

bone tunnel incision (see **Fig. 11**B) to retrieve the trailing end of the talar stem passing thread, which is then passed out the Y-graft delivery incision site.
- This trailing end of the talar passing thread is attached to the talar stem thread to allow delivery of the talar stem through the Y-graft delivery site incision and into the talar bone tunnel.
- Finally, the calcaneal stem of the Y-graft is delivered to the calcaneal tunnel in a similar manner through the calcaneal incision site (see **Fig. 11**B) by passing a mosquito forceps through the Y-graft delivery incision site and passed along the lateral wall of the calcaneus, being certain to pass under the peroneal tendons and Sural nerve to exit at the calcaneal incision to retrieve the trailing end of the calcaneal stem passing suture.
- This will allow the CFL portion of the Y-graft to pass along the lateral wall of the talus and calcaneus on a path nearly anatomic to the native CFL.

Fixation and tensioning of anatomic Y-graft to the bone tunnel

- With the ankle in neutral dorsiflexion, the Y-graft is balanced and tensioned by pulling the tension threads.
- Tension should be maintained on the sutures during interference screw insertion to prevent graft extrusion. Once all 3 stems of the anatomic Y-graft are fixed, the tensioning threads are removed, and the incision sites are closed using nylon sutures (**Fig. 12**A).
- The lower extremity is dressed and immobilized with a below-knee cast.

Pearls and Pitfalls

Table 1 outlines the pearls and pitfalls of percutaneous ankle reconstruction of lateral ligaments.

Postoperative Care

- The patient's operative limb is immobilized in a non–weight-bearing below-knee cast for a total of 6 weeks with weight bearing as tolerated. Alternatively, a more aggressive rehab approach has been used by Masato Takao with a similar Arthroscopic Ankle Reconstruction of Lateral Ligaments.[17]

Table 1	
Pearls and pitfalls of percutaneous ankle reconstruction of lateral ligaments	
Graft handling	1. Great care should be taken when harvesting autograft so as to get enough length.
	2. If allograft is used, it must be ordered properly and prepared before the surgery started with the exact measurements.
	3. After graft preparation cover it with wet gauze to keep it moist until ready for use.
Tunnel placement	1. Avoid tunnel fracture especially in fibula and talar neck.
	2. Always double check the tunnel trajectory on fluoroscopy before drilling.
Hindfoot alignment	In association with hindfoot varus there is a great strain on lateral ankle ligament. Always assess the foot before the surgery and do not hesitate to correct the hind foot varus in order to protect your ligament reconstruction.
Graft tensioning	1. Hold the ankle in neutral dorsiflexion.
	2. Avoid overtightening of the grafts and always check for the range of motion after graft placement.
Cast handling	Postoperative cast application, placed well-padded cast with the ankle in neutral position to reduce the strain on the grafts until healing.

- Suture removal and wound inspection usually done at 2 weeks postoperatively.
- Transition from cast to walking boot at 6 weeks postoperative for 4 weeks during which time a rehabilitation program is instituted focusing on restoration of motion, Achilles tendon stretching, proprioception training, and peroneal tendon strengthening.
- Athletic activity usually is within 6 to 9 months.

Complications

Early complications

- Nerve injury, in delivering the ATFL and CFL limbs or with tunnel construction on the talus and calcaneus
- Improper graft placement, especially placing the CFL limb over the peroneals
- Tunnel fracture in fibula or talus
- Poor graft fixation in the tunnel due to poor bone quality or improper sizing of the interference screws, or tunnel-graft ratio
- Infection
- Wound healing, albeit unlikely with percutaneous techniques
- Deep venous thrombosis

Late complications

- Joint stiffness
- Graft ingrowth failure

Outcome

- Anatomic reconstruction for failed chronic ankle instability is still preferred by most foot and ankle surgeons. It has good results in eliminating patient symptoms and facilitating return to function, in appropriate selected patients.
- ESSKA AFAS Ankle Instability Group, in 2016, published a systematic review. Six studies (2 Level III, 1 Level IV, and 3 Level V) were found in this review assessing minimally invasive lateral ligament reconstruction without the use of arthroscopy. All the included studies reconstructed both ATFL and CFL using auto and allograft by percutaneous technique. Xu and colleagues studied the difference between autograft and allograft and he concluded that the clinical outcome of the 2 grafts were both excellent with no significant difference identified. They also reported a relatively short recovery time for healing with minimal donor site problems in the autograft group. Young and colleagues described their inclusion criteria as previously failed reconstruction surgery, sever ankle instability (more than 15° of talar tilt, more than 10 mm of anterior drawer), general laxity of the ligaments, and body mass index higher than 25. They concluded that percutaneous reconstruction with allograft was effective as a salvage procedure for the treatment of severe and complicated CAI.
- It is recommended that surgeons currently using minimally invasive techniques for the treatment of CAI should do a prospective case series; comparative or randomized controlled trial too provides a higher quality of evidence on safety and efficacy.

ACKNOWLEDGMENTS

ESSKA AFAS Ankle Instability Group, The European Society of Sports Traumatolgy, Knee Surgery and Arthroscopy Ankle and Foot Associates Ankle Instability Group, comprises Jorge Batista, Thomas Bauer, James Calder, Woo Jin Choi, Ali Ghorbani,

Mark Glazebrook, Stéphane Guillo, Siu Wah Kong, Jon Karlsson, Jin Woo Lee, Peter G. Mangone, Frederick Michels, Andy Molloy, Caio Nery, Satoru Ozeki, Christopher Pearce, Anthony Perera, Hélder Pereira, Bas Pijnenburg, Fernando Raduan, James W. Stone, Masato Takao, and Yves Tourné.

REFERENCES

1. Brostrom L. Sprained ankles. V. Treatment and prognosis in recent ligament ruptures. Acta Chir Scand 1966;132(5):537–50.
2. Freeman MA. Instability of the foot after injuries to the lateral ligament of the ankle. J Bone Joint Surg Br 1965;47(4):669–77.
3. Kerkhoffs GM, Handoll HH, de Bie R, et al. Surgical versus conservative treatment for acute injuries of the lateral ligament complex of the ankle in adults. Cochrane Database Syst Rev 2007;(2):CD000380.
4. Pijnenburg AC, Bogaard K, Krips R, et al. Operative and functional treatment of rupture of the lateral ligament of the ankle. A randomised, prospective trial. J Bone Joint Surg Br 2003;85(4):525–30.
5. Takao M, Miyamoto W, Matsui K, et al. Functional treatment after surgical repair for acute lateral ligament disruption of the ankle in athletes. Am J Sports Med 2012;40(2):447–51.
6. Dierckman BD, Ferkel RD. Anatomic reconstruction with a semitendinosus allograft for chronic lateral ankle instability. Am J Sports Med 2015;43(8):1941–50.
7. Guillo S, Bauer T, Lee JW, et al. Consensus in chronic ankle instability: aetiology, assessment, surgical indications and place for arthroscopy. Orthop Traumatol Surg Res 2013;99(8 Suppl):S411–9.
8. Karlsson J, Lansinger O. Chronic lateral instability of the ankle in athletes. Sports Med 1993;16(5):355–65.
9. Lui TH. Arthroscopic-assisted lateral ligamentous reconstruction in combined ankle and subtalar instability. Arthroscopy 2007;23(5):554.e1-5.
10. Takao M, Oae K, Uchio Y, et al. Anatomical reconstruction of the lateral ligaments of the ankle with a gracilis autograft: a new technique using an interference fit anchoring system. Am J Sports Med 2005;33(6):814–23.
11. Acevedo JI, Mangone P. Ankle instability and arthroscopic lateral ligament repair. Foot Ankle Clin 2015;20(1):59–69.
12. Guillo S, Archbold P, Perera A, et al. Arthroscopic anatomic reconstruction of the lateral ligaments of the ankle with gracilis autograft. Arthrosc Tech 2014;3(5): e593–8.
13. Espinosa N, Smerek J, Kadakia AR, et al. Operative management of ankle instability: reconstruction with open and percutaneous methods. Foot Ankle Clin 2006; 11(3):547–65.
14. Kim HN, Dong Q, Hong DY, et al. Percutaneous lateral ankle ligament reconstruction using a split peroneus longus tendon free graft: technical tip. Foot Ankle Int 2014;35(10):1082–6.
15. Wang B, Xu XY. Minimally invasive reconstruction of lateral ligaments of the ankle using semitendinosus autograft. Foot Ankle Int 2013;34(5):711–5.
16. Youn H, Kim YS, Lee J, et al. Percutaneous lateral ligament reconstruction with allograft for chronic lateral ankle instability. Foot Ankle Int 2012;33(2):99–104.
17. Matsui K, Takao M, Miyamoto W, et al. Early recovery after arthroscopic repair compared to open repair of the anterior talofibular ligament for lateral instability of the ankle. Arch Orthop Trauma Surg 2016;136(1):93–100.

18. Takao M, Glazebrook M, Stone J, et al. Ankle arthroscopic reconstruction of lateral ligaments (Ankle Anti-ROLL). Arthrosc Tech 2015;4(5):e595–600.

19. Matsui K, Oliva XM, Takao M, et al. Bony landmarks available for minimally invasive lateral ankle stabilization surgery: a cadaveric anatomical study. Knee Surg Sports Traumatol Arthrosc 2017;25(6):1916–24.

20. Glazebrook M, Stone J, Matsui K, et al. Percutaneous ankle reconstruction of lateral ligaments (Perc-Anti RoLL). Foot Ankle Int 2016;37(6):659–64.

21. Kelikian A, Sarrafian SK. Sarrafian's anatomy of the foot and ankle: descriptive, topographic, functional. Philadelphia: Lippincott, Williams & Wilkins, Wolters Kluwer; 2011.

22. Clanton TO, Campbell KJ, Wilson KJ, et al. Qualitative and quantitative anatomic investigation of the lateral ankle ligaments for surgical reconstruction procedures. J Bone Joint Surg Am 2014;96(12):e98.

23. Taser F, Shafiq Q, Ebraheim NA. Anatomy of lateral ankle ligaments and their relationship to bony landmarks. Surg Radiol Anat 2006;28(4):391–7.

Malalignment and Lateral Ankle Instability

Causes of Failure from the Varus Tibia to the Cavovarus Foot

Fabian Krause, MD*, Angela Seidel, MD

KEYWORDS

- Varus malalignment • Cavovarus foot • Lateral ankle instability • Failure

KEY POINTS

- A varus malalignment of the tibia or the hindfoot is a biomechanical risk factor for chronic lateral ankle instability.
- Consequences of a varus malalignment of the lower leg are asymmetric loading of the hindfoot joints, recurrent ankle sprains, and in the long term, chronic lateral ankle instability and ankle arthritis.
- Lateral ligament repair or reconstruction is more likely to fail if the varus malalignment is not corrected.
- When evaluating patients with lateral ankle instability, a high index of clinical suspicion for lower leg varus malalignment and subsequent biomechanics should be maintained.

INTRODUCTION

Varus malalignment of the tibia or the hindfoot has been acknowledged to be a biome-chanical risk factor for chronic lateral ankle instability.[1–4] Patients with chronic lateral ankle instability often demonstrate tibia or hindfoot varus alignment on clinical and radiographic examination, and, when lateral ankle ligament repair or reconstruction is performed without correction of the malalignment, patients may have ongoing pain and recurrent instability.[5]

Although most varus tibia alignment is congenital (supramalleolar, distal third) or of posttraumatic cause (distal third and diaphyseal), the cavovarus deformity is either idiopathic or induced by an underlying neuropathic disease. Consequences of the malalignment of the varus tibia and of the varus hindfoot are asymmetric loading of

Disclosure Statement: The authors have nothing to disclose.
Department of Orthopaedic Surgery, Inselspital, University of Berne, Freiburgstrasse, Berne 3010, Switzerland
* Corresponding author.
E-mail address: FABIAN.KRAUSE@INSEL.CH

Foot Ankle Clin N Am 23 (2018) 593–603
https://doi.org/10.1016/j.fcl.2018.07.005
foot.theclinics.com

the hindfoot joints, recurrent ankle sprains, long-term chronic lateral ankle instability, and anteromedial ankle arthritis.[6] Varus hindfoot alignment can occur in isolation or as part of a subtle or obvious cavovarus deformity.

To avoid failure of operative treatment of lateral ankle instability, not only a thorough clinical and radiographic examination should be completed but also a complete understanding of the dynamic and static components of the malalignment and their biomechanical effects is crucial.

The purpose of this article is to draw attention to the importance of tibial and hindfoot malalignment in combination with lateral ankle instability. Missing the varus malalignment on clinical and radiological examination may contribute to failure of lateral ankle ligament repair or reconstruction.

PREDISPOSING BIOMECHANICS AND NEUROMUSCULAR ISSUES

Both varus tibia alignment and the cavovarus deformity move the weight-bearing axis toward the medial side of the ankle and raise the contact stress in the medial joint compartment, increasing the potential for premature cartilage degeneration.[7,8] In forefoot-driven hindfoot varus type of cavovarus feet, the plantarflexion of the first ray leads to hindfoot varus and forefoot adduction and to relative dorsiflexion of the talus within the ankle mortise. Residual dorsiflexion is thereby restricted and may cause anterior ankle impingement. Therefore, the contact stress in the cavovarus deformity is seen in the anteromedial ankle as opposed to the elevated medial contact stress in the exclusive coronal plane varus tibia alignment. With increasing anteromedial cartilage wear, caused by either elevated contact stress in the long-term or recurrent sprains with osteochondral lesions, the talus tilts into the anteromedial cartilage defect and consequently aggravates the varus malalignment.

Any varus malalignment of the lower leg medializes the Achilles tendon insertion at the calcaneal tuberosity and thereby the direction of tendon traction. The often shortened and medialized Achilles tendon pull provokes an inversion moment at heel strike, exposing the lateral restraints to increased strain and risk of failure.[9] Either due to the neuropathic underlying disease or recurrent lateral ankle sprains, the peroneus brevis tendon is commonly weak and degenerated, becoming incompetent and unable to sufficiently counteract an impending ankle sprain.

A plantarflexed first metatarsal consequent to peroneus longus overdrive is considered to be the primary deforming force of the most common forefoot-driven cavovarus deformity.[10] When the plantarflexion increases and the remaining ankle dorsiflexion is progressively reduced, the plantarflexion vector of the peroneus longus tendon is enabled, further flexing the first metatarsal. Subsequently, the tibialis anterior dorsiflexion vector is diminished, exacerbating the problem.

Mostly because of the plantarflexed first ray, the talocalcaneal angle in the cavovarus deformity is narrowed, moving the navicular to a position superior to the cuboid instead of medial to it.[11] The hindfoot rests locked in inversion throughout the gait cycle, restricting hindfoot eversion at heel strike and impairing stress dissipation.[11] In addition to overload of the lateral foot border, metatarsalgia, and plantar fasciitis, the locked inverted midfoot increases the risk of lateral ankle sprain.

Neuropathic cavovarus feet usually demonstrate a progressive muscle imbalance comprising a weak peroneus brevis and tibialis anterior muscle but a relatively strong peroneus longus, tibialis posterior, and triceps surae muscle.[12] Because of functional instability, the likelihood of recurrent lateral ankle sprains even after bony and ligamentous reconstruction is higher than in patients with competent muscles. Particularly in the progressive neuropathic diseases, additional tendon transfers (ie, tibialis posterior to the dorsum of the foot) and occasionally realigning midfoot and hindfoot fusions are required for appropriate stability. Because neuropathic nerves may be thickened in these patients, it is advocated to decompress the neurovascular bundle by a flexor retinaculum release after moderate to strong lateralizing calcaneal osteotomies in these patients.[6]

ASSESSMENT

Omitting the assessment of hindfoot alignment can lead to failure of lateral ligament repair or reconstruction.[13,14] For evaluation of hindfoot and tibia alignment, the patients are disrobed, standing barefoot, and examined from the back by the examiner. A physiologic hindfoot lies in a slight valgus of about 5° to 10°. A clinically straight hindfoot often actually represents a radiographic varus alignment. The peek-a-boo sign, observed from the front of the patient, represents a hindfoot varus.[10] The arch height is assessed from the side. Limited ankle dorsiflexion is often seen on range-of-motion assessment. Isolated gastrocnemius or combined triceps surae contracture is evaluated with the knee extended and flexed (Silfverskjöldt test). Posttraumatic rotational tibial deformities are best assessed with the patient lying prone and the lower leg bent 90° in the knee. The Coleman-block test allows determination of flexible and fixed deformities. The sole of the foot is examined for first ray and lateral border callosities, indicating overload. Ankle stability is tested by anterior drawer and talar tilt test and compared with the contralateral side. In addition to a full neurologic assessment, muscle power, particularly weakness of the peroneus brevis and tibialis anterior tendon, is distinguished.

Complementing clinical assessment, weight-bearing anteroposterior and lateral radiographs of the foot and ankle are usually sufficient to evaluate the obvious varus hindfoot. In subtle deformities, a hindfoot alignment view in comparison with the contralateral side may be helpful. Posttraumatic tibial deformities require full-length radiographs of the lower leg and occasionally computed tomography (CT) for assessment of bony morphology and rotational alignment. MRI or single-photon emission computed tomography-CT is often required to evaluate ligament competence, soft tissue and synovial inflammation or impingement, osteochondral lesions, and ankle arthritis.

STANDARD PROCEDURES IN CAVOVARUS RECONSTRUCTION

1. Lateralizing calcaneal osteotomy (**Fig. 1**)
2. Peroneus longus to brevis tendon transfer
3. First metatarsal or medial cuneiform (reversed Cotton osteotomy) dorsiflexion osteotomy
4. Lateral ligament repair (Broström-Gould) or anatomic autograft or allograft reconstruction (ie, gracilis tendon)

In a biomechanical study, it has been demonstrated that translational lateralizing osteotomies (ie, lateral sliding or Z-shaped with additional lateralization of the calcaneal tuberosity) more effectively neutralize the (antero-) medial elevated ankle pressure than isolated rotational osteotomies (ie, lateral closing "Dwyer" or Z-shaped without additional lateralization of the calcaneal tuberosity, "Pisani," or "Malerba").[6]

ASSOCIATED PROCEDURES IN CAVOVARUS RECONSTRUCTION

1. Ankle arthroscopy for osteochondral lesions, osteophytes, and synovitis
2. Peroneal tendon repair
3. Other tendon transfer in neuropathic cavovarus deformities

4. Claw toe reconstruction
5. Jones procedure
6. Supramalleolar valgus osteotomy in advanced ankle arthritis (alone or in combination), 2° to 5° overcorrection in medial moderate and advanced ankle arthritis[15]

A

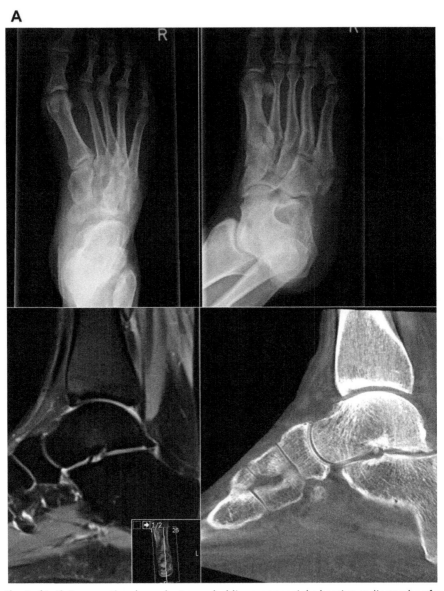

Fig. 1. (A–C) Preoperative dorsoplantar and oblique non-weight-bearing radiographs of a 34 year-old male mechanic with chronic lateral instability and a cavovarus deformity; CT and MRI show initial anteromedial ankle degeneration (A). Intraoperative radiographs of 8-mm lateralizing calcaneal slide osteotomy, 4-mm first metatarsal dorsiflexion osteotomy (reversed Cotton osteotomy), peroneus longus to peroneus brevis tendon transfer, and Broström-Gould repair (B). Eighteen months postoperative dorsoplantar and lateral weight-bearing radiographs of the foot with a not fully corrected talo-first metatarsal angle but symptom-free patient with a stable hindfoot (C).

B

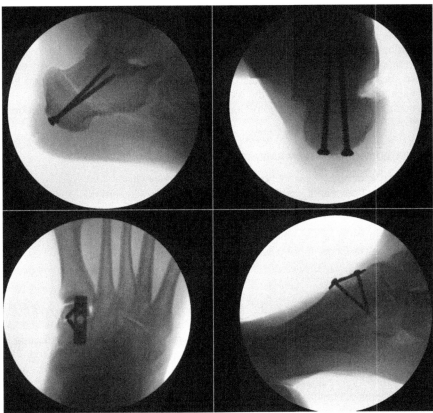

Fig. 1. (*continued*).

C

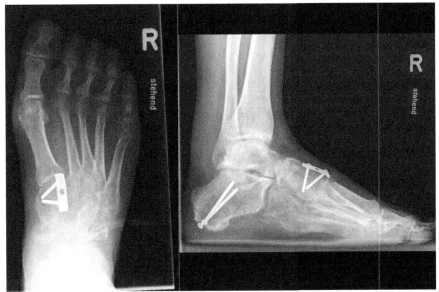

Fig. 1. (*continued*).

STANDARD PROCEDURES IN VARUS TIBIA

1. Supramalleolar valgus osteotomy for malalignment in the distal tibia, 2° to 5° over-correction in medial moderate and advanced ankle arthritis (**Fig. 2**)[15]
2. Two- or 3-dimensional diaphyseal tibia correction at the center of rotation and angulation for malalignment in the diaphyseal tibia
3. Lateral ligament repair (Broström-Gould) or anatomic autograft or allograft reconstruction (ie, gracilis tendon)

ASSOCIATED PROCEDURES IN VARUS TIBIA

1. Ankle arthroscopy for osteochondral lesions and synovitis
2. Lateralizing calcaneal osteotomy in advanced ankle arthritis (alone or in combination)
3. Peroneal tendon repair
4. Tibia lengthening or shortening
5. Bone reconstruction in bony defects, osteitis, or nonunion

DISCUSSION

Varus malalignment of the tibia or the hindfoot alone can lead to (antero-) medial ankle arthritis.[6] The likelihood to develop ankle arthritis is higher if the lateral ankle is additionally chronically unstable. Conversely, lateral ligament repair or reconstruction is more likely to fail if the varus tibia or hindfoot malalignment is not corrected. The importance of malalignment correction in unstable ankles is reflected in the literature in level IV evidence radiological and clinical studies.

A comparison of standard radiographs of 95 patients undergoing surgery for lateral ankle instability with a control group revealed that the surgical group had a higher frequency of cavovarus feet.[1] This relationship was substantiated by Fortin and colleagues,[16] who obtained clinical and radiographic measurements from 10 subjects with chronic lateral ankle instability and severe degenerative changes. Interestingly, all 10 subjects were determined as having a cavovarus deformity. After surgical correction of the deformity, all subjects had resolution of pain and instability. The investigators concluded that correction of the cavovarus foot deformity in patients with lateral ankle instability may help to normalize forces across the ankle, aiding in the effectiveness of lateral soft tissue reconstruction. Van Bergeyk and colleagues[4] retrospectively used CT imaging to analyze hindfoot alignment in the coronal plane and determined that those suffering from chronic ankle instability demonstrated a trend toward increased varus alignment of the hindfoot.

Louwerens and colleagues[17] reported that in 33 patients with chronic lateral ankle ligament instability, the cavovarus deformity was commonly found on clinical examination, whereas there was no significant correlation of the clinical deformity and radiographic foot anatomy.

In a recent clinical study, Araoye and colleagues[18] performed 20 lateral sliding calcaneal osteotomies in 119 patients (17%) in addition to different types of lateral ligament repair achieving an 89% success rate.

In a case series of 13 patients with longstanding cavovarus deformities and mild to moderate anteromedial ankle arthritis, the combined bony and soft tissue reconstruction of the deformity led to good outcome without progressive arthritis.[19] Although no lateral ligament repair or reconstruction was performed even in the presence of preoperative lateral ligament instability in 7 patients, no patient reported ongoing instability postoperatively. In 2 case series of Takakura and colleagues[15] and Tanaka and

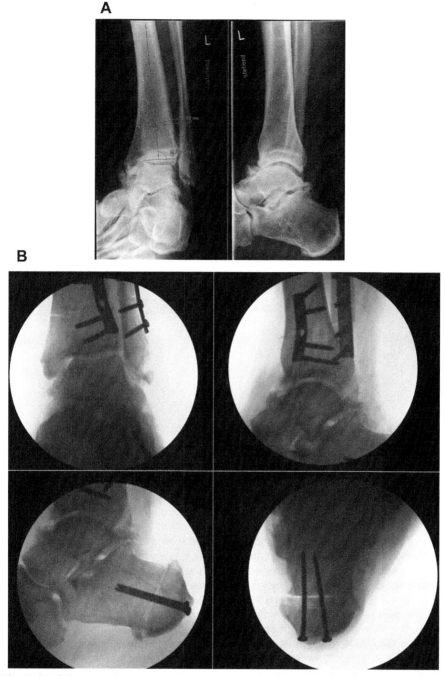

Fig. 2. (A–C) Preoperative anteroposterior and lateral ankle weight-bearing radiographs of a 48 year-old male handball player with chronic lateral instability, varus tibial plafond, and advanced medial ankle arthritis (A). Intraoperative radiographs of 6° lateral closing wedge supramalleolar osteotomy, 6-mm lateralizing calcaneal slide osteotomy, and Broström-Gould repair, broken drill bit after microfracturing of the medial talus (B). One-year postoperatively, anteroposterior and lateral ankle weight-bearing radiographs with not fully corrected talar tilt but improved symptoms (C).

C

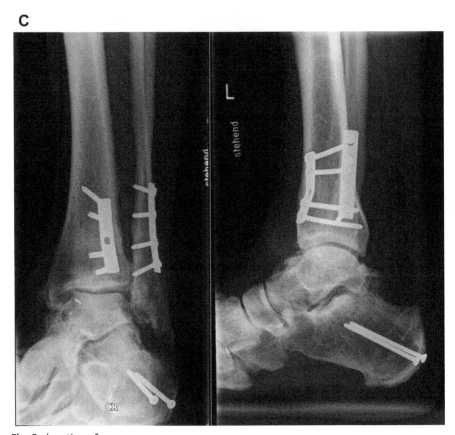

Fig. 2. (*continued*).

colleagues,[20] varus malalignment of the tibial plafond was corrected by medial opening supramalleolar tibial and fibular osteotomy, whereas the lateral ligaments were addressed only in 7%. At mean follow-up of 8 years, durable symptom relief without ankle instability was seen. Failures were noted in patients who had complete obliteration of the ankle joint space. The investigators recommended an overcorrection of 2° to 5° when moderate to advanced ankle arthritis is present.

If lateral stability is achieved exclusively with realignment but without ligament repair or reconstruction, the latter 3 studies emphasize the importance of hindfoot realignment. However, the patients in these studies already had ankle arthritis and were older and less active. In younger, more active patients without arthritis, the authors recommend to restore both alignment and ligamentous hindfoot stability.

Vienne and colleagues[21] published a case series of 8 patients with a cavovarus deformity and at least one prior failed lateral ligament stabilization. After cavovarus reconstruction with lateralizing calcaneal osteotomy (8), transfer of peroneus longus to peroneus brevis tendon (8), or ligament reconstruction (4, modified Broström-technique), overall satisfaction was 100% at an average follow-up of 37 months.

The evidence for the relationship of failed lateral ligament repair/reconstruction and hindfoot varus is poor and consists of one level IV case series. Strauss and colleagues[5] reviewed 160 patients with chronic lateral ankle ligament instability. Associated pathologic conditions were peroneal tendon injuries in 28%, os trigonum symptoms in 13%, lateral gutter ossicles in 10%, and anterior tibial spurs in 3%; hindfoot varus was seen in 8% of these patients. The most common cause for failure of ligament reconstruction was omission to realign the hindfoot varus (28% of the patients with failed surgery).

Literature review indicates that patients with chronic lateral ankle instability and tibia or hindfoot varus alignment likely require a realigning osteotomy to avoid ligament reconstruction failure caused by mechanical malalignment.[22,23] The overall success rate of lateral ligament repair or reconstruction in the current literature is 90% to 95%,[24–26] but likely lower when varus tibia or hindfoot is not corrected. Those patients with a physiologic alignment but generalized hyperlaxity, longstanding instability, high functional demands, poor soft tissues, or failed repair benefit from alternative procedures, such as combined mild calcaneal osteotomy and soft tissue reconstruction or augmented reconstruction perhaps with one of the tendon procedures, and gastrocnemius recession.[27]

Besides varus lower leg and hindfoot alignment, other causes for failure of repaired or reconstructed lateral ligaments are as follows:

1. Errors in graft placement and fixation
2. Reinjury
3. Residual subtalar instability[28]
4. Ligamentous laxity
5. Longstanding instability
6. High functional demand
7. Overtightening of the graft (subtalar and ankle joint loss of motion and impingement pain[27])

The bony correction of varus lower leg and varus hindfoot requires a comprehensive understanding of the underlying pathologic condition and thorough preoperative planning of the amount of correction and operative steps. Although an overcorrection of the varus tibia can result in overload of the medial midfoot and hindfoot tendons and ligaments, fatigue fracture, or nonunion, an overcorrection of a varus hindfoot or cavovarus deformity has not yet been reported. In most instances, however, a bony undercorrection, potentially contributing to another failure, is more likely.

SUMMARY

A lower leg or hindfoot varus malalignment is a frequently encountered but underestimated cause of chronic ankle instability and ankle arthritis in the long term. When evaluating patients with ankle instability, a high index of clinical suspicion for tibia and hindfoot varus malalignment and resultant biomechanics should be maintained. Management of lateral ankle instability in the presence of varus malalignment must comprise a generous indication for accurate hindfoot realignment. In young and active patients, realignment should be combined with formal lateral ligamentous repair.

REFERENCES

1. Larsen E. Static or dynamic repair of chronic lateral ankle instability. A prospective randomized study. Clin Orthop Relat Res 1990;(257):184–92.
2. Sugimoto K, Samoto N, Takakura Y, et al. Varus tilt of the tibial plafond as a factor in chronic ligament instability of the ankle. Foot Ankle Int 1997;18(7):402–5.
3. Scranton PE Jr, McDermott JE, Rogers JV. The relationship between chronic ankle instability and variations in mortise anatomy and impingement spurs. Foot Ankle Int 2000;21(8):657–64.

4. Van Bergeyk AB, Younger A, Carson B. CT analysis of hindfoot alignment in chronic lateral ankle instability. Foot Ankle Int 2002;23(1):37–42.

5. Strauss JE, Forsberg JA, Lippert FG 3rd. Chronic lateral ankle instability and associated conditions: a rationale for treatment. Foot Ankle Int 2007;28(10): 1041–4.

6. Krause F, Windolf M, Schwieger K, et al. Ankle joint pressure in pes cavovarus. J Bone Joint Surg Br 2007;89(12):1660–5.

7. Tarr RR, Resnick CT, Wagner KS, et al. Changes in tibiotalar joint contact areas following experimentally induced tibial angular deformities. Clin Orthop Relat Res 1985;(199):72–80.

8. Ting AJ, Tarr RR, Sarmiento A, et al. The role of subtalar motion and ankle contact pressure changes from angular deformities of the tibia. Foot Ankle 1987;7(5): 290–9.

9. Giannestras NJ. Foot disorders. Medical and surgical management. Philadelphia: Lea & Febiger; 1967.

10. Manoli A 2nd, Smith DG, Hansen ST Jr. Scarred muscle excision for the treatment of established ischemic contracture of the lower extremity. Clin Orthop Relat Res 1993;(292):309–14.

11. Aminian A, Sangeorzan BJ. The anatomy of cavus foot deformity. Foot Ankle Clin 2008;13(2):191–8, v.

12. Krause FG, Wing KJ, Younger AS. Neuromuscular issues in cavovarus foot. Foot Ankle Clin 2008;13(2):243–58, vi.

13. Ortiz C, Wagner E, Keller A. Cavovarus foot reconstruction. Foot Ankle Clin 2009; 14(3):471–87.

14. Desai S, Grierson R, Manoli A. The cavus foot in athletes: fundamentals of examination and treatment. Oper Tech Sports Med 18(1):27–33.

15. Takakura Y, Tanaka Y, Kumai T, et al. Low tibial osteotomy for osteoarthritis of the ankle. Results of a new operation in 18 patients. J Bone Joint Surg Br 1995;77(1): 50–4.

16. Fortin PT, Guettler J, Manoli A 2nd. Idiopathic cavovarus and lateral ankle instability: recognition and treatment implications relating to ankle arthritis. Foot Ankle Int 2002;23(11):1031–7.

17. Louwerens JW, Ginai AZ, van Linge B, et al. Chronic instability of the foot and foot geometry: a radiographic study. Foot 1996;6(6):13–8.

18. Araoye I, De Cesar Netto C, Cone B, et al. Results of lateral ankle ligament repair surgery in one hundred and nineteen patients: do surgical method and arthroscopy timing matter? Int Orthop 2017;41(11):2289–95.

19. Krause FG, Henning J, Pfander G, et al. Cavovarus foot realignment to treat anteromedial ankle arthrosis. Foot Ankle Int 2013;34(1):54–64.

20. Tanaka Y, Takakura Y, Hayashi K, et al. Low tibial osteotomy for varus-type osteoarthritis of the ankle. J Bone Joint Surg Br 2006;88(7):909–13.

21. Vienne P, Schoniger R, Helmy N, et al. Hindfoot instability in cavovarus deformity: static and dynamic balancing. Foot Ankle Int 2007;28(1):96–102.

22. Colville MR. Surgical treatment of the unstable ankle. J Am Acad Orthop Surg 1998;6(6):368–77.

23. Tourne Y, Mabit C. Lateral ligament reconstruction procedures for the ankle. Orthop Traumatol Surg Res 2017;103(1S):S171–81.

24. Baumhauer JF, O'Brien T. Surgical considerations in the treatment of ankle instability. J Athl Train 2002;37(4):458–62.

25. Kramer D, Solomon R, Curtis C, et al. Clinical results and functional evaluation of the Chrisman-Snook procedure for lateral ankle instability in athletes. Foot Ankle Spec 2011;4(1):18–28.
26. Yasui Y, Murawski CD, Wollstein A, et al. Operative treatment of lateral ankle instability. JBJS Rev 2016;4(5) [pii:01874474-201605000-00006].
27. DiGiovanni CW, Brodsky A. Current concepts: lateral ankle instability. Foot Ankle Int 2006;27(10):854–66.
28. Sammarco GJ, Carrasquillo HA. Surgical revision after failed lateral ankle reconstruction. Foot Ankle Int 1995;16(12):748–53.

Revision of Surgical Lateral Ankle Ligament Stabilization

Joseph T. O'Neil, MD, Gregory P. Guyton, MD*

KEYWORDS

- Lateral ankle ligaments • Instability • Failed stabilization
- Revision ankle stabilization

KEY POINTS

- Recurrent ankle instability in the setting of a previous surgical stabilization can be a complex and difficult problem to treat. Large-scale trials or series involving the patient population with failed surgery are lacking.
- Patients with recurrent ankle instability following a previous surgical stabilization should be evaluated for a joint hypermobility disorder and appropriately counseled.
- Patients should also be evaluated for other predisposing factors for failure of surgical ankle stabilization, including hindfoot varus, first ray plantarflexion, or midfoot cavus.
- The described technique seeks to capitalize on the potential benefits of both tenodesis and bone-to-bone suture tape augmentation in this high-risk group. A semitendinosis allograft is used to eliminate the morbidity of a split harvest of the peroneus brevis tendon.

INTRODUCTION

Ankle sprains continue to be among the most common musculoskeletal injuries, accounting for as many as 40% of all athletic injuries.[1,2] Furthermore, lateral ankle sprains account for 85% of ankle injuries,[3] caused by an inversion force to a plantar-flexed foot.[4] However, most patients who sustain an ankle sprain experience improvement of their symptoms with nonoperative treatment modalities, such as bracing and physical therapy, without developing symptoms of chronic ankle instability. Despite the success of nonoperative management, a small subset of patients eventually requires surgical intervention to restore stability to the ankle. Indications for surgery generally include mechanical instability with demonstrable laxity of the ankle joint on examination or functional instability, where patients subjectively report a sensation of ankle instability in the absence of a clear mechanical problem.

Financial Disclosures: The authors have nothing to disclose.
Department of Orthopaedic Surgery, MedStar Union Memorial Hospital, Baltimore, MD, USA
* Corresponding author. c/o Lyn Camire, MA, ELS, Editor, Department of Orthopaedic Surgery, MedStar Union Memorial Hospital, 3333 North Calvert Street, Suite 400, Baltimore, MD 21218.
E-mail address: lyn.camire@medstar.net

Surgical treatment of ankle instability has evolved through the years. Nilsonne and Elmslie were 2 of the earliest to report on the surgical treatment of ankle instability. In 1932, Nilsonne[5] described tenodesis of the peroneus brevis to the lateral periosteum of the distal fibula. In 1934, Elmslie[6] reported on 4 patients in whom he reconstructed the anterior talofibular ligament (ATFL) as well as the calcaneofibular ligament (CFL) using a fascia lata graft. In 1966, Broström[7] advocated direct anatomic suture repairs of the ATFL and CFL, inspired by the results published by Stener and others regarding suture repair of the metacarpophalangeal ligaments in the hand. Broström reported a success rate of approximately 85% with a straightforward soft tissue imbrication of the ATFL, and his results remain the standard for direct anatomic repair. Karlsson and colleagues[8] recommended routine inclusion of the CFL and shortening of the ligaments while reattaching them to the fibula at their anatomic origins using a bone trough and sutures because they noted that the ATFL and CFL were often attenuated and scarred rather than simply disrupted. Gould and colleagues[9] also described a modification of the Broström procedure, which involved mobilizing the superior margin of the inferior extensor retinaculum and suturing it to the repaired margin of the ATFL after a standard direct repair. This augmentation was found to improve resistance to direct inversion stress and limit excessive subtalar motion while maintaining normal anatomic relationships and subtalar joint function. In addition, the morbidity associated with the harvest of tendon grafts was eliminated. Finally, Glas and colleagues[10] and Sjølin and colleagues[11] reported another variation in which a standard direct repair was performed, followed by elevation of distally based periosteal flaps, which were then turned down over the suture line to reinforce the repair.

Although rare, recurrent instability can occur early or late after a stabilization procedure. Early recurrent instability is generally caused by an acute injury, whereas late recurrent instability can be caused by chronic repetitive minor trauma. Several factors have been shown to predispose patients to failure of operative stabilization, particularly ligamentous laxity, high functional demand, and a cavovarus deformity.[7–9,12–16]

The quality of the residual ankle ligaments and surrounding soft tissue plays a major role in the success of procedures for treating ankle instability. Excessive ligamentous laxity may be related to diseases of abnormal collagen structure, such as Marfan and Ehlers-Danlos syndromes. Marfan syndrome is a heritable disorder linked to a mutation of the FBN1 gene, which is responsible for the synthesis of fibrillin-1. The syndrome is characterized by tall stature, aortic root dilatation, joint hypermobility, optic lens dislocation, and striae.[17] Ehlers-Danlos syndrome (EDS) is another heritable disorder associated with fragile hyperelastic skin and joint hypermobility. It is currently classified in a system that contains 13 subtypes, with an extensive overlap in features. It results from a mutation in one of more than a dozen genes. The specific gene that is affected determines the subtype of EDS. Inheritance can be either autosomal dominant or recessive, and some cases result from a sporadic mutation. Most subtypes are inherited in an autosomal dominant fashion. A diagnosis can generally be made with a detailed history and physical examination, but can be confirmed with genetic testing or a skin biopsy.[18] Benign joint hypermobility syndrome represents a variety of undetermined genetic deficiencies involving genes that encode for the protein constituents of ligamentous tissue. Generalized ligamentous laxity can also be an acquired condition as the result of various disorders, including rheumatic fever, chronic alcoholism, and hyperparathyroidism.[19]

The degree of joint laxity can be characterized with either the Beighton score, which measures joint hyperextensibility, or the Brighton score, which takes both joint mobility and skin abnormalities into account.[20,21] Carter and Wilkinson[22] developed the initial classification of joint laxity in 1964 based on their observations of children with congenital dislocation of the hip. Beighton and Horan[23] then modified the Carter-Wilkinson criteria to assist in evaluating patients with joint laxity and EDS. Their scale has become the standard measure of joint laxity and has been used in multiple studies to evaluate the presence and extent of joint hypermobility.[24–27] It is a 9-point scale, with a higher score indicating greater hypermobility. The items that make up the scale include passive hyperextension of the small finger (measured bilaterally with one point per side), passive thumb apposition to the forearm (measured bilaterally), elbow hyperextension (measured bilaterally), knee hyperextension (measured bilaterally), and standing trunk flexion with the knees fully extended. A score ≥4 is generally accepted as indicating increased joint laxity. Criteria for a positive sign, represented by a score of 1, include greater than 90° of small finger extension, being able to touch the forearm with the thumb, greater than 10° of elbow and knee hyperextension, and being able to place both palms flat on the floor while keeping the knees extended. The use of the Beighton scale has high intraobserver and interobserver reliability and reproducibility.[21,28]

The Brighton criteria were initially described in the rheumatology literature and use the Beighton score as well as additional criteria to characterize joint hypermobility.[29] It is most useful in individuals with low Beighton scores but with obvious signs and symptoms of joint hypermobility. To be diagnosed with joint hypermobility using the Brighton criteria, patients must meet one of the following combinations: 2 major criteria, one major and 2 minor criteria, 4 minor criteria, or 2 minor criteria and a first-degree relative who has been diagnosed with EDS. The major criteria include a Beighton score ≥4 and arthralgia in ≥4 joints for ≥3 months. Minor criteria include a Beighton score of 1 to 3 (or 0–3 if older than 50 years of age); arthralgia in 1 to 3 joints for ≥3 months; back pain for ≥3 months; dislocation or subluxation of greater than 1 joint or the same joint more than once; ≥3 soft tissue injuries, tenosynovitis, or bursitis; Marfanoid habitus; thin, stretchy skin or abnormal scarring; ptosis, short-sightedness, or double vision; varicose veins; hernia; and rectal or uterine prolapse.

Ankle sprains and functional ankle instability are common in patients with joint hypermobility. The rate of excessive ankle joint laxity has been reported to be as high as 93% in patients with a hypermobility syndrome.[30] Decoster and colleagues[31] reported a higher incidence of ankle sprain in hypermobile athletes compared with their non-hypermobile counterparts (26.1% vs 9%). They noted that collegiate lacrosse players with hypermobility were more than twice as likely as their nonhypermobile counterparts to sustain an ankle sprain. The prevalence of joint hypermobility in patients undergoing ankle joint stabilization procedures has not been reported, but the presence of joint hypermobility is thought to negatively affect the outcomes of ankle stabilization procedures, although this remains to be definitively and objectively established.

WORKUP AND EVALUATION

A detailed history should always be obtained whenever a patient who has undergone lateral ankle stabilization presents with a complaint of recurrent instability. It should be determined whether the recurrence of instability came about as the result of an acute traumatic episode or whether it has resulted from a series of repetitive episodes. In addition, it should be determined whether the patient thought their initial surgery was a success and whether they experienced relief of their instability after their initial procedure. Inquiring about their procedure and postoperative rehabilitation may also provide helpful information. When available, the operative report from their initial procedure should be reviewed. The patient should also be asked about all nonoperative treatment completed since the recurrence of instability, particularly with regards to physical therapy and bracing.

The physical examination should begin with evaluation of the patient's weight-bearing alignment and an assessment of gait. Malalignment in the form of hindfoot varus, first ray plantarflexion, or midfoot cavus can predispose patients to repetitive lateral ankle injuries and be a cause of early operative failure if not properly addressed at the time of surgery. Range of motion of the ankle, subtalar, and talonavicular joints should be assessed. In particular, an unrecognized subtalar coalition may represent a potential additional risk factor for instability. Crepitus and/or pain with passive ankle motion may be indicative of intra-articular pathologic condition. Any tenderness along the ankle joint line and/or sinus tarsi should also be noted. Many patients will have a joint effusion, often due to one or more sequelae of ankle instability, such as synovitis, osteochondral lesions, or loose bodies. Palpation of the peroneal tendons should be performed to identify any tenderness, swelling, or instability. Muscle strength testing should be done, with particular attention paid to the strength of the peroneal tendons. Manual anterior drawer and talar tilt testing are important in evaluating the integrity of the lateral ankle ligaments. The anterolateral drawer test as described by Miller and colleagues[32] has been shown to detect more subtle degrees of ankle instability. The surgeon should pay particular attention and rule out deltoid instability as well as subtalar instability. The patient should also be examined for generalized ligamentous laxity and asked whether there is a family history of hypermobility disorders.

Radiographic assessment should include weight-bearing anteroposterior, mortise, and lateral ankle radiographs. The presence of any hardware, such as suture anchors, as well as bone tunnels from the patient's previous procedures should be noted, paying careful attention to their placement. Anterior drawer and talar tilt stress views can also be obtained, either manually or using a Telos device (Austin & Associates, Fallston, MD, USA), although their reproducibility and reliability are suspect.[33] If needed, comparison views of the contralateral ankle can be obtained. Because there is no definite value that confirms instability, comparison views can be helpful. It has been suggested that the anterior drawer should measure less than 10 mm or should be within 3 to 5 mm of the measurement in the contralateral ankle.[2] Talar tilt values can vary widely, from 5° to 23°. An absolute talar tilt of greater than 10° or 5° more than the contralateral ankle is consistent with laxity.[2,4] One of the primary benefits of stress radiography is to assist in making the often subtle diagnosis of subtalar

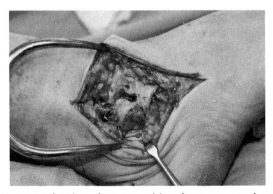

Fig. 1. The inferior peroneal retinaculum, comprising short separate sheaths for the longus and brevis tendons, may be released to allow the tendons to be mobilized.

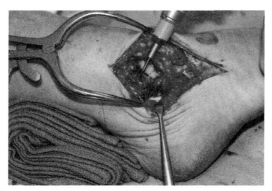

Fig. 2. A 4.0-mm burr is used to create a tunnel from the midportion of the ATFL origin on the fibula coursing distally and posteriorly.

instability, and they can be obtained if there is suspicion for subtalar instability.[34,35] These views are generally obtained with the ankle in dorsiflexion and 30° of internal rotation and the x-ray tube angled 45° cephalad. Medial displacement of the calcaneus of more than 5 mm is suggestive of pathologic laxity.[36]

MRI can also be helpful, particularly with regard to evaluating for chondral injuries and surrounding soft tissue structures, such as the peroneal tendons. However, the quality of the MRI scan varies for formally evaluating the lateral ligamentous structures, particularly in the setting of previous surgery. The presence of metallic suture anchors will also create a large amount of artifact, which can further distort the quality of the images.

SURGICAL TECHNIQUES

Many types of ankle ligament reconstructions have been described, all of which have different effects on ankle motion and mechanics. Surgical treatment options can generally be grouped into the following categories: direct anatomic repair with and without augmentation, nonanatomic reconstruction using tenodesis, and near anatomic reconstruction using tenodesis. Direct anatomic repair techniques with and without augmentation were discussed above in the introduction and are considered appropriate for primary procedures. The reported advantages of anatomic repair include ease of the procedure, restoration of normal anatomy and joint kinematics,

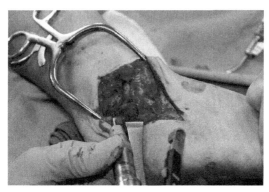

Fig. 3. The hindfoot may need to be inverted and the peroneal tendons protected with a retractor to achieve the angle necessary for this maneuver.

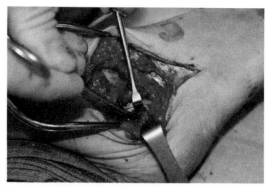

Fig. 4. The site of the CFL insertion on the lateral calcaneus is approximately 2 cm distal to and slightly posterior to the distal tip of the fibula.

and maintenance of ankle and subtalar motion.[7,9,14] In addition, there is no morbidity associated with harvesting of tendon grafts. The main disadvantage is the reliance on potentially weak or attenuated local soft tissue.[12]

Indications for nonanatomic augmented reconstruction using tenodesis include a history of failed Broström procedure, significantly attenuated soft tissues, or a genetic hypermobility disorder.[19] The most popular procedures have traditionally used the peroneus longus or brevis tendons.[19] Nilsonne[5] described tenodesing the peroneus brevis to the lateral periosteum of the distal fibula in 1932. Elmslie[6] reported on 4 patients in whom he reconstructed the ATFL as well as the CFL using a fascia lata graft in 1934.

It was not until 1952 that Watson-Jones[37] described detaching the entire peroneus brevis tendon proximally and then routing it through the fibula from posterior to anterior and securing it to the talar neck using drill holes. Initial studies using this procedure showed good to excellent short-term outcomes in 80% to 85% of patients, all for primary repairs.[37–44] The main issue with this reconstruction was that it did not replicate the anatomy of the CFL. In addition, although it led to a dramatic improvement in preventing internal rotation and anterior subluxation of the talus, it also was associated with a substantial loss of subtalar motion.[45–47]

Evans[48] described a similar procedure in 1953, which involved routing the entire peroneus brevis tendon through an oblique hole in the distal fibula and resuturing it

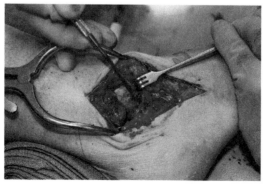

Fig. 5. A location just anterior to the cartilage of the lateral talus is chosen. If necessary, the attenuated ATFL may be split to gain access.

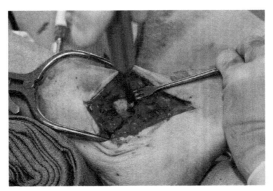

Fig. 6. The hole and tap should be drilled an additional 5 mm beyond the length of the screw to allow for oversinking of the screw.

to itself proximally, leaving its distal insertion on the base of the fifth metatarsal intact. Early clinical studies with short-term follow-up have reported good subjective results after the procedure.[44,48–54] However, residual anterior talar instability and reduced subtalar motion were observed.

Chrisman and Snook[55] reported a modification of the original Elmslie procedure in 1969, in which they used a split peroneus brevis tendon transfer with the proximal part of the graft routed through a tunnel in the anterolateral neck of the talus and passed from anterior to posterior through the fibula and then inferiorly into the calcaneus. This technique was reported to have several advantages over the other early nonanatomic reconstructions.[16] The split graft did not sacrifice a tremendous amount of peroneal strength, and its position was considered more anatomic because it reconstructed both the ATFL and the CFL.[46] The initial 4 clinical series of Chrisman-Snook reconstructions reported greater than 90% good to excellent results, all in primary repairs.[56–59] Snook and colleagues[59] revisited the procedure in 1985 and described modifications that consisted of drill holes in the calcaneus to secure the graft, tenodesis of the graft end to the lateral malleolus rather than the fifth metatarsal base, and the use of mild rather than forced eversion when tensioning the graft. They reported 93% good to excellent results. However, this technique also led to restriction of subtalar motion.

The focus then shifted to anatomic tendon reconstructions without sacrificing anatomy or kinematics. In 1995, Colville and Grondel[60] introduced a reconstruction in

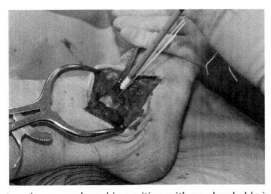

Fig. 7. The suture tape is now anchored in position with an absorbable interference screw.

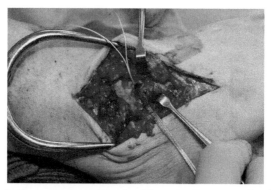

Fig. 8. In addition to the suture tape, 2 leads of the retention suture for the anchor tip pass through the cannulated interference screw.

which a split peroneus brevis tendon was used to augment the repair of the ATFL and CFL. After anatomic repair, the split tendon is anchored distally at its insertion and routed through bone tunnels in the calcaneus, fibula, and talus and sutured to itself with the foot in eversion. Subsequent studies confirmed maintenance of normal ankle kinematics and subtalar motion compared with both standard and modified Broström repairs.[45,61] Several more studies have also reported success using variations of this anatomic technique.[15,36,60,62–64] Graft placement and correct tensioning are considered to be the most important factors in determining success of the procedure.[15,61,62] Current consensus suggests the graft should be tensioned with the foot in neutral to slight valgus to avoid overtightening.[12,15,36,47,62,65]

Augmentation using a suture tape, or bone-to-bone suture augmentation, has been introduced recently for treatment in both primary and revision lateral ligament reconstructions. Some biomechanical studies have reported mechanical superiority of augmentation using bone-to-bone suture augmentation.[66–68] However, clinical evidence remains sparse.[69] Cho and colleagues[70] found bone-to-bone suture augmentation of a modified Broström procedure provided satisfactory clinical outcomes with a low recurrence rate of instability for the treatment of chronic lateral ankle instability in patients with generalized ligamentous laxity. In addition, the higher initial stability of the ligament repair with bone-to-bone suture augmentation may allow for an earlier rehabilitation program with a lower risk of ligament elongation. Cho and colleagues[71]

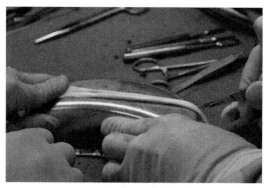

Fig. 9. A semitendinosis allograft is prepared and carefully split along its fibers to a thickness of 5 mm.

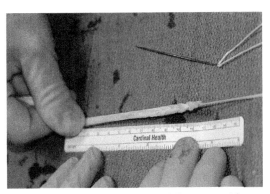

Fig. 10. The semitendinosis allograft is whip-stitched for 3 cm with a no. 2 UHMWPE core suture at one end.

also looked at the use of bone-to-bone suture augmentation in the setting of revision modified Broström procedure. They found bone-to-bone suture augmentation in the revision setting produced satisfactory intermediate outcomes without the need for a tendon graft or other nonanatomic reconstruction. Bone-to-bone suture augmentation also allowed for an earlier rehabilitation program.

Revision surgery for a failed lateral ankle stabilization procedure can include surgical site infection, wound-healing complications, scar sensitivity, recurrent instability, and ankle and/or subtalar stiffness as well as nerve injury, most commonly branches of the superficial peroneal and sural nerves.[16,72] Particular attention should be paid to the patient's previous incisions, and a determination should be made as to whether they can be used or whether a new incision is necessary. The surgeon must also consider potential obstacles caused by suture anchors and/or bone tunnels that were used in the previous procedure.

AUTHORS' PREFERRED TECHNIQUE

Once the choice has been made to proceed with revision surgery, a decision should be made as to whether an arthroscopic evaluation is required. Komenda and Ferkel[73] reported a 93% rate of intra-articular pathologic condition diagnosed arthroscopically before an open lateral ligament stabilization procedure, with a 25% rate

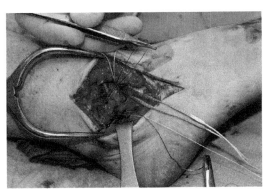

Fig. 11. The blunt suture end is passed retrograde through the convergent fibular tunnels to create a loop that exits through the ATFL origin.

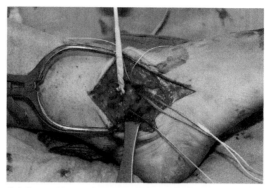

Fig. 12. The allograft is in position to be passed through the fibular tunnels leading with the previously whipstitched end.

of chondral pathologic condition.[73] O'Neill and colleagues[74] looked at the accuracy of MRI compared with the actual surgical findings in patients undergoing operative treatment of ankle instability. They found that radiologists identified only 39% of the chondral injuries seen arthroscopically, 56% of peroneal tendon tears, and 57% of intra-articular loose bodies. Overall sensitivity for a radiologist's ability to detect lesions was 45%. With regards to the attending surgeon's interpretation of the preoperative MRI, 47% of chondral injuries, 89% of intra-articular loose bodies, and 71% of peroneal tendon tears were identified, with an overall sensitivity of 63%. Their findings suggest that the sensitivity of MRI may not be adequate to detect lesions in patients undergoing ankle stabilization surgery. Thus, an arthroscopic evaluation of the ankle joint may be warranted before proceeding with a revision stabilization procedure. If intra-articular pathologic condition is noted, it should be appropriately addressed at that time.

Once any intra-articular pathologic condition has been dealt with, the choice of a surgical strategy to reconstruct a failed prior lateral ligament reconstruction presents numerous challenges and options. Although many methods of augmented repair and tenodesis have been described, they have largely been reported in the setting of primary lateral ankle ligament reconstructions. Large-scale trials or series involving the patient population with failed surgery are lacking; patients in this population would reasonably be expected to have an elevated incidence of genetic hypermobility conditions, behavioral factors, or anatomic variation that predispose them to failed surgical treatment. The

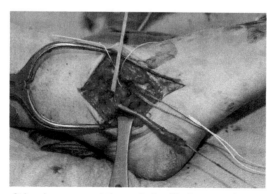

Fig. 13. The allograft has been passed through the fibular tunnels.

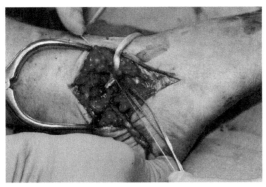

Fig. 14. The retention sutures from the previously placed interference screw are used in a short weave stitch to affix the midportion of the allograft into the small bone tunnel created by over-sinking the screw.

technique described here seeks to capitalize on the potential benefits of both tenodesis and bone-to-bone suture augmentation in this high-risk group.

The tenodesis originally described by Colville and Grondel[60] most nearly approximates the native anatomic structure of the ATFL and CFL. It offers, in theory, a smaller risk of diminished subtalar motion compared with other less anatomic tenodesis procedures. To eliminate the morbidity of a split harvest of the peroneus brevis tendon, a semitendinosis allograft is used.

Bone-to-bone suture tape augmentation provides an element of immediate stability that is not dependent on the quality of the patient's tissues as well as highly reproducible tensioning compared with biologic grafts. The technique presented here allows suture augmentation to overlie an anatomic allograft tenodesis procedure.

Surgical Technique

- The patient is positioned either in a full lateral position or with a bump underneath the ipsilateral hip. An extensile approach is made directly over the distal fibula and curving into the sinus tarsi to allow access to the anterior ankle and the peroneal sheath inferior to the superior peroneal retinaculum. The *inferior* peroneal retinaculum, comprising short separate sheaths for the longus and brevis tendons, may be released to allow the tendons to be mobilized (**Fig. 1**).

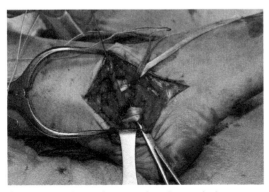

Fig. 15. The allograft is in a position to be passed underneath the peroneal tendons to avoid entrapment.

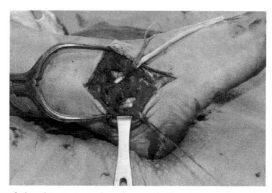

Fig. 16. The allograft has been passed underneath the peroneal tendons.

- The attenuated and previously repaired ATFL and CFL are taken down directly off of the fibula from the superolateral corner of the joint to the peroneal sheath. The fibular periosteum is not raised. A 4.0-mm burr is used to create a tunnel from the midportion of the ATFL origin on the fibula coursing distally and posteriorly (**Fig. 2**).
- A second converging tunnel is then made with the 4.0-mm burr from the CFL origin just posterior to the center of the tip of fibula. An adequate connection between the 2 burr passes is critical to ultimately pass the allograft tendon. All debris should be evacuated. The hindfoot may need to be inverted, and the peroneal tendons protected with a retractor to achieve the angle necessary for this maneuver (**Fig. 3**).
- With the inferior peroneal retinaculum released, the peroneal tendons can be mobilized anteriorly to gain access to the site of the CFL insertion on the lateral calcaneus. This is approximately 2 cm distal to and slightly posterior to the distal tip of the fibula (**Fig. 4**).
- The center of the ATFL insertion at the neck-body junction of the talus is localized. This is essentially midway between the anterolateral cartilage margin and the lateral talar process. A location just anterior to the cartilage of the lateral talus is chosen. If necessary, the attenuated ATFL may be split to gain access (**Fig. 5**).
- A pilot hole for the suture tape augmentation is drilled in this location aiming back toward the talar body by approximately 40°. This is followed by a tap for the

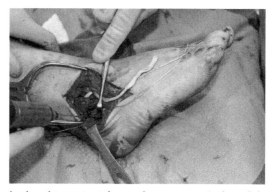

Fig. 17. Retraction is placed to protect the sural nerve posteriorly and the peroneal tendons anteriorly.

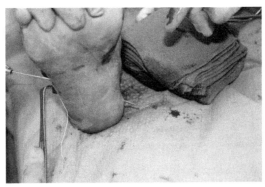

Fig. 18. A Beath pin is driven from the previously identified site of the CFL insertion obliquely across the foot to exit the skin along the inferomedial heel. Care must be taken to orient the pin obliquely to avoid the medial neurovascular bundle.

anchoring interference screw. The hole and tap should be drilled an additional 5 mm beyond the length of the screw to allow for oversinking of the screw (**Fig. 6**).

- The suture tape is now anchored in position with an absorbable interference screw. *Rather than leaving the screw flush with the surface, the screw is sunk to a depth of 5 mm below the cortex.* This creates a small channel in which to secondarily anchor the allograft tendon. In addition to the suture tape, 2 leads of the retention suture for the anchor tip pass through the cannulated interference screw (**Figs. 7** and **8**).
- A semitendinosis allograft is prepared and carefully split along its fibers to a thickness of 5 mm. It is whip-stitched for 3 cm with a no. 2 ultrahigh-molecular-weight polyethylene (UHMWPE) core suture at one end (**Figs. 9** and **10**).
- Any suture with a needle radius of curvature of approximately 1 cm is grasped by the sharp tip. The blunt end is passed retrograde through the convergent fibular tunnels to create a loop that exits through the ATFL origin (**Fig. 11**).
- The allograft is now passed through the fibular tunnels leading with the previously whipstitched end (**Figs. 12** and **13**).
- The allograft is positioned appropriately so that the whipstitched portion of the tendon will end up within the calcaneal tunnel beginning at the previously identified CFL insertion. The retention sutures from the previously placed interference screw are now used in a short weave-stitch to affix the midportion of the allograft into the small bone tunnel created by oversinking the screw (**Fig. 14**).

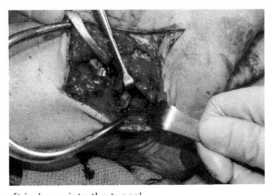

Fig. 19. The allograft is drawn into the tunnel.

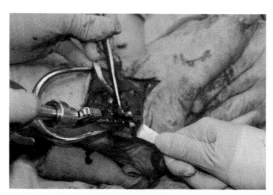

Fig. 20. The talus is held posteriorly into the ankle mortise, and the heel is held in approximately 10° of inversion while the allograft is tensioned through the lead suture out the medial heel.

- *The allograft is now passed underneath the peroneal tendons to avoid entrapment* (**Figs. 15** and **16**).
- Retraction is placed to protect the sural nerve posteriorly and the peroneal tendons anteriorly. A Beath pin is driven from the previously identified site of the CFL insertion obliquely across the foot to exit the skin along the inferomedial heel. Care must be taken to orient the pin obliquely to avoid the medial neurovascular bundle (**Figs. 17** and **18**).
- The end of the allograft is sized, and the minimum size of reamer required to pass it is chosen. An oblique tunnel through the calcaneus is then drilled over the Beath pin, with care taken not to breach the skin medially. The allograft is then drawn into the tunnel. The talus is held posteriorly into the ankle mortise, and the heel is held in approximately 10° of inversion while the allograft is tensioned through the lead suture out the medial heel. A 15-mm interference screw is now placed in the calcaneal tunnel to hold the graft in place. The bone in this portion of calcaneal tuberosity may be soft; as such, the screw should be sized 0.5 mm to 1.0 mm larger than the reamed tunnel to ensure purchase (**Figs. 19–21**).
- The suture tape is now applied to the lateral aspect of the fibula, just behind the tunnels, and under suitable tension with the ankle in 20° of plantarflexion. This

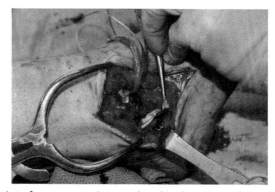

Fig. 21. A 15-mm interference screw is now placed in the calcaneal tunnel to hold the graft in place.

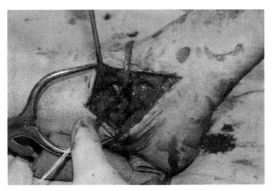

Fig. 22. The suture tape is applied to the lateral aspect of the fibula just behind the tunnels under suitable tension with the ankle in 20° of plantarflexion.

location is less anatomic than the anterior margin of the fibula, but still provides excellent augmentation for this most common position of ankle inversion injury. The tape will be slightly less tight when the ankle is dorsiflexed, but the ankle benefits from additional bony stability of the wider portion of the talus in the mortise in this position. The suture tape is secured with an additional small interference screw (**Figs. 22** and **23**).

- If desired, the excess length of the allograft may also be doubled back and sutured to the fibular periosteum in cases where the native tissues are extremely deficient (**Fig. 24**). Any usable components of the native ATFL and CFL are now incorporated into the reconstruction by repairing them to the fibular periosteum as well.

Aftercare

Unless concurrent peroneal repair has been undertaken, there is little benefit to immediate mobilization in the setting of revision lateral ankle ligament reconstruction. To diminish potential risk to the repair from a possible genetic collagen disorder or non-compliant patient behavior, non-weight-bearing immobilization in a cast or boot is recommended for 4 weeks after the procedure. This immobilization is followed by 4 weeks of progressive weight-bearing in a walking boot and the institution of physical therapy with an initial restriction of no greater than 15° of passive inversion.

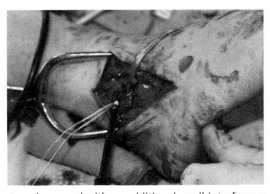

Fig. 23. The suture tape is secured with an additional small interference screw.

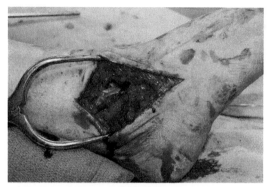

Fig. 24. If desired, the excess length of the allograft may also be doubled back and sutured to the fibular periosteum in cases where the native tissues are extremely deficient.

SUMMARY

Revision of a failed surgical lateral ankle instability stabilization procedure can present numerous challenges, with very few studies present in the literature on revision procedures. The greatest challenges involve patient factors, including the presence of generalized joint hypermobility with associated poor quality of soft tissue, behavioral noncompliance, and anatomic variation that can predispose one to a poor outcome.

The technique described here offers anatomic reconstruction of the ATFL and CFL, while minimizing the risk of reduced subtalar range of motion, as originally described by Colville and Grondel.[60] The use of a semitendinosis allograft avoids both the morbidity of peroneal tendon harvest and the use of potentially poor quality host tissue. The addition of a bone-to-bone suture tape augmentation allows for immediate stability and highly reproducible tensioning, while also avoiding reliance on suspect host tissue.

Further studies are needed to characterize reasons for failure of surgical stabilization of the lateral ankle ligaments as well as establish the optimum treatment methods for such patients. Although this is a rare problem, it presents major challenges. However, the technique described here can help to mitigate many of the problems inherent with this patient population and may allow for reliable and reproducible outcomes.

REFERENCES

1. Berlet G, Anderson RB, Davis W. Chronic lateral ankle instability. Foot Ankle Clin 1999;4:713–28.
2. Colville MR. Surgical treatment of the unstable ankle. J Am Acad Orthop Surg 1998;6:368–77.
3. Maffulli N, Ferran NA. Management of acute and chronic ankle instability. J Am Acad Orthop Surg 2008;16:608–15.
4. Frey C. Ankle sprains. Instr Course Lect 2001;50:515–20.
5. Nilsonne H. Making a new ligament in ankle sprain. J Bone Joint Surg 1932;14:380–1.
6. Elmslie RC. Recurrent subluxation of the ankle-joint. Ann Surg 1934;100:364–7.
7. Brostrom L. Sprained ankles. VI. Surgical treatment of chronic ligament ruptures. Acta Chir Scand 1966;132:551–65.
8. Karlsson J, Bergsten T, Lansinger O, et al. Reconstruction of the lateral ligaments of the ankle for chronic lateral instability. J Bone Joint Surg Am 1988;70:581–8.

9. Gould N, Seligson D, Gassman J. Early and late repair of lateral ligament of the ankle. Foot Ankle 1980;1:84–9.
10. Glas E, Paar O, Smasal V, et al. Periosteal flap reconstruction of the external ankle ligaments. Results of a follow-up study. Unfallchirurg 1985;88:219–22 [in German].
11. Sjølin SU, Dons-Jensen H, Simonsen O. Reinforced anatomical reconstruction of the anterior talofibular ligament in chronic anterolateral instability using a periosteal flap. Foot Ankle 1991;12:15–8.
12. Colville MR. Reconstruction of the lateral ankle ligaments. Instr Course Lect 1995; 44:341–8.
13. Fortin PT, Guettler J, Manoli A. Idiopathic cavovarus and lateral ankle instability: recognition and treatment implications relating to ankle arthritis. Foot Ankle Int 2002;23:1031–7.
14. Karlsson J, Bergsten T, Lansinger O, et al. Surgical treatment of chronic lateral instability of the ankle joint. A new procedure. Am J Sports Med 1989;17:268–73.
15. Sammarco GJ, Idusuyi OB. Reconstruction of the lateral ankle ligaments using a split peroneus brevis tendon graft. Foot Ankle Int 1999;20:97–103.
16. Sammarco VJ. Complications of lateral ankle ligament reconstruction. Clin Orthop Relat Res 2001;(391):123–32.
17. Wolf JM, Cameron KL, Owens BD. Impact of joint laxity and hypermobility on the musculoskeletal system. J Am Acad Orthop Surg 2011;19:463–71.
18. Lawrence EJ. The clinical presentation of Ehlers-Danlos syndrome. Adv Neonatal Care 2005;5:301–14.
19. Guyton GP. Chronic lateral ankle instability. In: Richardson EG, editor. Orthopaedic knowledge update foot and ankle 3. Rosemont (IL): American Academy of Orthopaedic Surgeons; 2003. p. 103–11.
20. Holbrook KA, Byers PH. Structural abnormalities in the dermal collagen and elastic matrix from the skin of patients with inherited connective tissue disorders. J Invest Dermatol 1982;79(Suppl 1):7s–16s.
21. Juul-Kristensen B, Rogind H, Jensen DV, et al. Inter-examiner reproducibility of tests and criteria for generalized joint hypermobility and benign joint hypermobility syndrome. Rheumatology (Oxford) 2007;46:1835–41.
22. Carter C, Wilkinson J. Persistent joint laxity and congenital dislocation of the hip. J Bone Joint Surg Br 1964;46:40–5.
23. Beighton P, Horan F. Orthopaedic aspects of the Ehlers-Danlos syndrome. J Bone Joint Surg Br 1969;51:444–53.
24. Aktas I, Ofluoglu D, Albay T. The relationship between benign joint hypermobility syndrome and carpal tunnel syndrome. Clin Rheumatol 2008;27:1283–7.
25. Dolan AL, Hart DJ, Doyle DV, et al. The relationship of joint hypermobility, bone mineral density, and osteoarthritis in the general population: the Chingford Study. J Rheumatol 2003;30:799–803.
26. Jonsson H, Valtysdottir ST, Kjartansson O, et al. Hypermobility associated with osteoarthritis of the thumb base: a clinical and radiological subset of hand osteoarthritis. Ann Rheum Dis 1996;55:540–3.
27. Rozen TD, Roth JM, Denenberg N. Cervical spine joint hypermobility: a possible predisposing factor for new daily persistent headache. Cephalalgia 2006;26: 1182–5.
28. Boyle KL, Witt P, Riegger-Krugh C. Intrarater and interrater reliability of the Beighton and Horan joint mobility index. J Athl Train 2003;38:281–5.
29. Grahame R, Bird HA, Child A. The revised (Brighton 1998) criteria for the diagnosis of benign joint hypermobility syndrome (BJHS). J Rheumatol 2000;27: 1777–9.

30. Kamanli A, Sahin S, Ozgocmen S, et al. Relationship between foot angles and hypermobility scores and assessment of foot types in hypermobile individuals. Foot Ankle Int 2004;25:101–6.
31. Decoster LC, Vailas JC, Lindsay RH, et al. Prevalence and features of joint hypermobility among adolescent athletes. Arch Pediatr Adolesc Med 1997;151:989–92.
32. Miller AG, Myers SH, Parks BG, et al. Anterolateral drawer versus anterior drawer test for lateral ankle instability: a biomechanical model. Foot Ankle Int 2016;37:407–10.
33. Frost SC, Amendola A. Is stress radiography necessary in the diagnosis of acute or chronic ankle instability? Clin J Sport Med 1999;9:40–5.
34. Ishii T, Miyagawa S, Fukubayashi T, et al. Subtalar stress radiography using forced dorsiflexion and supination. J Bone Joint Surg Br 1996;78:56–60.
35. Louwerens JW, Ginai AZ, Van Linge B, et al. Stress radiography of the talocrural and subtalar joints. Foot Ankle Int 1995;16:148–55.
36. Thermann H, Zwipp H, Tscherne H. Treatment algorithm of chronic ankle and subtalar instability. Foot Ankle Int 1997;18:163–9.
37. Watson-Jones R. Recurrent forward dislocation of the ankle joint. J Bone Joint Surg Br 1952;134:519.
38. Barbari SG, Brevig K, Egge T. Reconstruction of the lateral ligamentous structures of the ankle with a modified Watson-Jones procedure. Foot Ankle 1987;7:362–8.
39. Gillespie HS, Boucher P. Watson-Jones repair of lateral instability of the ankle. J Bone Joint Surg Am 1971;53:920–4.
40. Hedeboe J, Johannsen A. Recurrent instability of the ankle joint. Surgical repair by the Watson-Jones method. Acta Orthop Scand 1979;50:337–40.
41. Hendel D, Peer A, Halperin N. A simple operation for correction of chronic lateral instability of the ankle. Injury 1983;15:115–6.
42. Lucht U, Vang PS, Termansen NB. Lateral ligament reconstruction of the ankle with a modified Watson-Jones operation. Acta Orthop Scand 1981;52:363–6.
43. van der Rijt AJ, Evans GA. The long-term results of Watson-Jones tenodesis. J Bone Joint Surg Br 1984;66:371–5.
44. Zenni EJ Jr, Grefer M, Krieg JK, et al. Lateral ligamentous instability of the ankle: a method of surgical reconstruction by a modified Watson-Jones technique. Am J Sports Med 1977;5:78–83.
45. Bahr R, Pena F, Shine J, et al. Biomechanics of ankle ligament reconstruction. An in vitro comparison of the Brostrom repair, Watson-Jones reconstruction, and a new anatomic reconstruction technique. Am J Sports Med 1997;25:424–32.
46. Colville MR, Marder RA, Zarins B. Reconstruction of the lateral ankle ligaments. A biomechanical analysis. Am J Sports Med 1992;20:594–600.
47. Liu SH, Baker CL. Comparison of lateral ankle ligamentous reconstruction procedures. Am J Sports Med 1994;22:313–7.
48. Evans DL. Recurrent instability of the ankle – a method of surgical treatment. Proc R Soc Med 1953;46:343–4.
49. Karlsson J, Bergsten T, Lansinger O, et al. Lateral instability of the ankle treated by the Evans procedure. A long-term clinical and radiological follow-up. J Bone Joint Surg Br 1988;70:476–80.
50. Kristiansen B. Evans' repair of lateral instability of the ankle joint. Acta Orthop Scand 1981;52:679–82.
51. Orava S, Jaroma H, Weitz H, et al. Radiographic instability of the ankle joint after Evans' repair. Acta Orthop Scand 1983;54:734–8.

52. Silver CM, Deutsch SD. Evans repair of lateral instability of the ankle. Orthopedics 1982;5:51–6.

53. Tindall SF, Heaney SH. Repair of the lateral ligaments of the ankle by the Evans technique. J Bone Joint Surg Br 1976;58:133.

54. Vainionpaa S, Kirves P, Laike E. Lateral instability of the ankle and results when treated by the Evans procedure. Am J Sports Med 1980;8:437–9.

55. Chrisman OD, Snook GA. Reconstruction of lateral ligament tears of the ankle. An experimental study and clinical evaluation of seven patients treated by a new modification of the Elmslie procedure. J Bone Joint Surg Am 1969;51:904–12.

56. Rechtin GR, McCarroll JR, Webster DA. Reconstruction for chronic lateral instability of the ankle: a review of twenty eight surgical patients. Orthopedics 1982; 5:46–50.

57. Riegler HF. Reconstruction for lateral instability of the ankle. J Bone Joint Surg Am 1984;66:336–9.

58. Savastano AA, Lowe EB Jr. Ankle sprains: surgical treatment for recurrent sprains. Report of 10 patients treated with the Chrisman-Snook modification of the Elmslie procedure. Am J Sports Med 1980;8:208–11.

59. Snook GA, Chrisman OD, Wilson TC. Long-term results of the Chrisman-Snook operation for reconstruction of the lateral ligaments of the ankle. J Bone Joint Surg Am 1985;67:1–7.

60. Colville MR, Grondel RJ. Anatomic reconstruction of the lateral ankle ligaments using a split peroneus brevis tendon graft. Am J Sports Med 1995;23:210–3.

61. Schmidt R, Cordier E, Bertsch C, et al. Reconstruction of the lateral ligaments: do the anatomical procedures restore physiologic ankle kinematics? Foot Ankle Int 2004;25:31–6.

62. Acevedo JI, Myerson MS. Technique tip: modification of the Chrisman-Snook technique. Foot Ankle Int 2000;21:154–5.

63. Smith PA, Miller SJ, Berni AJ. A modified Chrisman-Snook procedure for reconstruction of the lateral ligaments of the ankle: review of 18 cases. Foot Ankle Int 1995;16:259–66.

64. Solakoglu C, Kiral A, Pehlivan O, et al. Late-term reconstruction of lateral ankle ligaments using a split peroneus brevis tendon graft (Colville's technique) in patients with chronic lateral instability of the ankle. Int Orthop 2003;27:223–7.

65. Sammarco GJ, Carrasquillo HA. Surgical revision after failed lateral ankle reconstruction. Foot Ankle Int 1995;16:748–53.

66. Schuh R, Benca E, Willegger M, et al. Comparison of Brostrom technique, suture anchor repair, and tape augmentation for reconstruction of the anterior talofibular ligament. Knee Surg Sports Traumatol Arthrosc 2016;24:1101–7.

67. Viens NA, Wijdicks CA, Campbell KJ, et al. Anterior talofibular ligament ruptures, part 1: biomechanical comparison of augmented Brostrom repair techniques with the intact anterior talofibular ligament. Am J Sports Med 2014;42:405–11.

68. Willegger M, Benca E, Hirtler L, et al. Biomechanical stability of tape augmentation for anterior talofibular ligament (ATFL) repair compared to the native ATFL. Knee Surg Sports Traumatol Arthrosc 2016;24:1015–21.

69. Cho BK, Park KJ, Kim SW, et al. Minimal invasive suture-tape augmentation for chronic ankle instability. Foot Ankle Int 2015;36:1330–8.

70. Cho BK, Park KJ, Park JK, et al. Outcomes of the modified Brostrom procedure augmented with suture-tape for ankle instability in patients with generalized ligamentous laxity. Foot Ankle Int 2017;38:405–11.

71. Cho BK, Kim YM, Choi SM, et al. Revision anatomical reconstruction of the lateral ligaments of the ankle augmented with suture tape for patients with a failed Brostrom procedure. Bone Joint J 2017;99-B:1183–9.
72. DiGiovanni CW, Brodsky A. Current concepts: lateral ankle instability. Foot Ankle Int 2006;27:854–66.
73. Komenda GA, Ferkel RD. Arthroscopic findings associated with the unstable ankle. Foot Ankle Int 1999;20:708–13.
74. O'Neill PJ, Van Aman SE, Guyton GP. Is MRI adequate to detect lesions in patients with ankle instability? Clin Orthop Relat Res 2010;648:1115–9.

Acute and Chronic Syndesmotic Injury
The Authors' Approach to Treatment

Michael Swords, DO[a,*], Jean Brilhault, MD, PhD[b,c],
Andrew Sands, MD[d]

KEYWORDS

- Syndesmosis • Ankle fracture • Fixation • Incisura • Ankle reconstruction
- Ankle arthroplasty • Wagstaffe • Chaput

KEY POINTS

- Syndesmosis injuries may at times be very subtle requiring thorough assessment of all ankle injuries.
- Failure to reduce and stabilize syndesmosis injuries leads to worse outcomes.
- Fractures of the posterior malleolus, Chaput tubercle of the tibia, and fracture of the Wagstaffe tubercle of the fibula may all represent osseous equivalents to syndesmotic injury and should be recognized and treated with stable internal fixation.
- Anatomic reconstruction of all components of the ankle injury results in improved clinical outcomes in both early and late presentation of syndesmotic rupture.
- The deltoid ligament, loss of the lateral plafond, syndesmotic widening, and fibular malunion must all be evaluated when performing total ankle arthroplasty when arthritis is due to a syndesmotic rupture resulting in coronal plane deformity.

INTRODUCTION
What Is the Syndesmosis?

The syndesmosis is the complex of osseous and ligamentous structures that maintain the relationship between the fibula and the tibia at the ankle level. The anterolateral (Chaput) tubercle of the tibia, anterior (Wagstaffe) tubercle of the fibula, and the incisura fibularis all contribute to the syndesmotic relationship. The incisura is not consistent in

Disclosure Statement: Michael Swords is a consultant for Depuy Synthes. Brilhault is a consultant for Newclip Technics, Wright Medical, Smith and Nephew and Integra Life Science.
[a] Orthopedic Surgery, Sparrow Hospital, Michigan Orthopedic Center, 2815 South Pennsylvania Avenue, Suite 204, Lansing, MI 48910, USA; [b] Service de Chirurgie Orthopédique, C.H.R.U. Tours, 1, Tours F-37000, France; [c] Service de Chirurgie Orthopédique, C.H.R.U. Tours, Université François-Rabelais de Tours, 37044 Tours Cedex 9, France; [d] Foot and Ankle Surgery, Weill Cornell Medical College, Downtown Orthopedic Associates, AO Foot and Ankle Expert Group, 170 William Street, New York, NY 10038, USA
* Corresponding author.
E-mail address: Foot.trauma@gmail.com

shape and may be either shallow or shallow concave.[1] The anterior inferior tibiofibular ligament (AITFL) originates from the anterolateral tubercle of the tibia (the Chaput tubercle) and attaches to the anterior tubercle of the fibula (Wagstaffe tubercle). The posterior inferior tibiofibular ligament (PITFL) extends from the posterior malleolus to attach along the posterior tubercle of the fibula. The interosseous membrane is located between the tibia and fibula and spans nearly the entire lower leg. The interosseous ligament (IOL) is found in the distal 1 cm of the lower leg and is contiguous with the interosseous membrane. As the number of ligaments that are ruptured increases, the ankle becomes increasingly less stable.[2] In a study performed by section of specific ligaments, Ogilvie-Harris and colleagues[3] found that the AITFL provided 35%, the transverse tibiofibular ligament or deep portion of the PITFL 33%, the IOL 22%, and the PITFL 9% of the overall stability. A second sectioning study resulted in significant syndesmotic widening occurring only after the IOL was sectioned.[4]

Why Repair the Syndesmosis?

Isolated malleolar fractures with syndesmotic injury have been reported to have worse functional outcomes (Short Musculoskeletal Function Assessment [SMFA]) at 1 year than patients who had a malleolar fracture without syndesmotic injury.[5] Sagi and colleagues[6] reported worse outcomes at 2 years on both the SMFA and Olerud-Molander in patients with syndesmotic malreduction, as confirmed by computed tomography (CT), than patients with an anatomic reduction. Weening and Bhondari[7] have shown that improved SMFA and Olerud-Molander scores were predicted by anatomic reduction of the syndesmosis on radiographic assessment.[7]

Small amounts of deformity can lead to significant problems with ankle function. Biomechanical studies have shown that lateral translation of 1 to 2 mm, shortening of 2 mm or more, and external rotation of 5° may result in altered pressure distribution.[8–10] Reconstruction is recommended when syndesmotic rupture is identified in both acute and chronic settings to prevent progression of arthritis and disability. In a successive series of patients undergoing ankle arthrodesis at a tertiary center, 20.3% of patients demonstrated widening of the ankle mortise.[11] Because of the high likelihood of the development of posttraumatic arthritis, or malalignment, chronic rupture of the syndesmosis should be identified and addressed to prevent long-term pain, disability, and progression of arthritis (**Fig. 1**).

Acute syndesmotic injury

Acute injuries to the syndesmosis may occur with a wide array of injuries to the lower extremity. Some syndesmotic injuries are obvious, but many are quite subtle and require due diligence to accurately diagnose the injury. Ankle injuries that may be otherwise amenable for nonsurgical treatment may be assessed in a variety of ways. External stress examination using radiographic imaging will provide information on the presence or absence of injury but may be too painful for patients to tolerate. A trial of weight bearing for 7 to 10 days may reveal instability on follow-up radiographs. In the setting of a fracture to the proximal fibula, tenderness about the distal leg or medial malleolus may indicate a Maisonneuve injury and should be evaluated.

Surgical treatment is indicated for bimalleolar, trimalleolar, and unstable lateral malleolus fractures. Syndesmotic instability is a surgical indication independent of fracture type. High fibula fractures are commonly associated with syndesmotic injury. The syndesmotic injury may be ligamentous or a result of an associated posterior malleolus fracture. When a posterior malleolus fracture is present, the posterior malleolus displaces superiorly following lateral malleolar displacement, as the PITFL tensions. In this scenario, the fibula fracture fails in tension and shortening; thus,

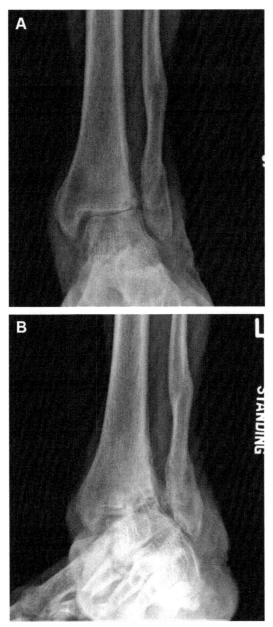

Fig. 1. Radiographs of an ankle 1 year after injury (*A*) and 2.5 years after injury (*B*) demonstrating rapid progression of arthritis from malunion of the fibula and rupture of the syndesmosis. Note rapid deterioration of the lateral tibia plafond resulting in increasing valgus of the ankle.

restoring length is critical. This restoration may be done with direct reduction of the fracture and rigid fixation, bridge plating, or an intramedullary device. Intramedullary devices work best in length-stable patterns, such as transverse or very short oblique fractures.

Although most surgeons understand the necessity to evaluate the stability of the syndesmosis in all operatively treated ankle fractures, it is important to recognize other injuries around the ankle that may result in syndesmosis disruption. Although rare, syndesmotic injury may also occur in the setting of distal tibia fractures, pilon fractures, talus fractures, and hindfoot injuries with associated dislocation (**Fig. 2**). Careful evaluation of the stability of the syndesmosis should be performed during surgery once fixation of these injuries has been achieved.

Surgical Technique for Acute Rupture

All components of the ankle fracture are addressed, reduced, and stabilized. Correct length, alignment, and rotation of the fibula are necessary before evaluating the syndesmosis.

Extreme proximal fibula fractures that result in shortening may be treated with a small incision at the level of the fracture for reduction and held with a pointed reduction clamp at the level of the fracture maintaining length and rotation. A Kirschner (K) wire may be placed just distal to the fracture from the fibula to the tibia to ensure length and rotation are maintained while the syndesmosis is repaired. Care must be taken to identify and protect the superficial peroneal nerve. In this setting, the syndesmosis is treated with two 4-mm-diameter positional screws placed through all 4 cortices through a small plate, typically a one-third tubular plate, to prevent

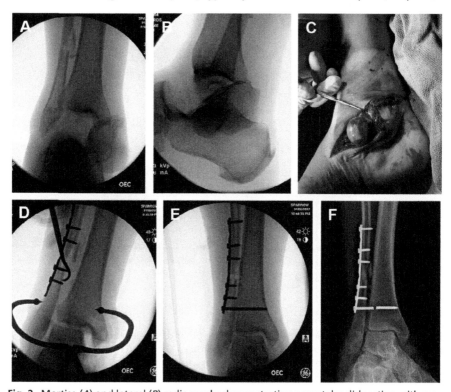

Fig. 2. Mortise (A) and lateral (B) radiographs demonstrating a pantalar dislocation with associated fibula fracture. The dislocation required open reduction (C). At the time of reduction, the fibula was repaired and the syndesmosis was found to be unstable (D). The syndesmosis was reduced and stabilized with a single 4-mm 4-cortex screw (E). The patient went on to union with asymptomatic hardware failure at the syndesmosis, which was retained (F).

shortening. After syndesmotic fixation is completed, the reduction clamp and K wire are removed.

In most Weber B fractures simply dissecting along the fracture line to the anterior aspect of the fibula will bring you to the incisura allowing direct evaluation. Often, when ruptured, the syndesmotic tissues will appear visibly torn and hemorrhagic.

It is important to remember instability of the syndesmosis may result in both widening in the coronal plane and instability in the sagittal plane, and both must be evaluated. If instability is noted, the syndesmotic relationship of the fibula and tibia at the incisura is assessed under direct visualization. Any loose debris or entrapped ligament is removed. The fibula is then reduced into the incisura under direct visualization with manual pressure and then held with a reduction clamp. The clamp is placed from the tip of the fibula to the tip of the medial malleolus, paralleling the transmalleolar axis. After reduction has been achieved, a K wire is placed above the anticipated level of syndesmotic fixation. This placement provides a second point of fixation preventing any potential alteration of the reduction from occurring at the time of insertion of syndesmotic fixation. Generally, a 4-mm solid positional screw is used to stabilize the syndesmosis and is inserted through all 4 cortices. The screw is placed parallel to the tines of the clamp, again following the transmalleolar axis to decrease the risk of loss of reduction. The screw is placed independent of the plate if a posterior antiglide technique has been used for fibula fixation, or through the plate if a lateral plate was used, as is often the case in higher fibula fractures. If comminution is present, the screw may be inserted through a plate, which will act as a washer preventing loss of fixation on the lateral side. Additional screws may be inserted as needed; but the more proximal a screw is placed, the increased likelihood it will break over time because of the normal rotational motion between the fibula and tibia stressing the implant over a greater distance between the tibia and fibula. Screws are not routinely removed.

Osseous Equivalents

Osseous equivalents of syndesmotic injury occur and should be treated with stable internal fixation in an anatomic fashion. Osseous equivalent injuries to the syndesmosis may include the following fractures:

- Fracture of the posterior malleolus
- Fracture of the Chaput tubercle of the tibia
- Fracture of the Wagstaffe tubercle of the distal fibula

Fracture of the posterior malleolus
Posterior malleolar injury represents instability of the bony attachment of the PITFL and necessitates direct anatomic fixation. Direct fixation of the posterior malleolus provides improved fixation strength when compared with syndesmotic fixation and is preferable.[12] Small fragments may be treated with lag screw fixation from posterior to anterior, but larger fragments should be treated with plate fixation. In most cases, an antiglide one-third tubular plate is used. Anterior to posterior screws are biomechanically inferior to posterior antiglide plating.[13]

Fracture of the Chaput tubercle of the tibia
Fractures of the Chaput tubercle of the tibia may result in failure of the AITFL. This fragment, although small, represents an avulsion of the tibial attachment of the syndesmosis and requires fixation. These injuries may be seen in isolation or as a component of a more complex injury. When present, it is necessary to address this injury with rigid

fixation. In most situations, lag screws inserted through a mini fragment plate are used to achieve necessary fixation.

Fracture of the Wagstaffe tubercle of the fibula

When addressing the lateral malleolus component in ankle injuries, it is crucial to evaluate for the presence of a fracture of the Wagstaffe tubercle. This fracture is often considered fracture comminution and left alone. This fragment represents avulsion of the fibular attachment of the AITFL and must be recognized and addressed at the time of fixation (**Fig. 3**). Anatomic reduction restores the appropriate tension and stability to the syndesmotic ligaments resulting in syndesmotic stability. Additionally, this fragment may be pulled medially by the AITFL and block standard syndesmotic reduction techniques. After the fibula fracture is reduced and stabilized, typically with a posterior antiglide plate, the Wagstaffe tubercle is reduced to the fibula and K wires are used to provide provisional fixation. The plate is then placed over the wires. Anterior to posterior screws are inserted through the plate. Appropriate screw length will result in stable bicortical fixation. Caution is necessary, as screws that are excessively long have the potential to irritate the peroneal tendons. This fixation will secure the fibular attachment of the AITFL and, if the fracture is large, the IOL. After fixation is complete, syndesmosis stability should be assessed. Similar to posterior malleolus fractures, typically no additional syndesmotic fixation is necessary after appropriate fixation of the Wagstaffe fracture.

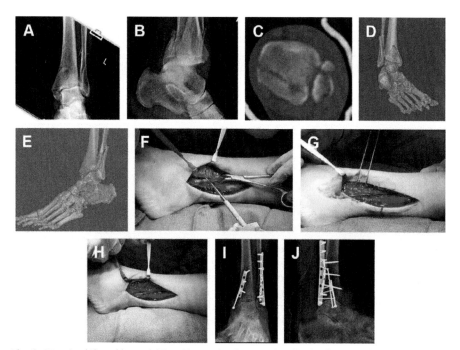

Fig. 3. Mortise (*A*) and lateral (*B*) radiographs show a trimalleolar fracture dislocation of the ankle. CT scan demonstrates a large posterior malleolus component (*C, D*) and fracture of the Wagstaffe tubercle of the fibula (*E*). A freer elevator is placed in the fracture line of the Wagstaffe tubercle (*F*). The fracture is reduced, and provisional fixation is achieved with K wires (*G*). A 2-mm plate is used for definitive fixation (*H*). Final radiographs demonstrate normal alignment of the syndesmosis by fixing all osseous elements, including the posterior malleolus and Wagstaffe tubercle (*I, J*).

Chronic syndesmotic rupture

Chronic syndesmotic rupture generally presents as persistent ankle pain after a history of injury. Generally the patient will have continued loss of function, which does not improve with time. Contracture of the Achilles or gastrocnemius, scar tissue, or patient guarding due to pain may all result in altered ankle motion. Motion should be examined and compared with the contralateral ankle both during preoperative evaluation as well as intraoperatively. Chronic syndesmotic rupture or malreduction must be considered when persistent pain is present after an ankle injury. Weight-bearing ankle radiographs, including anteroposterior (AP), lateral and mortise views are essential. Comparison views of the contralateral side may increase the likelihood of noticing subtle malalignment. CT allows the most accurate method of assessment in the chronic setting. In addition to evaluating the syndesmosis, CT is helpful in assessing the presence or absence of osteophytes, malunion of ankle fracture, and cystic changes, which may be features of arthritis. The goal is to provide treatment before significant ankle arthritis is present. A variety of scenarios may be the cause of chronic syndesmotic rupture including

1. Malunion of ankle fracture
2. Missed syndesmotic ligament injury
3. Malreduction at the time of fracture fixation
4. Loss of syndesmosis fixation before adequate healing

Malunion of the initial ankle fracture

Malunion of the initial ankle fracture injury may result in syndesmotic malalignment. Angular deformities tend to be easiest to correct, whereas rotation deformities are the most difficult. Rotational deformity is difficult to assess using standard fluoroscopy and may require direct visualization of the corresponding articular surfaces of the lateral shoulder of the talus and the distal tibia to best evaluate rotation.[14]

Closing wedge osteotomies are typically avoided, as they may result in shortening. Oblique osteotomies may restore length, alignment, and rotation through a single cut if made in the correct plane.[15] Obtaining length may be challenging, and a variety of techniques may be of assistance. A plate may be secured to the distal fragment first. A small distractor may be used to assist in obtaining appropriate length, and then fixation is inserted into the proximal end of the plate. Alternatively, a lamina spreader may be used to push the plate distal. A push screw is inserted 3 mm to 4 mm proximal to the plate. This screw must be bicortical to avoid a fracture from occurring. A depth gauge is used to measure the appropriate screw length, and then 6 mm is added to allow sufficient screw prominence to engage the lamina spreader. The lamina spreader is used to push the plate distal creating necessary length, and then fixation is placed in the proximal end of the plate. Regardless of which technique is used to obtain length, it is important to avoid introducing angular deformity as lengthening occurs. The fibula is a straight bone and should appear straight on both AP and lateral views.

Missed syndesmotic ligament injury

Syndesmotic rupture may be very subtle and may not be recognized or treated at the time of injury. Sagittal and rotational deformities may be difficult to recognize on standard radiographs. Films of the contralateral ankle may identify some small deformities as a result of missed syndesmotic rupture. A CT scan of both ankles is most effective in identifying deformity from missed syndesmotic injury and should be ordered when there is concern that a syndesmotic injury may have been missed.

Malreduction at the time of the syndesmotic fixation
Syndesmosis fixation is difficult. Even when recognized and treated carefully, malreduction may occur at a surprisingly high rate. Postoperative CT scans should be used to ensure appropriate reduction if uncertain. Intraoperative CT may aid in intraoperative reduction but is not available in most centers.

Loss of syndesmotic fixation before adequate healing
Loss of fixation may occur from the hardware breaking or loosening over time. Occasionally, this may occur when the surgeon removes the hardware before healing of the syndesmosis and may result in instability.

Numerous techniques have been described for repair of chronic syndesmotic rupture. All techniques involve debridement of the syndesmosis of scar tissue to allow reduction. This debridement is generally done in an open fashion but may be done arthroscopically.[16] The literature consists of case reports and small series. Techniques range from arthrodesis of the syndesmosis,[17–21] screw fixation after reduction,[18,22–24] and ligamentous reconstruction. Ligamentous procedures have also been described for late reconstruction of the syndesmosis.[25,26] Generally, all series report good results and improvement regardless of the technique used.

Surgical Technique for Treatment of Late Rupture of the Syndesmosis

Patients are placed in the supine position with a bump under the ipsilateral hip. In some cases, a posterior approach to the syndesmosis will be required, based on the preoperative CT scan; it will be necessary to position patients for improved access by using a larger bump. The leg is elevated on a positioning pillow to facilitate intraoperative imaging. A longitudinal incision is made down the lateral aspect of the fibula. Dissection is carried down to the fibula. If preexisting syndesmotic or fibular fixation is present, it is removed. Care is taken to look for, and protect, the superficial peroneal nerve, as the position of the nerve is variable.

Dissection is carried over the front of the fibula (**Fig. 4**A). The syndesmotic region is often full of posttraumatic scar tissue and may require debridement over approximately the distal 6 to 8 cm. Initially, dissection occurs over the fibula anteriorly and soft tissue is removed allowing the placement of a lamina spreader approximately 5 to 6 cm above the ankle joint. After the lamina spreader is placed, debridement continues distally toward the distal tibiofibular articulation. The lamina spreader is gradually moved distally to assist with the exposure. Bone is often present and may consist of generalized posttraumatic ossification of the syndesmotic region or bone fragments from the initial injury. The incisura region is debrided carefully to prevent injury to the articular cartilage found on the corresponding articular facets at the distal tibiofibular articulation. Osteophyte formation is common in the late reconstruction setting. Osteophytes may be present on the distal tibia, distal fibula, or both. The presence and location of osteophytes is determined from the preoperative CT scan. Osteophytes may be present posteriorly or anteriorly on either the distal fibula or tibia if translational malreduction in the sagittal plane is present or in the syndesmotic region itself. The osteophytes will need to be carefully removed with an osteotome. The syndesmosis is debrided carefully all the way down to the ankle joint until the articular cartilage of the talar dome is visible when looking distally between the fibula and tibia (**Fig. 4**B). A pituitary rongeur is very helpful for this portion of the procedure. Fluoroscopy may be used as the debridement of the syndesmotic region approaches the ankle joint to confirm the position and prevent accidental injury to the talar articular cartilage. Occasionally, the incision may need to be lengthened distally to remove any osteophytes present

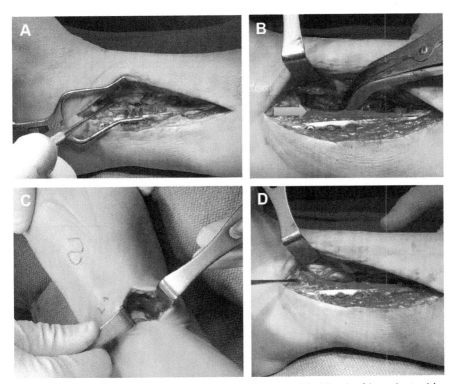

Fig. 4. The incisura is approached through the prior surgical incision in this patient with a neglected syndesmotic injury. The syndesmosis is clearly malaligned at the incisura (*A*). A lamina spreader is placed between the tibia and fibula, and all impediments of reduction are removed down to the ankle joint until the talar dome (*arrow*) is visible (*B*). A medial arthrotomy is made, and the ankle is cleaned of scar and any osteophytes (*C*). The fibula is reduced under direct visualization at the incisura (*D*). The prior plate was left on, as the original fracture of the fibula was well reduced and not fully healed.

at the anterior ankle level extending off the anterolateral aspect of the tibia or off the fibula.

After the syndesmotic region is clear of all impediments for reduction, the ankle joint is addressed. An anteromedial ankle arthrotomy is made just medial to the anterior tibialis. The ankle joint capsule is opened sharply. Most patients will have extensive scarring within the ankle joint. This portion of the procedure can also be completed through arthroscopic approaches. In the open setting, a thorough arthrolysis is performed removing any soft tissue obstruction in the medial gutter as well as across the anterior aspect of the ankle. Any osteophytes or loose ossific densities are removed (**Fig. 4**C). Patients often have diminished dorsiflexion at presentation, which may be a result of intra articular pathology such as scar tissue or osteophytes, generalized post traumatic scarring after injury, or equinus contracture. With the presence of osteophytes and scar tissue it is difficult to assess for the presence or absence of a contracture so they must be removed to allow for a more accurate assessment. The fibula is reduced back into the incisura (**Fig. 4**D). This is done with direct visualization and can generally be performed with manual pressure. A pointed reduction clamp is then placed from the tip of the lateral malleolus to the tip of the medial malleolus recreating the transmalleolar axis. A K wire is then placed above the level of anticipated syndesmotic fixation to prevent introduction of rotational deformity at the time of screw insertion. Before screw insertion, reduction is visually confirmed by looking at the relationship between the fibula and tibia. The mortise view is reviewed, and a lateral view may be obtained and compared with the contralateral ankle to help evaluate the fibular position in the sagittal plane by assessing the distance from the posterior cortex of the fibula to the posterior cortex of the fibula. Fixation generally consists of 4.0 cortical screws through all 4 cortices. In later presentations, individuals with larger body habitus, or in cases with a greater amount of fibular lengthening, an additional screw or two should be considered. Screw trajectory should parallel the tip to tip axis of the reduction clamp.

In cases of chronic syndesmotic malposition without fibular malunion, whereby fibular hardware is removed from the fibula, new fixation should be placed through a plate to avoid loss of fixation or fracture from occurring through the holes in the fibula left from the old fixation construct.

Postoperatively, patients are placed in a splint for 2 weeks and then in a fracture boot for the remainder of treatment. Non–weight bearing is maintained for 6 weeks. Screws are left in indefinitely and are only removed if the lateral hardware proves to be symptomatic and typically after a minimum of a year. The hardware is maintained in most patients.

Chronic Syndesmosis Rupture and Total Ankle Arthroplasty

In the presence of advanced ankle arthritis, ankle arthrodesis and ankle arthroplasty are the reconstruction options. With ankle arthrodesis, any malalignment or instability will be resolved by restoring appropriate alignment at the time of the arthrodesis, and stability is maintained over time by the union of the arthrodesis. If ankle arthroplasty is considered, staged or simultaneous treatment of ligamentous abnormalities must be performed to achieve the best possible results.[27–29]

If the additional procedures are time consuming and will add excessive length to both the tourniquet time and procedure consideration should be given to staging the ankle arthroplasty to decrease risk of wound complications.[30] There are no evidence-based guidelines available to help with the decision-making when performing ankle arthroplasty in the presence of these conditions. The primary goal of ankle arthroplasty is to restore normal anatomic alignment and balance the ankle joint.

In cases of posttraumatic ankle arthritis from syndesmotic injury and/or fibula mal reduction, it is important to assess 4 main parameters at the time of total ankle arthroplasty:

1. Medial deltoid ligament insufficiency
2. Lateral bone defect of the tibial plafond
3. Widening of the syndesmosis
4. Malunion of the fibula

Assessment of the deltoid

Assessment of the deltoid ligament is paramount in valgus ankle deformities. Deltoid insufficiency is common and must be addressed to stabilize the talus and prevent valgus ankle tilt and rotational instability. If the talar valgus is greater than 10° and the deltoid is grossly incompetent (medial talo-malleolar gapping), a staged procedure or ankle arthrodesis should be considered.

Lateral bone defect of the lateral plafond

Bone defects in the tibial plafond can often be managed with a cut performed at the proximal aspect of the defect, perpendicular to the shaft of the tibia. The proximal aspect of the defect is to the lateral plafond due to translation of the talus laterally from chronic injury to the syndesmosis leading to erosion. If this would result in a cut that is too proximal, syndesmotic arthrodesis is performed, either as a staged procedure or performed simultaneously, in order to provide stable lateral support to the tibial implant[31] (**Fig. 5**).

Widening of the syndesmosis
In cases with what seems to be isolated syndesmotic widening, debridement of the tibial fibular space and incisura is performed after performing the tibial cut. If syndesmotic reduction is achieved by joint distraction (a small laminar spreader may be used to distract the ankle), no fixation is necessary and the total ankle arthroplasty is performed. If this is not the case, the syndesmosis is formally reduced and held with screw fixation. Care must be taken at the time the screws are placed such that they will not impinge on the keel of the tibial implant (if there is one).

Malunion of the fibula
If the fibula is shortened because of malunion, the tibial cut is performed and then ligament balance is assessed by joint distraction. If a rectangular shape is present at the ankle joint, ligamentous stability is present and total ankle arthroplasty is performed as usual. If, when the joint is distracted, the shape is trapezoidal, the fibula is short and an osteotomy is performed through a direct lateral

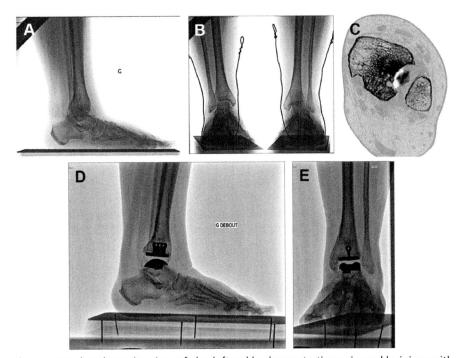

Fig. 5. Lateral and mortise view of the left ankle demonstrating prior ankle injury with widening of the syndesmosis and failure of the lateral plafond resulting in ankle valgus (A, B). CT demonstrating abnormal syndesmosis relationship with a bone fragment as well as widening (C). At the time of arthroplasty, the tibial cut is made at the level of the lateral plafond and is perpendicular to the long axis of the tibia, correcting the deformity. Lateral and mortise postoperative radiographs demonstrate correction of the malalignment at the time of total ankle arthroplasty (D, E).

approach. An oblique lengthening osteotomy is performed in order to obtain a rectangular bone gap between the tibial and the talus. The osteotomy is stabilized with a lateral plate and screw construct. In most cases, there is sufficient bone contact along the oblique osteotomy that bone graft is not necessary. If bone grafting is necessary, ample autograft material may be obtained from the resected tibial bone.

SUMMARY

Acute and chronic syndesmotic ruptures have a varied presentation and may be difficult to diagnose. A high index of suspicion is necessary. Treatment in both the acute and chronic rupture settings is of benefit and requires understanding of all contributing factors. Despite the varied pathology that may lead to syndesmotic rupture and the myriad approaches to treat these injuries, in both the acute and chronic setting, there is clear consensus that the best clinical outcomes are achieved with anatomic reconstruction.[7,32–34]

REFERENCES

1. Elgafy H, Semann HB, Blessinger B, et al. Computed tomography of normal distal tibiofibular Syndesmosis. Skeletal Radiol 2010;39(6):559–64.
2. Xenos JS, Hopkinson WJ, Mulligan ME, et al. Evaluation of the ligamentous structures, methods of fixation, and radiographic assessment. J Bone Joint Surg Am 1995;77(6):847–56.
3. Ogilvie-Harris DJ, Reed SC, Hedman TP. Disruption of the ankle Syndesmosis: biomechanical study of the ligamentous restraints. Arthroscopy 1994;10(5): 558–60.
4. Bachmann L, Seifert C, Zwipp H. Experimental and clinical diagnosis of ankle injuries with the Syndesmosis spreader. In: Schmidt R, Benesch S, Lipke K, editors. Chronic ankle instability. Ulm (Germany): Libri; 2000. p. 235–8.
5. Egol KA, Pahk B, Walsh M, et al. Outcome after unstable ankle fracture: effect of Syndesmosis stabilization. J Orthop Trauma 2010;24(1):7–11.
6. Sagi HC, Shah AR, Sanders RW. The functional consequence of Syndesmotic joint malreduction at a minimum 2-year follow-up. J Orthop Trauma 2012;26(7): 439–43.
7. Weening B, Bhondari M. Predictors of functional outcome following transsyndesmotic screw fixation of ankle fractures. J Orthop Trauma 2005;(2):102–8.
8. Ramsey PL, Hamilton W. Changes in the tibiotalar area of contact caused by lateral talar shift. J Bone Joint Surg Am 1976;58:356–7.
9. Zindrick MR, Hopkins DE, Knight GW, et al. The effect of lateral talar shift upon the biomechanics of the ankle joint. Orthopaedic Transactions 1985;9:332–3.
10. Thordarson DB, Motamed S, Hedman T, et al. The effect of fibular malreduction on contact pressures in an ankle fracture malunion model. J Bone Joint Surg Am 1997;79(12):1809–15.
11. Grass R, Herzmann K, Biewener A, et al. Injuries of the distal tibiofibular Syndesmosis. Unfallchirurg 2000;103:520–32 [in German].
12. Gardner MJ, Brodsky A, Briggs SM, et al. Fixation of posterior malleolus fractures provides greater syndesmotic stability. Clin Orthop Relat Res 2006;(447):165–71.
13. Bennett C, Behn A, Daoud A, et al. Buttress plating versus anterior-to-posterior lag screws for fixation of the posterior malleolus: a biomechanical study. J Orthop Trauma 2016;30(12):664–9.

14. Marmor M, Hansen E, Han HK, et al. Limitations of standard fluoroscopy in detecting rotational malreduction of the Syndesmosis in an ankle fracture model. Foot Ankle Int 2011;32(6):616–22.

15. Sangeorzan BJ, Sangeorzan BP, Hansen ST, et al. Mathematically directed single-cut osteotomy for correction of tibial malunion. J Orthop Trauma 1989; 3(4):267–75.

16. Espinosa N, Smerek JP, Myerson MS. Acute and chronic Syndesmosis injuries: pathomechanisms, diagnosis and management. Foot Ankle Clin 2006;11(3):639–57.

17. Outland T. Sprains and separations of the inferior tibiofibular joint without important fracture. Am J Surg 1943;59:320. N.S.

18. Harper M. Delayed reconstruction and stabilization of the tibiofibular Syndesmosis. Foot Ankle Int 2001;22(1):15–8.

19. Katznelson A, Lin E, Militiano J. Ruptures of the ligaments about the tibio-fibular Syndesmosis. Injury 1983;15(3):170–2.

20. Pena FA, Coetzee JC. Ankle syndesmosis injuries. Foot Ankle Clin 2006;11(1): 35–50, viii.

21. Van Dijk CN. Syndesmotic injuries. Tech Foot Ankle Surg 2006;5(1):34–7.

22. Mullins J, Sallis J. Recurrent sprains of the ankle joint with diastasis. J Bone Joint Surg 1958;40-B(2):270–3.

23. Beals T, Manoli A. Late Syndesmosis reconstruction: a case report. Foot Ankle Int 1998;19:485–7.

24. Swords MP, Sands AK, Shank JR. Late treatment of syndesmotic injuries. Foot Ankle Clin 2017;22(1):65–75.

25. Grass R, Rammelt S, Biewener A, et al. Peroneus longus ligamentoplasty for chronic instability of the distal tibiofibular Syndesmosis. Foot Ankle Int 2003; 24(5):392–7.

26. Yasui Y, Takao M, Miyamoto W, et al. Anatomical reconstruction of the anterior inferior tibiofibular ligament for chronic disruption of the distal tibiofibular Syndesmosis. Knee Surg Sports Traumatol Arthrosc 2011;19(4):691–5.

27. Haskell A, Mann RA. Ankle arthroplasty with preoperative coronal plane deformity: short -term results. Clin Orthop Relat Res 2004;424:98–103.

28. Hobson SA, Karantana A, Dhar S. Total ankle replacement in patients with significant pre-operative deformity of the hindfoot. J Bone Joint Surg Br 2009;91(4): 481–6.

29. Queen RM, Adams SB Jr, Viens NA, et al. Differences in outcomes following total ankle replacement in patients with neutral alignment compared with tibiotalar joint malalignment. J Bone Joint Surg Am 2013;95(21):1927–34.

30. Gross CE, Hamid KS, Green C, et al. Operative wound complications following total ankle arthroplasty. Foot Ankle Int 2017;38(4):360–6.

31. Parlamas G, Hannon CP, Murawski CD, et al. Treatment of chronic syndesmotic injury: a systematic review and meta-analysis. Knee Surg Sports Traumatol Arthrosc 2013;21(8):1931–9.

32. Scolaro JA, Marecek G, Barei DP. Management of syndesmotic disruption in ankle fractures: a critical analysis review. JBJS Rev 2014;2(12):1–10.

33. Jones CB, Gilde A, Sietsema DL. Treatment of syndesmotic injuries of the ankle: a critical analysis review. JBJS Rev 2015;3(10):1–15.

34. Schepers T, Dingemans SA, Rammelt S. Recent developments in the treatment of acute syndesmotic injuries. Fuß & Sprunggelenk 2016;14(2):66–78.

Medial Ankle Instability
The Deltoid Dilemma

Saud Alshalawi, MD[a], Ahmed E. Galhoum, MD, MRCS (England)[b],
Yousef Alrashidi, MD[c], Martin Wiewiorski, MD[d],
Mario Herrera, MD[e], Alexej Barg, MD[f],
Victor Valderrabano, MD, PhD[g],*

KEYWORDS

- Deltoid ligament • Medial ankle instability • Ankle instability • Ankle sprain
- Spring ligament

KEY POINTS

- The deltoid ligament complex is injured more commonly than expected.
- In medial ankle instability, a hindfoot valgus deformity of the foot can typically be corrected by activation of a functioning tibialis posterior muscle.
- Medial ankle instability (acute or chronic) can present as isolated lesions or combined with other lesions.
- Besides clinical examination, radiographs and MRI, ankle arthroscopy is encouraged to confirm the diagnosis and visualize the associated injuries.
- It is mandatory to support deltoid ligament repair by adding corrective osteotomies to reduce the strain in the deltoid ligament complex.

INTRODUCTION

Many orthopedic surgeons consider ankle instability almost a synonym for lateral instability of the ankle. This fact could reflect that medial ankle instability (MAI) is a controversial topic that is poorly discussed in literature. Severe ankle sprain may affect the medial ligament complex, whose deterioration and suboptimal treatment can

Disclosures: The authors have nothing to disclose in relation to this article.
[a] Prince Sultan Military Medical City, PO Box 13225-6604, Riyadh 12233, Saudi Arabia;
[b] Department of Orthopedic, Nasser Institute for Research and Treatment, Nile Corniche Street, Cairo 1351, Egypt; [c] Orthopaedic Department, College of Medicine, Taibah University, PO Box 30001, Medina 42353, Saudi Arabia; [d] Head Foot and Ankle Unit, Orthopaedic and Trauma Department, Kantonsspital Winterthur, Winterthur 8401, Switzerland; [e] Head Foot and Ankle Unit, Orthopaedic Department, University of La Laguna, Tenerife 38200, Spain; [f] Department of Orthopaedics, University of Utah, 590 Wakara Way, Salt Lake City, UT 84108, USA; [g] Orthopaedic Department, Swiss Ortho Center, Swiss Medical Network, Schmerzklinik Basel, Hirschgässlein 15, Basel 4010, Switzerland
* Corresponding author.
E-mail address: vvalderrabano@swissmedical.net

Foot Ankle Clin N Am 23 (2018) 639–657
https://doi.org/10.1016/j.fcl.2018.07.008
1083-7515/18/© 2018 Elsevier Inc. All rights reserved.

foot.theclinics.com

result in chronic *rotational ankle instability* (ie, combination medial and lateral ankle instability). In a prospective study, an arthroscopic exploration of the deltoid ligament done during treatment of chronic lateral ankle instability revealed that 20% of patients had a concomitant lesion of the deltoid.[1]

In this article, the authors aim to highlight the diagnosis and management of the different clinical presentations of MAI.

ANATOMY OF THE DELTOID LIGAMENT COMPLEX

The deltoid ligament complex is composed of a superficial layer, a deep layer, and the spring (calcaneonavicular) ligament. The spring ligament is often included with the deltoid ligament complex because it assists in stabilizing the medial ankle structures of the ankle joint through its connection to the deltoid by the tibiospring ligament (**Fig. 1**).

The superficial deltoid layer consists of 4 components.[2] Each component originates from the anterior colliculus of the medial malleolus and spans both the ankle joint and the subtalar joint:

- *Tibionavicular ligament* attaches to the dorsomedial surface of the navicular bone and creates the anterior part of the deltoid. Some of its fibers are attached to the spring ligament.
- *Tibiospring ligament* attaches to the spring ligament. It creates the most superficial connection to the superior edge of the plantar spring ligament.[2–4]
- *Tibiocalcaneal ligament* descends vertically to the sustentaculum tali, and a few of its fibers attach also to the spring ligament.
- *Superficial posterior tibiotalar ligament* originates from the posteromedial surface of the medial malleolus and passes backward and laterally to insert into the superoposterior surface of the talus.

The deep deltoid layer is shorter and thicker than the superficial layer and crosses only the ankle joint. It consists of the following ligaments[2,4]:

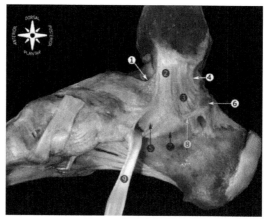

Fig. 1. Cadaveric anatomic dissection of the medial ankle ligament complex. (*1*) Tibionavicular ligament; (*2*) tibiospring ligament; (*3*) tibiocalcaneal ligament; (*4*) deep posterior tibiotalar ligament; (*5*) spring ligament complex; (*6*) medial talar process; (*7*) sustentaculum tali; (*8*) medial tolocalcaneal ligament; (*9*) posterior tibial tendon. (*Reprinted* by permission from Springer Nature: Knee Surgery, Sports Traumatology, Arthroscopy. Golanó P, Vega J, de Leeuw PAJ, et al. Anatomy of the ankle ligaments: a pictorial essay; 2010;18:557. ©2010)

- *Anterior tibiotalar ligament* arises from the anteromedial surface of the medial malleolus and attaches to the superoanterior surface of the talus.
- *Deep posterior tibiotalar ligament* is directly deep to the superficial posterior tibiotalar ligament and shares the same origins and insertions.
- Boss and Hintermann[4] found one variant band of the deep deltoid layer, which is *deep to the tibiocalcaneal ligament*.

Functionally, the calcaneonavicular or spring ligament belongs to the medial deltoid complex and consists of the following 2 components:

- *Superomedial calcaneonavicular ligament* arises from the middle facet of the subtalar joint and the superomedial part of the sustentaculum tali and inserts into the superomedial surface of the navicular. It is the strongest and the most medial component of the spring ligament. Some fibers of the ligament are also connected to the posterior tibial tendon. This ligament is covered with a fibrocartilage that "articulates" with the inferior aspect of the talar head.
- *Inferior calcaneonavicular ligament* lies more plantar and lateral. It arises from an area between the anterior and middle facets of the calcaneus and inserts on the inferior aspect of the navicular.

BIOMECHANICAL PROPERTIES

The deltoid ligament complex is an essential medial ankle joint stabilizer. Its disruption may laterally displace the talus or tilt it within the ankle mortise.[5] The superficial component has been shown to limit mainly external rotation and resist valgus stress of the ankle and hindfoot. The deep component resists mainly ankle eversion and lateral migration of the talus. Moreover, the deltoid is the primary stabilizer of the ankle against plantarflexion.[2,4,5]

Tibial rotation and foot inversion-eversion is affected by sectioning the medial ligaments only.[6,7] Therefore, the physiologic gait pattern depends highly on deltoid integrity.[8] A cadaver study by Earll and colleagues[9] found that sectioning of the superficial deltoid ligament will reduce the contact area up to 43%, and peak pressure increases up to 30%. Therefore, small alterations in the deltoid ligament complex lead to secondary lateral ankle instability, respective rotational ankle instability, and increased risk for ankle osteoarthritis (OA).[10,11]

MECHANISM OF INJURY OF ACUTE MEDIAL ANKLE INSTABILITY

Medial ankle sprains are widely thought to be rare. During the last decade, some studies have revealed that the deltoid ligament complex is injured more frequently than expected. The injury is thought to be a combination of eversion and external rotation of the hindfoot or the reverse, that is, inward body rotation on a fixed foot. With severe external rotation moments, the tibiofibular syndesmotic ligaments may be injured too.[1,12] Osteochondral lesions (OCL) of the ankle may typically be part of the acute medial ankle instability (AMAI).[13,14] Deltoid injuries occur commonly in relation to fractures such as Wb C/pronation external rotation or pronation abduction and less frequently with Wb B/supination external rotation ankle fractures.[6,15]

Progression and Pathologic Condition of Chronic Medial Ankle Instability

Persistent symptoms and repetitive ankle sprains are recognized as chronic ankle instability (CAI), which is mostly attributed to an initial acute injury. This popular explanation was linked to the mechanical CAI, which can be defined as an abnormal motion of the talus within the ankle joint complex due to pathologic ligament laxity/insufficiency. Furthermore, the impairment of proprioception around the ankle following acute injury[16] leads to functional CAI, which increases the strain on the ligaments chronically due to inadequate active muscle protection.[17,18]

Chronic mechanical instability may be the result of the following 2 contributing factors:

- *Ligamentous chronic mechanical instability* occurs due to pathologic laxity of the deltoid ligament complex itself following an injury. Some studies suggest that, after an anterior tibiofibular ligament (ATFL) rupture, there is an increase in the internal rotation of the hindfoot that further stresses the medial ankle ligaments and subsequently causes chronic rotational ankle instability (ie, combined lateral and medial instability).[12,19–21] In chronic rotational ankle instability, the talus falls medial with talonavicular subluxation. Such a talar position leads to lesions of the spring ligament and secondarily to flattening of the longitudinal medial arch of the foot (ie, an acquired pes planus).
- *Bony chronic mechanical instability* is favored by certain types of ankle morphologies. A wider talar dome and reduced talar coverage by the tibial plafond represent loss of congruency in chronic rotational ankle instability or chronic medial ankle instability (CMAI) subjects.[22–24]

Functional CAI is the result of 2 pathologic mechanisms. The first is the impairment of proprioceptive sensation, which is a result of damage to the mechanoreceptors of the ankle joint capsule and affects the stretch receptors of the ligaments.[25,26] The second mechanism is a slowed neuromuscular reflex, which exhibits reduced ligamentous responsiveness to inversion and eversion stimuli.[27,28] Failure to control position is the end stage, where CMAI patients have difficulty maintaining their position during single leg stance.[29,30]

PATIENT'S HISTORY

An acute injury of the deltoid ligament complex following a pronation (eversion) trauma usually presents with symptoms ranging from discomfort to a severely painful and swollen medial ankle with the inability to bear weight. The mechanism of trauma, level of daily activity, level of athletic activity, and any history of previous ankle sprain should be clarified.

Chronically, a deltoid ligament injury presents as a medial giving way, especially when walking on uneven ground. The patient usually complains of pain at the anteromedial part of the ankle joint, and sometimes the pain emanates laterally from subfibular impingement due to the hindfoot valgus. Mechanical symptoms like catching or locking may be present with development of intra-articular impingement (hypertrophic synovium, anteromedial osteophytes, OCLs). Any associated foot deformity or disease, history of ankle sprains, and the patient's activity level should also be clarified.

CLINICAL EXAMINATION

The clinical examination of MAI starts with careful bilateral inspection of the ankle in the standing, walking, and sitting position with a hanging relaxed leg. It is essential to assess for swelling, hematoma, malalignment, deformity, and scars. When a patient bears weight, asymmetrical planovalgus and abductus of the affected ankle and foot may indicate MAI.

Palpation should include medial and lateral ligaments and joint spaces in addition to palpating the syndesmosis, the posterior tibial, peroneal, and Achilles tendons. Typically, patients with MAI will show tenderness, mostly in the medial gutter, over the deltoid ligament and the spring ligament. Some patients may have tenderness along the posterior tibial tendon, because the incidence of MAI with posterior tibial tendon insufficiency (PTTI) is high.[1,12] In advanced cases, tenderness at the lateral ankle ligament (in rotational ankle instability) and subfibular area (due to hindfoot valgus) may be elicited.

The integrity of the superficial deltoid ligament can be evaluated on a relaxed sitting patient with hanging legs using the "external rotation test," whereas the deep deltoid can be assessed by the "eversion stress test." A combined eversion and external rotation stress test addresses both the deep and the superficial deltoid ligament. The anterior drawer test is also a valuable tool for diagnosing anteromedial subluxation in deltoid ligament insufficiency (**Box 1**).[1,12,31]

Most surgeons think that acquired adult flatfoot only occurs due to PTTI. Although true in many instances, some cases cannot be explained by this pathologic condition. Damage to the deltoid ligament complex can lead to a hindfoot valgus with a normal functioning posterior tibial muscle, that is, by isolated MAI. Often, however, both MAI and PTTI may coexist. To exclude PTTI, a single heel rise test is used. In the setting of a healthy posterior tibial tendon and muscle, the hindfoot reduces into varus on single heel rise from the excessive valgus position.

A variety of possible deltoid ligament injuries can occur due to involvement of the syndesmotic complex. Associated ankle fractures are common in acute presentations. Thus, attention should be paid to the presence of positive syndesmotic tests. Fractures associated with inversion or eversion trauma must be excluded clinically and radiologically.

Valderrabano and colleagues[32] classified clinical CMAI into 4 grades based on increasing severity and ligamentous damage (**Table 1**).

IMAGING
Conventional Radiographs

Adequate standard ankle radiographs (weight-bearing, if possible) are useful in acute cases to exclude widening of the medial ankle clear space, deltoid avulsion fragments, syndesmotic lesions, and ankle fractures. In chronic cases, the following weight-bearing radiographs are necessary:

- Ankle mortise view
- Foot dorsoplantar view
- Foot lateral view
- Hindfoot alignment (Saltzman) view

Box 1
Clinical manifestation of medial ankle instability

Symptoms and Signs

Giving way

Medial pain and instability during walking & sports

Medial tenderness (deltoid & spring ligament)

Asymmetric hindfoot valgus

Positive external rotation stress test

Positive eversion stress test

Positive anteromedial drawer test

Negative single heel rise test (hindfoot valgus on tiptoe)

Table 1 Clinical classification of chronic medial ankle instability						
	Giving Way	Hindfoot Valgus/ Pronation	Medial Ankle Pain	Anterolateral Ankle Pain	Posterior Tibial Dysfunction	Flexibility of Deformity
Grade I	+	+	+	(+)	−	Yes
Grade II	++	++	++	+	(+)	Yes
Grade III	+++	+++	+++	++	++	Yes
Grade IV	++++	++++	++++	+++	+++	No

Adapted from Valderrabano V, Hintermann B. Diagnostik und Therapie der medialen Sprunggelenkinstabilität. Arthroskopie 2005;18:112–8.

Besides pathologic pes planovalgus and abductus, other pathologic conditions, such as OCL, periarticular changes, bony impingements, accessory navicular, talocalcaneal coalition, and early osteoarthritic changes, will be evident in these studies. In some cases, contralateral imaging may be needed for comparison, particularly when assessing syndesmotic injuries.

The authors agree with other investigators that stress radiography is not useful as a diagnostic tool for CMAI or rotational ankle instability; stress radiography has a low sensitivity and may cause more local damage and consequently harm the patient.[1,12,13] In some cases, full limb radiography (orthoradiogram) may be needed to rule out genu valgum malalignment.

MRI

MRI is an important modality in the diagnosis of AMAI or CMAI that can identify the extent of the injury and associated pathologic conditions and is valuable in preoperative planning.[33–38] However, Yu and colleagues[33] found that 20% of patients had false negative MRI findings in the setting of acute deltoid ligament complex injury associated with ankle fractures. Thus, an elongated ligament, which is an important finding in MAI, cannot be visualized or diagnosed by MRI. The sensitivity and specificity of MRI to detect associated lesions, especially if chondral lesions are suspected, are 84% and 75%, respectively.[39]

In a retrospective review, 46 patients with CAI underwent MRI preoperatively and were treated surgically. All patients had an ATFL tear: 91% was involvement of the calcaneofibular ligament, 49% had posterior talofibular ligament (PTFL) involvement, and 72% had deltoid ligament injury. In this study, 23% of cases had superficial deltoid involvement; 6% had deep deltoid lesions, and 43% had injury to both components of the deltoid ligament.[38]

On MRI, the superficial deltoid may be found torn at its origin or more distally. Deltoid ligament tears occur most commonly at the proximal origin. The best view to evaluate the proximal tear is on axial images at the level of the tibial plafond, where the deltoid is detached from the medial malleolus. Deep deltoid involvement can be seen on coronal images, as either discontinuous or absent fibers. Deltoid tears located more distally or tears of the spring ligament are ideally seen in the sagittal plane.

Ultrasonography

Ultrasonography (US) plays a significant role in evaluating the ankle ligaments. The ligaments are hyperechoic when oriented parallel to the US beam. US is more useful in acute ligamentous injuries, with an accuracy up to 93.8% sensitivity and a 100% specificity in detecting ATFL tears when compared with MRI. In addition, dynamic US can be performed, assessing for ankle ligament stability and bony impingement in real time using joint stress maneuvers. However, a skilled and experienced operator is necessary to obtain such results.[40,41]

Computed Tomography Scan and Single-Photon Emission Computed Tomography–Computed Tomography

Computed tomography (CT) has limited value in diagnosing ankle ligamentous pathologic condition, but it is useful in identify associated pathologic conditions. Single-photon emission CT-CT may be needed in certain cases with persistent pain because it is very helpful in detecting ankle OCL pathologic condition, ankle OA, or subtalar joint OA, any of which could change the treatment protocol.[42]

Diagnostic Arthroscopic Examination

Arthroscopic examination detects deltoid ligament insufficiency and anatomic structural abnormalities of the unstable ankle (**Fig. 2**). In some cases, MAI is suspected clinically with negative imaging examinations, but arthroscopic assessment detects instability (**Fig. 3**). The authors recommend performing diagnostic ankle arthroscopy before a surgical repair/reconstruction of the ankle ligaments to support an MRI diagnosis, assess the deltoid ligament complex biomechanically intraoperatively, and visualize associated injuries, such as cartilage lesions.[12,13,43–45] Valderrabano and Hintermann[13] classified CMAI into 4 grades based on arthroscopic examination (**Table 2**).

TREATMENT OPTIONS
Acute Medial Ankle Instability

Isolated acute medial ankle instability
Nonoperative treatment The initial treatment of isolated AMAI (ie, all grades of ankle sprain) should aim at pain control with early stabilization and reduction of swelling (eg, by lymphatic drainage) for 1 to 2 weeks. PRICE (Protection, Rest, Ice, Compression, and Elevation) is encouraged in the initial treatment phase to achieve these goals.

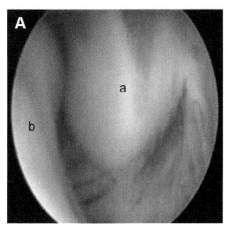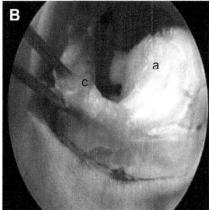

Fig. 2. Case of CMAI. A 20-year-old woman who sustained an eversion ankle sprain 8 months before and was complaining of medial ankle pain and giving way. The intraoperative situation demonstrated complete rupture of deltoid ligament complex. (*A*) Arthroscopic picture of the medial ankle. (*B*) Medial open: [a] Medial malleolus; [b] Talus; [c] Proximal tear of the deltoid ligament complex, that is, tibionavicular ligament and tibiospring ligament.

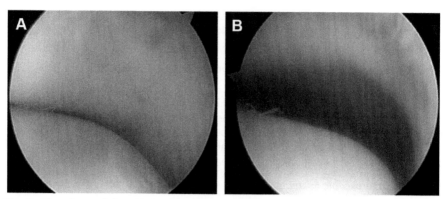

Fig. 3. Chronic medial ankle arthroscopy on the diagnostic arthroscopy. Arthroscopic anterior view of medial ankle demonstrates (*A*) no medial opening by relaxed arthroscopy and (*B*) wide medial gapping with the external-rotation and eversion stress test.

Soft ankle orthosis is indicated for simple sprains (grade I) until the patient becomes asymptomatic and has strengthened their ankle muscle, although more severe sprains (grades II–III) may require a stronger ankle brace or walker that provides substantial stabilization in order to avoid eversion. These patients have to wear the brace for 6 weeks, after which, they can prevent further ankle sprains by using insoles. Physiotherapy programs aimed at optimizing range of motion, neuromuscular training, and muscle force of the ankle (especially the posterior tibial muscle) should be implemented as early as possible. Physiotherapy may reduce CMAI, injury recurrence risk, and long-term complications (eg, chronic rotational ankle instability, OA).[10,46,47]

Operative treatment Grades II–III medial ankle sprain may require operative intervention only if the patient assessment reveals additional injuries, such as syndesmotic injuries, severe dislocation, OCLs, or fractures. In addition, AMAI in professional athletes should be carefully examined and surgery considered on a case-by-case basis.

Intraoperatively, the authors encourage surgeons to start with ankle arthroscopy to adequately assess deltoid ligament insufficiency and exclude other injuries. Then, deltoid ligament repair should be performed by direct suturing using intraosseous or anchor sutures. The spring ligament and the quality of PTT should be inspected and evaluated. In severe AMAI with an intraoperatively detected PTTI

Table 2
Arthroscopic classification of chronic medial ankle instability

	Superficial/ Ventral Deltoid	Deep/ Posterior Deltoid	Medial Malleolus Periosteal Scar	Medial Malleolus Osteophytes	Tibiotalar Distance (mm)	Lateral Ligament Lesion
Grade I	Elongation/partial tear/avulsion	Normal	+	+	2–5	No
Grade II	Rupture	Elongation/ partial tear	++	++	2–5	No
Grade III	Rupture	Elongation/ partial tear	+++	+++	<5	Yes
Grade IV	Rupture	Rupture	++++	++++	<5	Yes

Adapted from Valderrabano V, Hintermann B. Diagnostik und Therapie der medialen Sprunggelenkinstabilität. Arthroskopie 2005;18:112–8.

and known chronic flatfoot, the posterior tibial tendon may need to be augmented/ reconstructed (flexor digitorum longus [FDL] transfer) and supported by calcaneal osteotomy (OT) in a primary setting. Such a reconstruction would reduce the postoperative risk of a posttraumatic pes planovalgus and valgus ankle OA. For professional athletes, the authors recommend as little surgery as possible in order to maintain their competitive level.

Postoperative care consists of partial weight-bearing in a walker boot for 6 weeks and then physiotherapy for another 6 weeks while the patient wears an insole to prevent further ankle trauma.

Syndesmotic injury associated with acute medial ankle instability

High ankle sprains cause injury to the syndesmotic complex in almost 10% of all ankle sprains.[48] The diagnosis of syndesmotic injuries in the acute setting remains a challenge for surgeons. If the patient is suspected to have syndesmotic injury in the presence of normal standing radiographs, ankle MRI is indicated. Syndesmotic injuries have been classified into the 3 following grades[48]:

- o *Nonoperative treatment* is indicated in AMAI without significant hindfoot valgus combined with stable syndesmotic injury (grade I) or questionable stability (grade II). The treatment consists of a walker for 4 to 6 weeks and a physiotherapy training program.
- o *Operative treatment* is indicated in AMAI with asymmetric hindfoot valgus and the inability to bear weight due to lesions of the anterior inferior tibiofibular ligament and interosseous syndesmotic ligament (grade II–III). The authors encourage diagnostic ankle arthroscopy to assess the extent of deltoid ligament and syndesmosis injury and to confirm the diagnosis.[1,48–51] Recent studies suggest that ankle arthroscopy is a more sensitive modality than stress radiologic testing.[1,50] After ankle arthroscopy, surgical syndesmotic stabilization and deltoid ligament repair are done in the same setting (see surgical technique).

Ankle fractures associated with acute medial ankle instability

The necessity of deltoid ligament repair for injuries associated with a malleolar fracture remains controversial. Harper, de Souza and colleagues, and Johnson and Hill[52–54] reported on patients with ruptures of the deep deltoid ligament associated with ankle fractures, where fixation of the fracture was done without repairing the deltoid ligament. All patients showed "satisfactory" outcomes at their final outpatient visit. The investigators of these studies recommend that the repair of the deltoid ligament was not required if anatomic open reduction and internal fixation (ORIF) was achieved. However, all of these studies had a significant number of patients who had residual medial ankle pain.[33]

Yu and colleagues[33] reported on 131 patients with ankle fractures associated with deltoid ligament ruptures, which were repaired surgically. A significant improvement in all outcome values was noted after operative intervention when compared with the preoperative status.

Nonoperative treatment Undisplaced ankle fractures, such as a Wb A fracture, combined with AMAI are indicated for nonoperative treatment. Even a variable stability ankle fracture, such as a Wb B fracture, can be managed conservatively. The nonsurgical treatment of the ankle fractures combined with AMAI consists of a walker with 15-kg partial weight bearing for 6 weeks and a physiotherapy program.

Operative treatment Ankle fracture fixation and deltoid ligament repair should be considered for more unstable ankle fractures (displaced Wb B and Wb C fractures), tibial plafond fractures, talar fractures, or ankle OCL. In ankle fractures, the authors recommend starting with ankle arthroscopy to evaluate the joint and the deltoid ligament complex injury. After surgical fixation of the fracture, the medial deltoid ligament of ankle should be repaired also.

Adequate reduction of a medial malleolar fracture does not assure restoration of competence of the medial ligaments. Tornetta[55] demonstrated that distal injuries with a fracture width of less than 17 mm risked residual deltoid insufficiency despite satisfactory fragment fixation. In lateral unimalleolar fractures, if the lateral malleolus is well reduced, the medial ligament should heal adequately.[53] However, a persistent increase in the medial clear space (>3 mm) will require surgical exploration and deltoid repair.[56]

Chronic Medial Ankle Instability

Nonsurgical treatment of chronic medial ankle instability

Classically, CMAI patients should be conservatively managed for 3 to 6 months unless there is an associated pathologic condition that necessitates earlier surgical intervention. The aim of treatment is to stabilize the ankle on a well-aligned ankle and hindfoot and rehabilitate for asymptomatic function.

Physiotherapy The goal of physiotherapy is to address coordination and proprioceptive sensation as well as muscle strengthening (especially invertors). Good results of physiotherapy and rehabilitation were reported, specifically in those patients suffering from functional as compared with mechanical instability.[12,13,44,47] Proprioceptive training has been advised in literature to decrease the frequency of ankle sprains.[47,57]

Insoles The use of plantar insoles with medial arch support can help in the correction of hindfoot malalignment and pes planovalgus deformities. Hindfoot varus insoles break down such that in CMAI PTTI develops quickly. In addition, insoles improve functional stability by increasing plantar cutaneous sensation, which will improve postural control and reduce the risk of injury.[12,58]

Braces, tape, or orthoses The goal of the brace is to improve the biofeedback mechanism. Braces can augment stability by providing additional neurologic feedback through cutaneous and mechanoreceptors. Multiple studies have suggested that adequately applied braces or orthoses do not adversely affect performance.[44,59,60] The brace should be designed to allow dorsi/plantar flexion while resisting coronal and rotational loads. Patients should wear an appropriate brace until supervised rehabilitation is completed. Those patients who suffer from moderate or severe ankle sprains should use an orthosis for a minimum of 6 months. Athletes may need to wear it as usual in lightweight sports or competitive sports.

Stabilizing shoes Medial hindfoot stabilizing shoes should be used for severe case in which the patient is not fit for operative treatment. The patient should wear the shoes at all times.[13,31]

Operative treatment of chronic medial ankle instability

Indications Patients who fail to become asymptomatic with conservative measures are considered for operative treatment. Specifically, patients with ongoing medial instability on an almost daily basis, recurrent ankle sprains, persistent pain, worsening deformities (pes planovalgus), and limitations in their professional and recreational activities are indicated for surgical intervention. The aims of surgery are to reestablish joint stability, correct deformities (eg, hindfoot valgus or pes planovalgus et abductus), reduce risk for future ankle sprains, and thereby reduce damage to the cartilage.

Diagnostic arthroscopy As mentioned before, diagnostic arthroscopy is important as the last diagnostic tool before open ligament surgery. Arthroscopy is performed while the patient is supine and the knee is flexed 90°, putting the foot in a hanging position. The ankle joint is insufflated with normal saline solution. Standard ankle arthroscopy portals are used. The capsule is dissected bluntly to prevent damage to the neurovascular elements. Always introduce the blunt trocar and arthroscope (5-mm 30° standard arthroscope) in a dorsiflexed position to avoid iatrogenic cartilage damage. Enough intra-articular ankle distension is usually achieved by the hanging foot and the intra-articular fluid pressure; if not, more distension can be obtained by applying manual traction on the hindfoot. A systematic arthroscopic examination is performed to assess internal ankle joint structures. CMAI typically shows a so-called naked medial malleolus with detached anteromedial ligaments. The deltoid ligament complex is stressed by applying gentle external rotation or eversion pull of the ankle joint under arthroscopic control. If the foot is everted or pronated and the deltoid ligament allows significant medial gapping, the deltoid ligament is considered insufficient (see **Fig. 3**). The most common presentation of ligament involvement is the combined medial and lateral ligament lesion.[12,13,57]

Surgical approach A slightly curved 8- to 10-cm incision is made, starting 2 to 4 cm proximal to the tip of the medial malleolus and aiming toward the tuberosity of the navicular bone. After fascial dissection, the anterior aspect of the deltoid ligament is exposed. A longitudinal incision of the tendon sheath facilitates the assessment of the posterior tibial tendon and exploration of the spring ligament. The posterior vessels and nerve should be protected. After plantarly retracting the posterior tibial tendon, the spring ligament is judged. The level of deltoid tear should be identified and evaluated. When there is concomitant lateral ankle instability, a lateral approach to the ankle should be done to repair the ATFL and CFL as well.

Surgical ligament repair techniques The technique for medial ligament reconstruction that is likely to produce the best outcome should be selected. The treatment options depend on the level of ligament injury[31] and local soft tissue status (**Table 3**). The primary option is to tension the deltoid from distal to proximal and attach it to the medial malleolus by transosseous sutures or anchors, provided that the deltoid tissue quality is sufficient. If the soft tissues are inadequate for a stable direct repair, augmentation reconstruction options are the alternative, such as (**Fig. 4**): periosteal flaps, and free autograft reconstruction from sources such as the plantaris longus (hamstring tendon or the FDL).[61–66] In the authors' practice, the tissues usually are mostly adequate for primary repair; the interosseous suture is the more common option selected.

Reconstruction of type I lesion (most common) The anterior border of the medial malleolus is exposed and refreshed to create a rough surface suitable for ligament reattachment. Two drill holes are made in the medial malleolus at 5 to 6 mm from

Table 3
Surgical anatomic location classification of chronic medial ankle instability

Type I lesion	Proximal tear/avulsion of the deltoid ligament; most common
Type II lesion	Intermediate tear of the deltoid ligament
Type III lesion	Distal tear/avulsion of the deltoid and spring ligament

Adapted from Valderrabano V, Hintermann B. Diagnostik und Therapie der medialen Sprunggelenkinstabilität. Arthroskopie 2005;18:112–8.

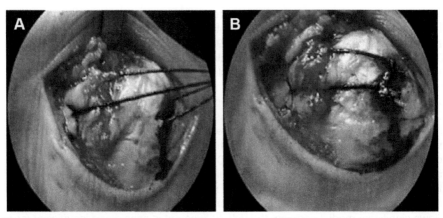

Fig. 4. Primary repair of proximal deltoid ligament tear. (*A*) The transosseous sutures pulling on the tibionavicular and tibiospring ligaments. (*B*) Tight and stable reconstruction after suturing the sutures.

the tip. Two intraosseous sutures (Vicryl 2) are inserted; the first is to shorten the tibionavicular and tibiospring fibers and the second is to shorten the anterior part of the deep deltoid ligament. These sutures should be tightened at 90° of ankle dorsiflexion. If the repair and ligaments remnants are weak, a periosteal flap is reflected from the medial aspect of the tibia to reinforce the repaired ligaments.

Reconstruction of type II lesion The degenerative and insufficient ligament tear is refreshed and debrided. End-to-end sutures are applied to the torn ligament. When there is a large gap, intraosseous sutures to the medial malleolus should be added. Additional soft tissue and a periosteal flap may be needed to augment the repaired ligament.

Reconstruction of type III lesion If necessary, the tear is debrided. Then 2 Vicryl sutures are inserted into the spring ligament side by side. A periosteal flap is added to the repair in cases of insufficient soft tissue remnants.

Additional surgeries
Reconstruction of the affected ligaments alone has been successful in inherently well-aligned feet; however, this is not the same in cases with longstanding hindfoot valgus and forefoot abduction. With these deformities, the achieved ligament repair tends to fail once the patients resume full physical and sports activity.[1,19,43,66] These cases require either a lateral calcaneal lengthening OT or a medial sliding calcaneal OT to correct hindfoot valgus and forefoot abduction or hindfoot valgus only, respectively.

The *lateral calcaneal lengthening OT* is performed with an oscillating saw parallel to the posterior facet of the subtalar joint at the floor of sinus tarsi and almost perpendicular to the plantar aspect of the foot. As the OT is widened by a K-wire spreader, the hindfoot valgus and forefoot abduction deformity of the foot are corrected. A tricortical iliac crest autograft or an allograft is shaped to the proper length and width required and placed into the OT site. The OT is protected by one 3.5-mm AO screw or 5.0 cannulated compression screw or even a plate (**Fig. 5**).

For *the medial sliding calcaneal OT*, an incision oblique over the lateral wall of the tuber calcanei is performed, avoiding the sural nerve and peroneal tendons. Under Hohmann hook protection, the OT is performed by an oscillating saw on the lateral, the dorsal, and plantar cortex and then at the end also on the medial cortex of the

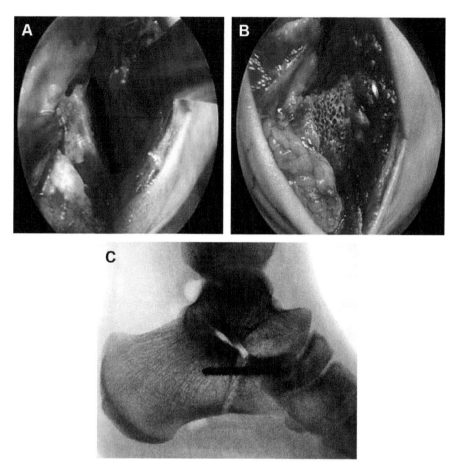

Fig. 5. Lateral calcaneal lengthening OT. (*A*) Intraoperative image of the open wedge of the lateral calcaneal lengthening OT. (*B*) Introduced allograft. (*C*) Radiograph with the screw crossing and stabilizing the OT.

calcaneus. The proximal "fragment" of the calcaneus is mobilized and displaced medially as needed to correct the hindfoot valgus. The proximal fragment is fixed temporarily in the new position by 2 K-wires and compressed by dorsiflexing the ankle. After checking with fluoroscopy, the ideal position of the K-wires, and measurement of the screw length, 2 cannulated screws are introduced over the K-wires for OT fixation. As an alternative to the double screw fixation, a plate may also be used.

Reconstruction of the lateral ankle ligaments is mandatory when rotational ankle instability is present. The surgery is mainly performed by primary repair or by augmentation with a plantaris tendon autograft.[13,19,43,44,66]

OCL of the ankle are commonly associated with MAI and should be managed concomitantly with medial ankle ligament repair.[14] In the senior author's case, treatment of OCL is done in a single-step cartilage repair by autologous matrix-induced chondrogenesis (AMIC).[67]

The *posterior tibial tendon* should be routinely evaluated intraoperatively. If the tendon has some degenerative changes, debridement of the tendon is performed. If the tendon is elongated and not functioning, shortening of the tendon or FDL transfer can be considered.

A *talonavicular or triple arthrodesis* may be indicated when medial instability is severely advanced with a stiff hindfoot valgus.[13,65] If there is lateral ankle valgus OA, supramalleolar OT might be indicated. Any other associated lesions should be managed simultaneously with ligament repair to enhance good surgical outcomes (**Table 4**).

Treatment protocol after medial ankle ligament complex repair For the first 6 postoperative weeks, the physiotherapy program treatment focuses on lymphatic drainage (PRICE therapy) and gently improving the range of motion of the ankle. The ankle is protected by a high-shaft stabilizing walker with partial weight-bearing 15 kg until 6 weeks. The authors recommend applying a 90° splint during bedtime for the first 6 weeks as well.

After 6 weeks, the authors recommend using a more flexible stabilizing shoe for another 6 weeks and later on a varus insole. The physiotherapy program should be started in the form of proprioception, coordination, and muscle strengthening exercises. In the case of any additional surgeries, rehabilitation programs might be prolonged.

SURGICAL OUTCOMES
Acute Medial Ankle Instability

Yu and colleagues[33] reported on 131 patients with ankle fracture associated with deltoid ligament ruptures that were identified and repaired operatively. The average American Orthopaedic Foot and Ankle Society (AOFAS) score was 93.4 points at the last visit (preoperative was 64.0). The mean visual analogue scale was 1.2 points, and the mean 36-item short form health survey score was 79 points. Significant improvement was observed in all of the 3 aforementioned measures following surgical treatment.

Chronic Medial Ankle Instability

Hintermann and colleagues[12] reported the outcome of a prospectively evaluated 54 cases with CMAI. The investigators found an increase in the average AOFAS Hindfoot

Table 4		
The most common associated injuries of medial ankle instability and recommended treatment		
Type of MAI	Associated Injuries	Additional Treatment Combined Medial Ankle Ligament Repair
AMAI	Ankle fracture with dislocation	ORIF
	Syndesmotic injury	Syndesmotic stabilization (rope technique or syndesmotic screw)
CMAI	Hindfoot valgus	Medial sliding calcaneal OT
	Hindfoot valgus & forefoot abduction	Lateral calcaneal lengthening OT
	Severe pes planus	Cotton OT
	Genu valgum	Knee varus producing OT
	Medial and lateral (rotation) instability	Repair/reconstruction medial and lateral
	OCL	Repair by AMIC technique
	Posterior tibial tendon insufficient	Debridement/FDL transfer
	Bony impingements	Resection
	Gastrocnemius-soleus complex contraction	Strayer procedure
	Syndesmotic injury	Syndesmotic stabilization
	Talonavicular joint or subtalar joint OA	Talonavicular or triple arthrodesis
	Lateral ankle OA	Supramalleolar OT
	Ankle OA	Total ankle arthroplasty
	Talocalcaneal coalition	Resection
	Tarsal tunnel syndrome	Release

score from 42.0 points (before operative treatment) to 91.5 points with an average follow-up of 4.4 years (range 2.0–6.6 years). Forty-eight cases (89%) showed good/ excellent clinical results, fair in 4 cases (7%), and poor in 1 case (2%).

DISCUSSION

The incidence of isolated deltoid ligament injuries occurring in all ankle sprains has been reported as 3% to 4%.[68] However, it was found that 23% of patient had isolated CMAI. Recent studies have shown that the medial ligament complex (isolated or combined with lateral ligament injury) is injured more frequently than expected, and the occurrence in acute and chronic presentations must be considered.

Controversy exists regarding the need for repair of the deltoid ligament complex during management of AMAI combined with ankle fracture fixation. Yu and colleagues[33] found that there is a significant improvement of surgical outcome measures after repair of the deltoid ligament complex in AMAI. However, more investigations are needed.

Uncorrected hindfoot valgus or pes planovalgus et abductus is the most common cause of recurrence of CMAI. A hindfoot OT is considered in the case of concomitant hindfoot deformity. Reconstruction of the injured ligaments was shown to be effective in well-aligned feet to decrease the load on the medial ankle ligament complex.[1,12,19,43,44]

Although the ankle joint is generally found to have low incidence of OA, there is evidence that the ankle joint is more vulnerable to arthritic changes following severe ligamentous injury than previously thought. It has been found that 13% to 16% of posttraumatic ankle OA are caused by ligamentous injury.[10,11] In the same study, findings further show that injury to the lateral ankle ligaments is the main predisposing factor for developing OA (85% due to lateral ligament lesions). However, 12% of OA cases are due to medial ligament lesions, and 3% are due to combined medial and lateral ligament lesions. The latency time for developing OA is shorter in medial ligament lesions, that is, AMAI, and CMAI lead to faster onset of severe ankle OA. The latency time to develop ligamentous ankle OA may be influenced by the level/severity of cartilage damage that occurred at the time of injury.[10]

SUMMARY

The medial ankle ligament complex is an important medial stabilizer of the ankle and hindfoot. The superficial components of the deltoid limit external rotation, whereas the deep components also prevent eversion of the ankle joint. The spring ligament is a part of this complex. The mechanism of injury is suspected to be a combination of eversion and external rotation of the foot. Besides clinical examination and radiographs, MRI is indicated for persistent instability symptoms. Ankle arthroscopic examination is encouraged to confirm the diagnosis and visualize the associated injuries.

Acute Medial Ankle Instability

Injury of the deltoid ligament can present with an acute clinical picture (swelling, hematoma), and the inability to bear weight. Acute medial ankle sprains can also be associated with other lesions such as syndesmotic injury or ankle fracture. The initial treatment of isolated deltoid ligament complex injury is nonoperative and often successful. Deltoid ligament repair is indicated in failed nonoperative treatment. If the other associated injuries necessitate surgical intervention, then the medial ligament complex might be repaired also. Adequate reduction of ankle fracture does not assure restoration of competence of the deltoid ligament. Significant improvement was seen in clinical measures after deltoid ligament repair and stabilization of the ankle fracture or syndesmotic injury in the same sitting.

Chronic Medial Ankle Instability

In chronic presentations, the criteria for CMAI are a feeling of giving way, pain over the medial gutter of the ankle, and a hindfoot valgus deformity that can typically be corrected by the tibialis posterior muscle. Failure to become asymptomatic with conservative measures, persistence of clinical instability, increased deformities, and limitation of professional and sports activities are indications for surgical intervention. If the soft tissues are inadequate for a stable repair, reconstruction options are appropriate. It is mandatory to support deltoid ligament repair or reconstruction by adding corrective osteotomies to reduce the strain in the medial ligament. Any associated injuries (eg, lateral ligament injury, PTTI, or OCL) should be also addressed.

REFERENCES

1. Hintermann B, Boss A, Schäfer D. Arthroscopic findings in patients with chronic ankle instability. Am J Sports Med 2002;30(3):402–9.
2. Milner CE, Soames RW. The medial collateral ligaments of the human ankle joint: anatomical variations. Foot Ankle Int 1998;19(5):289–92.
3. Pankovich AM, Shivaram MS. Anatomical basis of variability in injuries of the medial malleolus and the deltoid ligament. I. Anatomical studies. Acta Orthop Scand 1979;50(2):217–23.
4. Boss AP, Hintermann B. Anatomical study of the medial ankle ligament complex. Foot Ankle Int 2002;23(6):547–53.
5. Close JR. Some applications of the functional anatomy of the ankle joint. J Bone Joint Surg Am 1956;38-A(4):761–81.
6. Heim D, Schmidlin V, Ziviello O. Do type B malleolar fractures need a positioning screw? Injury 2002;33(8):729–34.
7. Grath GB. Widening of the ankle mortise. A clinical and experimental study. Acta Chir Scand Suppl 1960;(Suppl 263):1–88.
8. Hintermann B, Sommer C, Nigg BM. Influence of ligament transection on tibial and calcaneal rotation with loading and dorsi-plantarflexion. Foot Ankle Int 1995;16(9):567–71.
9. Earll M, Wayne J, Brodrick C, et al. Contribution of the deltoid ligament to ankle joint contact characteristics: a cadaver study. Foot Ankle Int 1996;17(6): 317–24.
10. Valderrabano V, Hintermann B, Horisberger M, et al. Ligamentous posttraumatic ankle osteoarthritis. Am J Sports Med 2006;34(4):612–20.
11. Valderrabano V, Horisberger M, Russell I, et al. Etiology of ankle osteoarthritis. Clin Orthop Relat Res 2009;467(7):1800–6.
12. Hintermann B, Valderrabano V, Boss A, et al. Medial ankle instability an exploratory, prospective study of fifty-two cases. Am J Sports Med 2004;32(1):183–90.
13. Valderrabano V, Hintermann B. Diagnostik und Therapie der medialen Sprunggelenkinstabilität. Arthroskopie 2005;18(2):112–8.
14. Taga I, Shino K, Inoue M, et al. Articular cartilage lesions in ankles with lateral ligament injury. An arthroscopic study. Am J Sports Med 1993;21(1):120–6 [discussion: 126–7].

15. Riegels-Nielsen P, Christensen J, Greiff J. The stability of the tibio-fibular syndesmosis following rigid internal fixation for type C malleolar fractures: an experimental and clinical study. Injury 1983;14(4):357–60.

16. Freeman M. Instability of the foot affer injuries to the lateral ligament of the ankle. Bone Joint J 1965;47(4):669–77.

17. Freeman M, Dean M, Hanham I. The etiology and prevention of functional instability of the foot. Bone Joint J 1965;47(4):678–85.

18. Tropp H. Commentary: functional ankle instability revisited. J Athl Train 2002; 37(4):512–5.

19. Alrashidi Y, Stelzenbach C, Herrera-Perez M, et al. Anatomical ligament reconstruction in rotational chronic ankle instability. Foot Ankle Surg 2016; 22(2 Suppl 1):49.

20. Kjærsgaard-Andersen P, Wethelund J-O, Helmig P, et al. The stabilizing effect of the ligamentous structures in the sinus and canalis tarsi on movements in the hindfoot An experimental study. Am J Sports Med 1988;16(5):512–6.

21. DiGiovanni BF, Fraga CJ, Cohen BE, et al. Associated injuries found in chronic lateral ankle instability. Foot Ankle Int 2000;21(10):809–15.

22. Frigg A, Magerkurth O, Valderrabano V, et al. The effect of osseous ankle configuration on chronic ankle instability. Br J Sports Med 2007;41(7):420–4.

23. Frigg A, Frigg R, Hintermann B, et al. The biomechanical influence of tibio-talar containment on stability of the ankle joint. Knee Surg Sports Traumatol Arthrosc 2007;15(11):1355–62.

24. Magerkurth O, Frigg A, Hintermann B, et al. Frontal and lateral characteristics of the osseous configuration in chronic ankle instability. Br J Sports Med 2010;44(8): 568–72.

25. Willems T, Witvrouw E, Verstuyft J, et al. Proprioception and muscle strength in subjects with a history of ankle sprains and chronic instability. J Athl Train 2002;37(4):487.

26. Forkin DM, Koczur C, Battle R, et al. Evaluation of kinesthetic deficits indicative of balance control in gymnasts with unilateral chronic ankle sprains. J Orthop Sports Phys Ther 1996;23(4):245–50.

27. Vaes P, Duquet W, Van Gheluwe B. Peroneal reaction times and eversion motor response in healthy and unstable ankles. J Athl Train 2002;37(4):475.

28. Raugust J. The effect of functional ankle instability on peroneal reflex latency. University of Alberta Health Sciences Journal 2006;3:16–9.

29. Rose A, Lee RJ, Williams RM, et al. Functional instability in non-contact ankle ligament injuries. Br J Sports Med 2000;34(5):352–8.

30. Bernier JN, Perrin DH, Rijke A. Effect of unilateral functional instability of the ankle on postural sway and inversion and eversion strength. J Athl Train 1997;32(3): 226.

31. Hintermann B. Medial ankle instability. Foot Ankle Clin 2003;8(4):723–38.

32. Valderrabano V, Paul J, Knupp M, et al. AKUTE UND CHRONISCHE OSG-INSTABILITÄT. GOTS-Expertenmeeting 2012;(Sprunggelenksinstabilität):43–56.

33. Yu G-R, Zhang M-Z, Aiyer A, et al. Repair of the acute deltoid ligament complex rupture associated with ankle fractures: a multicenter clinical study. J Foot Ankle Surg 2015;54(2):198–202.

34. Ramsey PL, Hamilton W. Changes in tibiotalar area of contact caused by lateral talar shift. J Bone Joint Surg Am 1976;58(3):356–7.

35. Crim J. Medial-sided ankle pain. Magn Reson Imaging Clin N Am 2017;25(1): 63–77.

36. Chun K-Y, Choi YS, Lee SH, et al. Deltoid ligament and tibiofibular syndesmosis injury in chronic lateral ankle instability: magnetic resonance imaging evaluation at 3t and comparison with arthroscopy. Korean J Radiol 2015;16(5):1096–103.
37. O'Neill PJ, Van Aman SE, Guyton GP. Is MRI adequate to detect lesions in patients with ankle instability? Clin Orthop Relat Res 2010;468(4):1115–9.
38. Crim JR, Beals TC, Nickisch F, et al. Deltoid ligament abnormalities in chronic lateral ankle instability. Foot Ankle Int 2011;32(9):873–8.
39. Park H-J, Cha S-D, Kim S, et al. Accuracy of MRI findings in chronic lateral ankle ligament injury: comparison with surgical findings. Clin Radiol 2012;67(4):313–8.
40. Henari S, Banks LN, Radiovanovic I, et al. Ultrasonography as a diagnostic tool in assessing deltoid ligament injury in supination external rotation fractures of the ankle. Orthopedics 2011;34(10):e639–43.
41. Peetrons PA, Silvestre A, Cohen M, et al. Ultrasonography of ankle ligaments. Can Assoc Radiol J 2002;53(1):6.
42. Leumann A, Valderrabano V, Plaass C, et al. A novel imaging method for osteochondral lesions of the talus—comparison of SPECT-CT with MRI. Am J Sports Med 2011;39(5):1095–101.
43. Alrashidi Y, Stelzenbach C, Herrera-Perez M, et al. Chronic rotational ankle instability- a case series study. Sports Orthop Traumatol 2015;31(3):200–5.
44. Galhoum AE, Wiewiorski M, Valderrabano V. Ankle instability: anatomy, mechanics, management and sequelae. Sports Orthop Traumatol 2017.
45. Guillo S, Bauer T, Lee J, et al. Consensus in chronic ankle instability: aetiology, assessment, surgical indications and place for arthroscopy. Orthop Traumatol Surg Res 2013;99(8):S411–9.
46. Hoiness P, Glott T, Ingjer F. High-intensity training with a bi-directional bicycle pedal improves performance in mechanically unstable ankles–a prospective randomized study of 19 subjects. Scand J Med Sci Sports 2003;13(4):266–71.
47. Eils E, Rosenbaum D. A multi-station proprioceptive exercise program in patients with ankle instability. Med Sci Sports Exerc 2001;33(12):1991–8.
48. Gerber JP, Williams GN, Scoville CR, et al. Persistent disability associated with ankle sprains: a prospective examination of an athletic population. Foot Ankle Int 1998;19(10):653–60.
49. Wolf BR, Amendola A. Syndesmosis injuries in the athlete: when and how to operate. Curr Opin Orthop 2002;13(2):151–4.
50. Takao M, Ochi M, Oae K, et al. Diagnosis of a tear of the tibiofibular syndesmosis. Bone Joint J 2003;85(3):324–9.
51. Stoffel K, Wysocki D, Baddour E, et al. Comparison of two intraoperative assessment methods for injuries to the ankle syndesmosis: a cadaveric study. J Bone Joint Surg Am 2009;91(11):2646–52.
52. Johnson DP, Hill J. Fracture-dislocation of the ankle with rupture of the deltoid ligament. Injury 1988;19(2):59–61.
53. Harper MC. The deltoid ligament. An evaluation of need for surgical repair. Clin Orthop Relat Res 1988;(226):156–68.
54. de Souza LJ, Gustilo RB, Meyer TJ. Results of operative treatment of displaced external rotation-abduction fractures of the ankle. J Bone Joint Surg Am 1985;67(7):1066–74.
55. Tornetta P 3rd. Competence of the deltoid ligament in bimalleolar ankle fractures after medial malleolar fixation. J Bone Joint Surg Am 2000;82(6):843–8.
56. Maynou C, Lesage P, Mestdagh H, et al. Is surgical treatment of deltoid ligament rupture necessary in ankle fractures? Rev Chir Orthop Reparatrice Appar Mot 1997;83(7):652–7.

57. Czajka CM, Tran E, Cai AN, et al. Ankle sprains and instability. Med Clin North Am 2014;98(2):313–29.
58. Augustin JF, Lin SS, Berberian WS, et al. Nonoperative treatment of adult acquired flat foot with the Arizona brace. Foot Ankle Clin 2003;8(3):491–502.
59. Baier M, Hopf T. Ankle orthoses effect on single-limb standing balance in athletes with functional ankle instability. Arch Phys Med Rehabil 1998;79(8):939–44.
60. Robbins S, Waked E, Rappel R. Ankle taping improves proprioception before and after exercise in young men. Br J Sports Med 1995;29(4):242–7.
61. Boyer MI, Bowen V, Weiler P. Reconstruction of a severe grinding injury to the medial malleolus and the deltoid ligament of the ankle using a free plantaris tendon graft and vascularized gracilis free muscle transfer: case report. J Trauma 1994;36(3):454–7.
62. Hintermann B, Valderrabano V, Kundert HP. Lengthening of the lateral column and reconstruction of the medial soft tissue for treatment of acquired flatfoot deformity associated with insufficiency of the posterior tibial tendon. Foot Ankle Int 1999;20(10):622–9.
63. Ellis SJ, Williams BR, Wagshul AD, et al. Deltoid ligament reconstruction with peroneus longus autograft in flatfoot deformity. Foot Ankle Int 2010;31(9):781–9.
64. Deland JT, de Asla RJ, Segal A. Reconstruction of the chronically failed deltoid ligament: a new technique. Foot Ankle Int 2004;25(11):795–9.
65. Knupp M, Lang TH, Zwicky L, et al. Chronic ankle instability (medial and lateral). Clin Sports Med 2015;34(4):679–88.
66. Wiewiorski MJ, Alrashidi Y, Stelzenbach C, et al. Anatomical lateral and medial ligament reconstruction in rotational chronic ankle instability. Foot Ankle Orthopaedics 2016;1(1). 2473011416S2473000003.
67. Valderrabano V, Miska M, Leumann A, et al. Reconstruction of osteochondral lesions of the talus with autologous spongiosa grafts and autologous matrix-induced chondrogenesis. Am J Sports Med 2013;41(3):519–27.
68. Brostrom L. Sprained ankles. VI. Surgical treatment of "chronic" ligament ruptures. Acta Chir Scand 1966;132(5):551–65.

Spring Ligament Instability

Gonzalo F. Bastias, MD[a,b,c,]*, Miki Dalmau-Pastor, PhD, PT, DPM[d,e,f],
Claudia Astudillo, MD[g], Manuel J. Pellegrini, MD[c,h,i]

KEYWORDS

- Spring ligament • Calcaneonavicular ligament • Adult acquired flatfoot deformity
- Pes planus • Posterior tibial tendon insufficiency

KEY POINTS

- The spring ligament complex plays a fundamental role in the static stability of the talonavicular joint and the medial longitudinal arch.
- Isolated injury or secondary failure in the context of posterior tibial tendon insufficiency has been related to flatfoot deformity.
- Spring ligament repair and augmentation or reconstruction techniques focus on deformity correction and restoring the medial arch and have been progressively included in the treatment of flexible flatfoot deformity treatment algorithms.
- Restoring normal function of the spring ligament complex has been associated with a decrease in the need for nonanatomic procedures, such as lateral column lengthening and hindfoot fusions.

INTRODUCTION

The complexity of the pathologic process that leads to flatfoot deformity has been only partially understood. The crucial role of spring ligament complex (SLC), however, within this process has recently evolved. Several reasons can explain this situation, which can be summarized in an improvement in anatomic knowledge and

Disclosure Statement: Dr M.J. Pellegrini is a paid consultant for Arthrex. Dr G.F. Bastias, Dr M. Dalmau-Pastor, and Dr C. Astudillo have nothing to disclose.
[a] Department of Orthopedic Surgery, Clinica Las Condes, Estoril 450, Las Condes, Santiago 7591047, Chile; [b] Foot and Ankle Unit, Complejo Hospitalario San José, San José 1196, Santiago 8380419, Chile; [c] Department of Orthopedic Surgery, Universidad de Chile, 1027 Independencia, Santiago 8380453, Chile; [d] Human Anatomy and Embryology Unit, Experimental Pathologies and Therapeutics Department, Universitat de Barcelona, Feixa Larga s/n, 08907, Hospitalet de Llobregat, Barcelona 08907, Spain; [e] Health Sciences Faculty of Manresa, Universitat de Vic-Central de Catalunya, Sagrada Família, 7. 08500 Vic, Barcelona, Spain; [f] Groupe de Recherche et d'Etude en Chirurgie Mini-Invasive du Pied, 2 Rue Georges Negrevergne, Merignac 33700, France; [g] Department of Radiology, Clinica Las Condes, Estoril 450, Las Condes, Santiago 7591047, Chile; [h] Department of Orthopedic Surgery, Hospital Clinico Universidad de Chile, Santos Dumont 999, Independencia, Santiago 8380456, Chile; [i] Clinica Universidad de los Andes, Plaza 2501, Santiago 7620157, Chile
* Corresponding author. Estoril 450, Las Condes, Santiago, Chile.
E-mail address: gbastias@clinicalascondes.cl

Foot Ankle Clin N Am 23 (2018) 659–678
https://doi.org/10.1016/j.fcl.2018.07.012
1083-7515/18/© 2018 Elsevier Inc. All rights reserved.

understanding of the close SLC to deltoid complex relationship and by outstanding advances in biomechanics concepts.

These reasons have led to an optimization of flatfoot treatment strategies. In addition to bony realignment, these treatment strategies focus on a renewed interest in SLC and medial soft tissue reconstruction to obtain an adequate correction of the talonavicular deformity and restoration of the medial longitudinal arch.

ANATOMY

The SLC is a group of ligaments that connect the sustentaculum tali of the calcaneus and the navicular bone. The main function of the SLC is to support the head of the talus, an important part of the articular surface of the talocalcaneonavicular joint, commonly referred to as acetabulum or coxa pedis.[1] The dorsal portion of the ligament is covered by fibrocartilage and articulates through a small triangular surface located at the medial side of the head of the talus.[2]

The SLC is formed by 2 distinct ligamentous bands: the superomedial calcaneonavicular (SMCN) ligament and the inferomedial calcaneonavicular (ICN) ligament (**Fig. 1**). Due to the intrinsic difficulty in dissecting this area, however, the

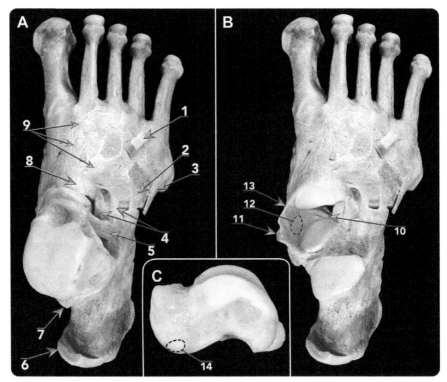

Fig. 1. Osteoarticular dissection of the SLC. (*A*) Superior view of the foot. (*B*) Superior view of the foot with the talus removed. (*C*) Medial view of a right talus. 1, Peroneus tertius tendon. 2, Dorsolateral calcaneocuboid ligament. 3, Peroneus brevis tendon. 4, Bifurcate ligament (calcaneonavicular and calcaneocuboid components). 5, Cervical ligament. 6, Calcaneal tendon. 7, Posterolateral talar tubercle. 8, Dorsal talonavicular ligament (cut). 9, Dorsal tarsal ligaments. 10, Inferior calcaneonavicular ligament. 11, Tibialis posterior tendon. 12, Fibrocartilaginous area of the SMCN ligament. 13, SMCN ligament. 14, Articular surface of the talus for the SMCN ligament.

fibrocartilaginous nature of the dorsal part of the ligaments, and the indivisibility of its distinct components, different descriptions are available in the literature.[3-6] These include 1 study describing a third additional component or midplantar oblique (MPO) ligament as a distinct part of the SLC.[7] Other cadaveric studies include the tibiospring component of the medial collateral ligament of the ankle (deltoid ligament) as part of the SLC, because this fascicle is one of the origins of the SMCN ligament, highlighting the intimate functional relationship between both complexes.[6,8]

The SMCN ligament is a quadrangular structure originating from the anterior and medial margins of the sustentaculum tali and at the anterior margin of the anterior articular surface of the calcaneus. From these points, it directs anteriorly to insert at the margin of the posterior articular surface of the navicular, specifically at the dorsal, medial, and plantar margins of its medial third. The medial portion of this ligament is in close relation with the posterior tibialis tendon (PTT), whereas its lateral portion articulates with the head of the talus.

The ICN ligament is a trapezoidal ligament that holds the inferior part of the talar head (**Fig. 2**). It originates from the coronoid fossa of the calcaneus, which is a small fossa on the sustentaculum tali, between the anterior and middle calcaneal articular surfaces. From this point, it directs medially to insert on the plantar aspect of the navicular, where it is in continuity with the SMCN ligament (**Fig. 3**). A medial and a lateral fascicle can be differentiated in this ligament.

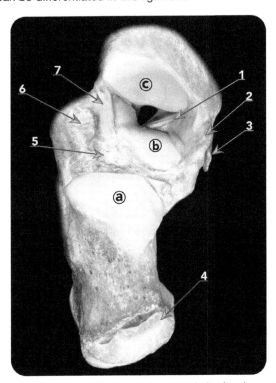

Fig. 2. Superior view of the talocalcaneonavicular joint (talus has been removed) and the SLC. a, Posterior subtalar articular surface of the calcaneus. b, Anterior subtalar articular surface of the calcaneus. c, Posterior articular surface of the navicular. 1, Inferior calcaneonavicular ligament. 2, SMCN ligament. 3, Tibialis posterior tendon. 4, Calcaneal tendon. 5, Interosseous talocalcaneal ligament (cut). 6, Cervical ligament (cut). 7, Calcaneonavicular component of the bifurcate ligament.

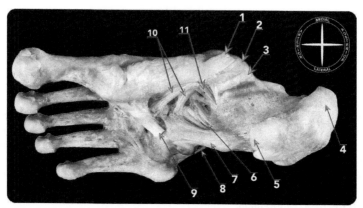

Fig. 3. Plantar view of an osteoarticular dissection of the SLC. 1, Tibialis posterior tendon. 2, SMCN ligament. 3, Sustentaculum tali. 4, Calcaneal tendon. 5, Plantar aponeurosis. 6, Plantar calcaneocuboid ligament. 7. Long plantar ligament. 8. Peroneus brevis tendon. 9, PL tendon. 10, Expansions of tibialis posterior tendon. 11. Inferior calcaneonavicular ligament.

BIOMECHANICS

The acetabulum pedis is conformed by the SLC, the anterior and middle facets of the calcaneus, and the proximal portion of the navicular. This structure provides static stability to the talar head and hence to the talonavicular joint. Moreover, is believed to provide medial longitudinal arch support and to provide kinetic coupling between the hindfoot and the forefoot.[4,9,10]

A cadaveric study by Reeck and collaborators,[11] however, demonstrated that contact forces in the calcaneonavicular ligament are much lower than in other talar articulations. Despite these findings, medial orientation must contribute to stabilize the talar head against medial subluxation.

Histologic reports have shown that the fibrocartilaginous plate of the SMCN ligament is likely formed secondary to repetitive loads it sustains. Likewise, the ICN ligament presents organized longitudinal fibers to resist tensile forces.[4]

CLINICAL PRESENTATION
Isolated Spring Ligament Rupture

Isolated injuries to the SLC in the presence of a normal PTT are uncommon. They usually result in an acquired flatfoot deformity presenting acutely but in some cases manifestations can be insidious and not easily related to a traumatic event. Patients commonly relate eversion injuries of the hindfoot sustained during physical activities progressing to a unilateral planovalgus deformity. Most of these cases are misdiagnosed as medial ankle sprains before developing the characteristic components of the flatfoot deformity: hindfoot valgus, loss of midfoot arch, and forefoot abduction.[12] Even though most of the clinical findings may mimic the classic PTT insufficiency presentation, there are some distinguishing features that can guide the diagnosis.

In a series of 9 cases, Tryfonidis and colleagues[13] described a characteristic clinical sign in patients with SLC insufficiency. Patients retained ability to perform a single leg, tiptoe standing on the affected side with partial restoration of medial arch but with persistent forefoot abduction and heel valgus. In addition, they reported that all their patients presented with tenderness anterior to the medial malleolus in contrast to the posterior-inferior tenderness typically found in PTT rupture and dysfunction. Other investigators have described a more plantar location of the pain, between the sustentaculum tali and the navicular.[9,12]

Differential diagnosis includes acute tears of the superficial deltoid ligament, most commonly at its navicular insertion, but they can also be found at its medial malleolus origin.[14] In the authors' experience, it is not possible to clinically differentiate an acute injury of the SLC from lesions of the deltoid complex. It has been well established that both structures share anatomic components and function as a unit.[6] Although the definitive diagnosis is usually done intraoperatively, the authors suggest the use of MRI to confirm the location of the injury in patients with acute flatfoot deformity.

Role in Acquired Adult Flatfoot Deformity Secondary to Posterior Tibial Tendon Insufficiency

Multiple studies have demonstrated that PTT insufficiency by itself is not capable of producing acquired adult flatfoot deformity (AAFD), even though it is the main dynamic stabilizer of the medial arch of the foot. As part of a progressive pathologic process, dysfunction of the PTT increases stress over the medial structures of the foot and ankle, leading to failure of the SLC and development of talonavicular deformity.[15,16] Tears or attenuation of the SLC, most commonly of the SMCN portion, can be found in more than 70% of the patients with some degree of deformity secondary to PTT insufficiency.[17,18] Diagnosis of this injury has been typically done with MRI evaluation and intraoperative inspection. On the other hand, the role of clinical examination assessing SLC involvement in patients with AAFD secondary to PTT dysfunction is unclear and literature on the matter is scarce.

Pasapula and collaborators[19] described the neutral heel lateral push test to determine SLC integrity. They examined 21 cadaveric specimens to assess the lateral translation of the midfoot when applying a lateral force to the medial midfoot with graduated anterograde and retrograde defunctioning of the PTT and flexor digitorum longus (FDL) tendon. In all specimens, a significant displacement occurred after the SLC was released regardless of the dissection sequence. The investigators concluded that the SLC is the most important ligament preventing lateral translation of the midfoot. They described a clinical test consisting of holding the heel in a neutral position and applying a lateral force to the medial midfoot. A firm endpoint is suggestive of SLC integrity, whereas lateral translation without endpoint suggests injury to the SLC. Clinical validation of this clinical sign, however, is still lacking. In the context of AAFD secondary to PTT insufficiency, clinical determination of SLC injury is currently not reliable.

IMAGING STUDIES
Radiographs

Standard weight-bearing x-ray evaluation continues to be the initial study for evaluation of flatfoot deformity. Despite that radiological findings do not differ from the typical characteristics described for PTT insufficiency, Williams and collaborators[20] reported there was a significant association between an increased Meary talus-first metatarsal angle (over 5°) and SLC injury on MRI.

Ultrasound

Due to the advances in MRI imaging techniques and their dependency on operator experience, ultrasound is usually not included in the first line of study when suspecting an SLC injury. Potential limitations are that it only allows the visualization only of the SMCN component of the SLC with a limited soft tissue contrast. It can be a useful tool, however, for detecting abnormalities in the PTT, frequently associated with SLC pathology.[1,15]

The correct visualization of the SMCN ligament is usually obtained with the probe placed inferior to the medial malleolus, with one end placed over the sustentaculum tali and the other end slightly tilted superiorly over the talar head toward the supero-medial aspect of the navicular bone. The normal appearance is a hyperechoic fibrillar structure.

Ultrasound signs of abnormality are loss of normal fibrillar internal structure, marked widening or flattening, a defect or gap, and increased vascularity on Doppler examination.[13]

MRI

MRI is the modality of choice for the evaluation of the SLC by providing an excellent visualization of its tridimensional orientated structure, which allows for assessment of the extent of injury. In addition, MRI is useful to diagnose adjacent abnormalities involving the soft tissue structures of the medial side of the ankle, such as deltoid ligament, flexor retinaculum, and PTT. It also depicts other potential sources of chronic medial ankle pain that are part of the differential diagnosis: tarsal tunnel syndrome, accessory flexor muscles, and subtalar coalition among others.[21]

Spring ligament is often abnormal in patients with acquired flat foot deformity, whether acute or chronic deformity, in isolation or associated with talonavicular dislocation, deltoid ligament, and PTT abnormalities.[21]

SMCN is best visualized in coronal and axial planes (**Figs 4**A, B). Studies have reported that the normal thickness is between 2 mm and 4 mm.

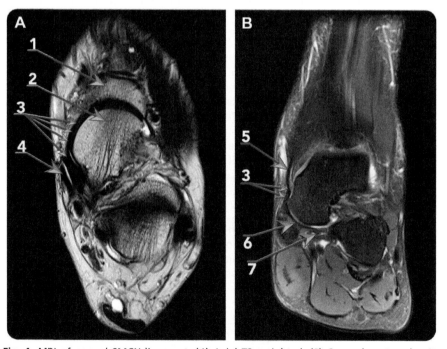

Fig. 4. MRI of normal SMCN ligament. (*A*) Axial T2 weighted. (*B*) Coronal proton density with fat suppression (PD FS) of the ankle. 1, Navicular bone. 2, Talar head. 3, SMCN ligament. 4, Posterior tibial tendon. 5, Tibiospring ligament. 6, MPO band. 7, ICN band.

Different MRI signs of abnormal features of the SMCN have been described.[1,10,22–24] The most common reported signs are increased signal on proton density with fat suppression (PD FS) or T2-weighted sequences, thickening greater than 5 mm, thinning less than 2 mm, and partial or complete discontinuity, including defects in the junction of tibiospring ligament with the SMCN ligament (**Figs. 5–7**).

ICN and MPO portions are best visualized in the axial plane but are also seen in sagittal and coronal images[10] (**Fig. 8**). MPO band is the thinnest portion, with a mean thickness of 2.8 mm (range:1–5 mm). It looks striated in T1-weighted and T2-weighted images with alternating layers of fibers bundles and fat.[22,23]

ICN band is short and thick, separated from the MPO band by fat and the spring ligament recess, and runs slightly oblique to the long axis of the foot. It has intermediate signal in T1-weighted and T2-weighted images and a mean thickness of 4 mm (2–6 mm). Pathology affecting these bands is infrequently reported.[23]

TREATMENT

Management of SLC injuries are immersed in conventional flatfoot deformity treatment strategies, including medializing sliding calcaneal osteotomy, lateral column lengthening, and FDL transfer. All these procedures aim to reduce the stress on the medial structures but none of them manages to reconstitute the plantar arch in a satisfactory way.[16]

Repair or reconstruction of the SLC has usually been reported as an adjunctive procedure in stage IIB flatfoot deformity before progression to later stages and severe collapse of the midfoot and rigidity develops.[17] Furthermore, some investigators have proposed that SLC reconstruction may avoid the need of nonanatomic procedures like lateral column lengthening and even subtalar and midfoot fusions in severe

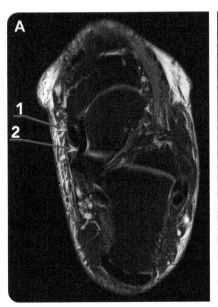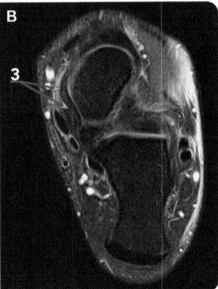

Fig. 5. MRI of SMCN ligament thickening. (*A and B*) Axial PD FS. 1, Posterior tibial tendon. 2, SMCN thickened. 3, SMCN thickened and increased in signal. (*B*) Note the surrounding edema due to chronic stress to the soft tissue.

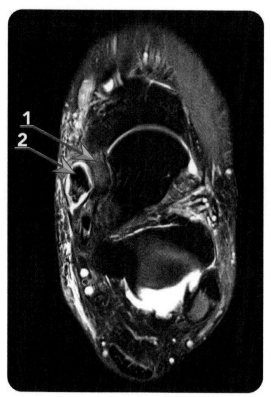

Fig. 6. MRI of SMCN ligament with marked thickening and increased signal. Axial PD FS. 1, SMCN. 2, Posterior tibial tendon with degeneration and tenosynovitis.

deformities.[25] Including SLC repair, however, did not significantly enhance bony correction in a flatfoot cadaveric model under cyclic loading.[26]

The investigators suggest that the presence of SLC injuries are habitual when midfoot abduction (>5° anteroposterior talar—first metatarsal angle and/or >30% talar head uncoverage) and/or talonavicular sag (>5° lateral talar—first metatarsal angle) are present. Surgeons must be prepared to perform a repair or reconstruction of the SLC if confirmed during inspection.

Isolated SL injuries are amenable for repair or reconstruction without adjunctive procedures. Several reports have demonstrated excellent results with isolated procedures after acute tears. Chronic isolated lesions associated with attenuation of the medial structures, however, may require additional procedures in a similar fashion as flatfoot reconstruction, even in the absence of PTT pathology.[27]

Adequate intraoperative visualization of the SLC can be demanding but it is imperative for diagnosis confirmation and for appropriate repair or reconstruction, independent of the surgical technique. Orr and Nunley[27] suggest positioning the ankle and hindfoot in full inversion with plantar retraction of the PTT. This provides excellent visualization of the superomedial portion and most of the middle and inferior portions of the SLC.

Direct Repair

SLC tears are frequently the result of a chronic degenerative process, resulting in an attenuation of the tissue that makes repairing it unpredictable.[5] Macklin Vadell and

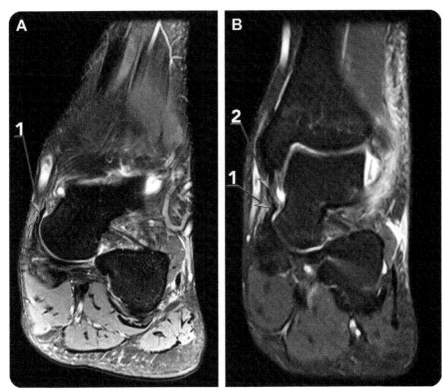

Fig. 7. MRI of Partial rupture of the SMCN ligament. (*A and B*) Coronal PD FS. 1, SMCN. 2, Tibiospring ligament. (*B*) Note also in (*B*) tibiospring ligament rupture, disruption of deep components of deltoid ligament and lateral soft tissue edema.

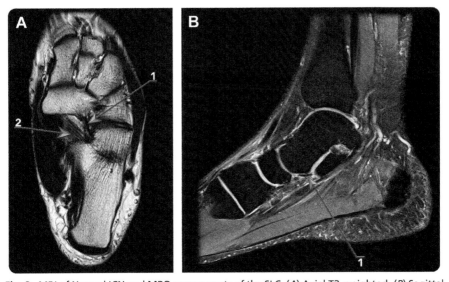

Fig. 8. MRI of Normal ICN and MPO components of the SLC. (*A*) Axial T2-weighted. (*B*) Sagittal PD FS. 1, ICN band. 2, MPO band.

Colleagues, however, recommend resecting the lesions ends and suturing the remaining portions with reabsorbable stiches for lesions smaller than 1 cm. For larger lesions, a Z-shortening tenotomy of the PTT can be added to the procedure, to protect the repair.[9]

Other techniques described for direct repair include advancement and reinsertion through transosseus navicular drill holes, plication of the talonavicular capsule, and re-tensioning in vest-over-pants fashion.[12,28]

Recently, Lui[29] described an endoscopic technique for repairing the superficial deltoid ligament and the SLC. Repair is performed through a PTT endoscopy and/or talonavicular arthroscopy, depending on the compromise of the tibiospring or SMCN ligament. The advantage of this method is limited soft tissue dissection, but caution must be paid to not injuring the medial plantar nerve. Clinical results remain to be reported (**Fig. 9**).

Reconstruction

Strategies oriented to reconstruct the SLC rely on the principle that native tissues are usually degenerated and attenuated and not suitable for repair. Thus, reconstruction with tendon autograft or allograft theoretically could better withstand stress forces across the talonavicular joint and maintain correction of the deformity.

Several options have been described to reconstruct the SLC, mainly on cadaveric studies. Deland and collaborators[30] described a deltoid ligament bone-block graft taken from the medial malleolus that preserved the insertion of superficial portion of the ligament at the sustenculum tali. The bone-block was attached to the navicular after correction of the longitudinal arch with manipulation. This technique was able to partially correct the deformity under radiological examination but was not clinically successful.[16] Thordarson and colleagues,[31] on the other hand, created a flatfoot deformity model on 6 fresh-frozen cadavers and compared the use of peroneus longus (PL), tibialis anterior, and Achilles tendon transfers under cyclical loads. Reconstruction with PL tendon provided significantly greater correction in the sagittal and transverse planes across most loads. The other techniques performed poorly with premature failure and loss of correction at lower loads. Despite its success in the laboratory, this procedure was not applied in the clinical setting.

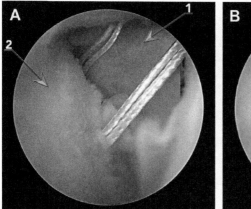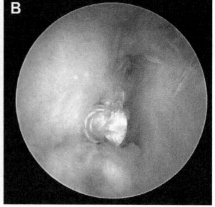

Fig. 9. (*A*) Tibialis posterior tendon (1) endoscopy with assessment of the tibiospring ligament. The SLC corresponds to the medial wall of the tendon sheath (2). If a tear is present, the talar head will be exposed. (*B*) Repair is performed by using a CPR Viper suture passer preloaded with a no. 2 FiberWire suture. (*Courtesy of* Dr Hector Masaragian MD, Buenos Aires, Argentina.)

Choi and colleagues[32] proposed an anatomic approach to SLC reconstruction that also used the PL tendon and compared 3 reconstructive variations to recreate the SLC on a cadaveric flatfoot model: superomedial, plantar, and combined reconstruction techniques. The combined superomedial/plantar passage of the tendon through the calcaneus and navicular was shown more effective than either of the other 2 simple approaches, correcting the talonavicular joint from an abducted to and adducted position and the subtalar joint from an everted to an inverted position. The investigators concluded that the combined PL technique recreates the normal anatomic restraints of the native SLC while successfully correcting the deformity. They express a minor concern on the effects of losing the PL effect as a plantar flexor of the first ray but highlighting the positive effect on the rebalancing of the foot secondary to the elimination of the abducting and eversion forces of the PL.

Williams and collaborators[25] published a clinical series on SLC reconstruction. They reported on 13 patients (14 feet) undergoing flatfoot surgery with SLC reconstruction using a PL tendon transfer for those cases in which lateral column lengthening failed to correct forefoot abduction. Decision to reconstruct the spring ligament was taken intraoperatively after bony procedures using fluoroscopy and simulating weight bearing to assess persistent talonavicular abduction (more than $30°$) or talonavicular sag (more than $10°$). The PL tendon was harvested proximal to the extensor retinaculum, left attached to the base of the first metatarsal, and retrieved through a medial approach. The graft was then passed from dorsal to plantar through a navicular bone tunnel. Fixation of the proximal end of the graft was done differently according to the characteristics of the talonavicular deformity. If significant plantar sag was found in addition to the abduction deformity, a calcaneal hole was created and used for fixating the graft at this level, thus reducing both components of the deformity (10 patients). In cases of presentation only with abduction deformity, however, a tibial drill hole was made to fixate the graft more proximally (4 patients). The American Orthopedic Foot and Ankle Society (AOFAS) Hindfoot score increased significantly from 43.1 preoperatively to 90.3 postoperatively. All radiological measurements had significant improvement. Eleven patients had excellent satisfaction results and 2 patients reported good results (3 feet). Eversion strength remained normal in all but 1 case.

The fact that patients received different concomitant procedures like FDL transfer, medializing calcaneal osteotomy, or first tarsometatarsal fusion makes it difficult to identify the real effect of the SLC reconstruction. Nevertheless, the outcomes were comparable to other reports, including patients undergoing lateral column lengthening or medializing calcaneal osteotomy with FDL transfer without SLC reconstruction.[33] Moreover, the investigators advocate the use of reconstruction of the SLC complex in the context of severe flatfoot deformity to avoid double arthrodesis or triple arthrodesis of the hindfoot.

Baxter and colleagues[34] compared 3 different reconstruction techniques with PL tendon on a flatfoot model without bony procedures or tendon transfers. The investigators compared an anatomic double bundle technique with 2 nonanatomic reconstructions (talonavicular and tibionavicular configurations). Anatomic reconstruction provided the least amount of correction of the midfoot deformity and had no effect correcting hindfoot valgus. There was a graded effect between deformity correction and proximal fixation of the reconstruction, with the tibionavicular technique providing the most correction of hindfoot valgus, even though it had no interface with the calcaneus. The investigators concluded that reconstructive techniques that included the tibial attachment better corrected midfoot and hindfoot deformity in comparison to anatomic reconstruction and similarly to deltoid complex reconstruction.[35]

Flexor hallucis longus (FHL) tendon autograft reconstruction was described by Lee and Yi on 23 patients.[36] This tendon was selected because of its origin from the deep posterior compartment of the leg, similar to the PTT. The investigators harvested the FHL tendon at the level of the first metatarsophalangeal joint and passed it from plantar to dorsal through the medial cuneiform and then reoriented it in a plantar direction through the navicular and finally passed it from medial to lateral through the sustenculum tali. Clinical outcomes were reported at an average of 8.2 months' follow-up, with an improvement of the AOFAS ankle-hindfoot score from 72.6 preoperatively to 86.4 postoperative. Radiographic parameters were also improved by this reconstruction technique. According to the investigators, this technique reestablishes the static support of the SLC, provides a dynamic midfoot support, and thus eliminates the need for a concomitant FDL transfer.

The use of autologous PTT also has been recently described.[3,37] The rationale behind this alternative approach is to use the diseased PTT that is usually resected during flatfoot reconstruction, and avoid sacrificing a healthy tendon (PL, TA, and FHL). Rysmann and Jeng[37] described a single bundle procedure, consisting of a proximal release of the PTT while maintaining an intact distal attachment. The proximal stump is then passed through a single bone tunnel in the sustenculum tali and tensioned to resemble the SLC. The investigators present results on 3 patients that were reconstructed via this technique in conjunction with medializing calcaneal osteotomy, FDL transfer, and gastrocnemius recession. At 1-year average follow-up, they report excellent radiologic results without evidence of persisting pain over the reconstruction site secondary to leaving the degenerated PTT. The investigators recommend using an alternate reconstruction technique in cases of a PTT that is absent or unusable.

Repair and Augmentation

New alternatives of treatment to complement and reinforce direct repair of the SLC have appeared with development of modern systems for soft tissue augmentation. Tendon harvesting performed during reconstruction can be related to morbidity and loss of strength.[5] Additionally, augmentation techniques may reduce the need of demanding reconstructive techniques and subsequently, the need for tendon harvesting.

Acevedo and Vora[38] described an augmentation technique with FiberTape (Arthrex, Naples, Florida) that replicates both the SMCN and ICN bands of the SLC in association with additional adjunctive bony procedures. The proximal limb (double) is secured at the level of the sustentaculum tali using an interference screw. A single limb is used to replicate the SMCN band by advancing the FiberTape from dorsal to plantar in the medial pole of the navicular. The second limb is then passed from plantar to dorsal, replicating the ICN ligament, in conjunction with the FDL longus tendon transfer. Both FiberTape limbs and the transferred tendon are then secured with another interference screw. The investigators reported the results in 26 patients with only one case presenting radiologic failure. Furthermore, they reported greater correction of the medial arch when using this technique than when performing FDL transfer and medializing osteotomy alone. The advantage of this technique is that it avoids the need of drill multiple tunnels around the sustentaculum tali and potentially decreases the necessity of additional lateral column procedures or subtalar arthroereisis by dramatically improving talar head coverage. Long-term correction of the medial arch using direct repair and augmentation is still to be determined.

Palmanovich and colleagues[39] described a direct repair with nonabsorbable suture followed by reinforcement with FiberTape passed through drilled tunnels in the sustentaculum tali and the navicular, forming a **Fig. 8**. The remaining limbs were anchored to the medial malleolus to reconstruct the anterior fibers of the deltoid ligament. In a subsequent article,[40] the investigators reported the results of their technique in 5 patients with isolated SLC injury. All patients had clinical improvement and were able to perform single heel rise at 1 year follow-up. The AOFAS ankle-hindfoot score also showed improvement from 55.8 before surgery to 97.6 postoperatively during the first year after surgery. No improvement was noted after 1-year follow-up and no clinical recurrence was observed at 5 years' to 10 years' follow-up.[40]

AUTHORS' PREFERRED METHOD OF TREATMENT

The authors propose that isolated injuries or attenuation of the medial soft tissue restraints that produce talonavicular abduction and, in particular, hindfoot valgus should be addressed by direct repair and augmentation not only of the SLC but also the deltoid complex (**Fig. 10**). This concept relies on the SLC and deltoid ligament not only sharing anatomic components but also functioning as a biomechanical unit.[6] Both clinical and biomechanical studies have highlighted the importance of including the deltoid complex in the reconstructive plan, especially in the context of AAFD secondary to PTT insufficiency.[15,25,34,39,40] The authors present a combined augmentation technique that includes acting on both the SLC and deltoid ligament complex. In this setting, Nery and colleagues[41] recently reported satisfactory results on 10 patients operated using this concept. In the AAFD setting, the authors perform this technique in conjunction with lateral column lengthening and/or medializing calcaneal osteotomy with FDL transfer.

Combined Anatomic Spring and Deltoid Ligament Augmentation Associated with Flexor Digitorum Longus Transfer

The patient is placed in the supine position with a thigh tourniquet. If indicated, a lateral column lengthening and/or medializing calcaneal osteotomy are performed

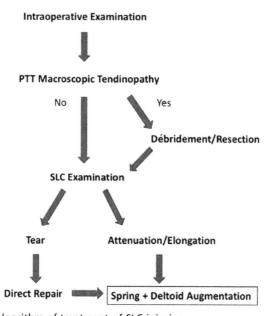

Fig. 10. Author's algorithm of treatment of SLC injuries.

in a conventional manner first. A medial incision is carried out from 2 cm proximal to the tip of the medial malleolus, just behind the posterior border of the tibia and directed toward the navicular tuberosity. After blunt dissection of the subcutaneous tissue, the flexor retinaculum is opened and the PTT is inspected. All macroscopic tendinopathy is resected. There are situations, however, in which part of the navicular insertion can be retained, in particular in those patients with low-quality residual medial ligaments.[37] Careful examination of the SLC and direct repair is performed if any identifiable tear is present. In most cases, global attenuation of the medial tissues is present, so the authors proceed to the combined augmentation procedure (**Fig. 11**A, B).

Dissection of the FDL tendon is then carried out distally where it is just before the knot of Henry. The distal free end of the tendon (1 cm) is prepared using a Krackow technique with FiberLoop suture (Arthrex), and its diameter is measured using a Bio-Tenodesis (Arthrex) guide (**Fig. 11**C).

The authors proceed to locate the sustentaculum tali, where the first blind tunnel is going to be drilled. This tunnel will be shared by the tibiocalcaneal arm of the deltoid ligament and spring ligament internal brace. A 1.35-mm Kirschner (K)-wire is inserted in the sustentaculum tali, angled 15° plantarly and slightly posterior to avoid the subtalar joint. Position can be checked under fluoroscopy prior to drilling with a 3.4-mm cannulated drill.

The next step is to elevate the medial ligament complex from the medial malleolus in a Brostrom fashion, following the osseous contour from medial to lateral and leaving tibial periosteum proximally, for a pants-over-vest repair at the end of the procedure. The tibial blind tunnel will be created in the intercollicular groove using a 3.4-mm drill bit angling proximally and then tapped with the 4.75-mm SwiveLock Tap (Arthrex). Then, a 3.5-mm corkscrew anchor is placed in the anterior colliculus in preparation for retightening of the entire medial ligament complex (**Fig. 12**).

To prepare the talar tunnel, the deltoid ligament is retracted distally to locate the insertion of the deep deltoid ligament in the talus. Talar blind tunnel preparation is performed in the same way than tibial tunnel was prepared. Angulation toward the talar body is necessary to achieve optimal purchase. After preparation is completed, the deltoid ligament is retracted proximally and a stab incision is performed immediately over the talar tunnel position, to maintain the internal brace augmentation superficially to the retightened medial ligament and mark the location of the talar tunnel underneath (**Fig. 13**).

The last tunnel to be prepared is the navicular tunnel. After placing a K-wire in an adequate position in the navicular by leaving at least 1 cm of bone from the medial border, the authors drill with a cannulated 5.0-mm drill from dorsal to plantar. Drill

A   **B**   **C**

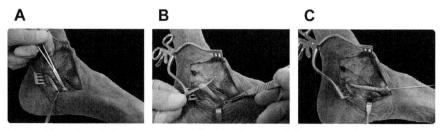

Fig. 11. Dissection of the FDL tendon. (*A*) Identification of the FDL tendon at the plantar aspect of the foot. (*B*) Distal end harvested just before Henry knot. (*C*) 1 cm from the free-end of this tendon is prepared with a Krackow suture.

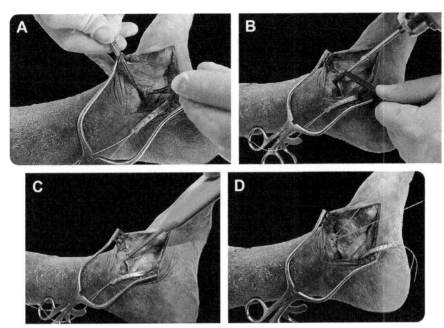

Fig. 12. Medial malleolus tunnel preparation. (*A*) Dissection of the medial ligament complex from the medial malleolus. (*B*) Tibial blind tunnel is placed in the intercollicular groove. (*C*) Tapering of the tibial blind tunnel. (*D*) Insertion of a 3.5-mm anchor at anterior colliculum.

size should be selected considering bone quality and FDL tendon diameter. In cases of adequate bone quality, the authors recommend drilling 0.5 mm over tendon size (**Fig. 14**).

Once all 4 blind tunnels have been adequately drilled and tapped, the authors perform the medial Brostrom-type retightening, by performing a Mason-Allen stitch using FiberWire (Arthrex) sutures loaded in the 3.5-mm corkscrew anchor. The foot should be maintained in inversion while the knots are being tied (**Fig. 15**).

After the medial Brostrom has been completed, augmentation with internal brace is performed. The first step of the ligament repair starts with the insertion of a 4.75-mm × 15-mm SwiveLock loaded with a FiberTape and inserted into the intercolicular tunnel of the tibial malleolus.

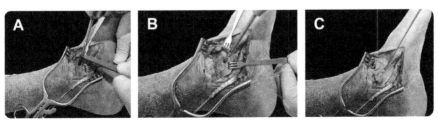

Fig. 13. Talar tunnel preparation. (*A*) Retraction of the deltoid ligament distally and drilling of the talar tunnel with angulation toward the talar body. (*B*) Tapering of the talar tunnel. (*C*) After preparation is completed, the deltoid ligament is retracted proximally and a stab incision is performed immediately over the talar tunnel position.

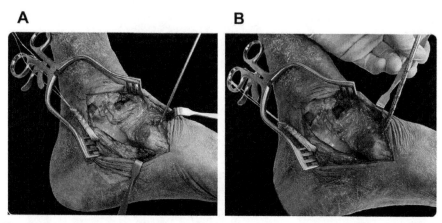

Fig. 14. Navicular tunnel preparation. (*A*) Placing of a K-wire leaving at least 1 cm of bone from the medial border. (*B*) Drilling with a cannulated 5.0-mm drill from dorsal to plantar.

One of the bands of the FiberTape already anchored to the medial malleolus is passed through the 4-mm PEEK Eyelet of a 4.75-mm × 13.5-mm SwiveLock and placed into the talus. Care is taken not to overtighten this augmentation, by placing a clamp underneath the tape and marking the amount of tape that is driven into the tunnel. This step completes the tibiotalar arm of the deltoid ligament augmentation.

Next, the tibiocalcaneal arm of the FiberTape (already anchored to the tibial malleolus) is passed through the 4-mm PEEK Eyelet of a 3.5-mm × 13.5-mm SwiveLock in which another no. 2 FiberTape was mounted. This additional step is used for SLC augmentation. This anchor is placed in the sustentaculum tunnel, taking the same precautions not to overtighten the repair and holding the foot in neutral dorsiflexion and slight external rotation. This step completes the deltoid ligament augmentation (**Fig. 16**).

The final step is the SLC augmentation with the FDL tendon transfer. As the last step of the procedure, both bands of the FiberTape attached to the sustentaculum are passed through the bone tunnel at the navicular bone. One of them is

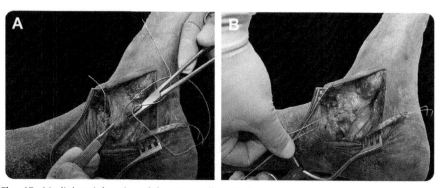

Fig. 15. Medial retightening. (*A*) Mason-Alley stitch using the 3.5 mm anchor previously placed at the medial malleolus. (*B*) Retightening with the foot placed in inversion.

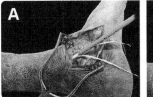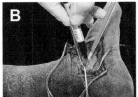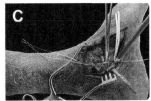

Fig. 16. Deltoid ligament augmentation. (*A*) Insertion of a SwiveLock with a FiberTape at the tibial tunnel. (*B*) One of the bands of the FiberTape already anchored to the tibial malleolus is placed into the talus tunnel. (*C*) The other band is placed on the sustentaculum tunnel with another SwiveLock with a mounted FiberTape for SLC augmentation.

from dorsal to plantar and the other is passed together with the FDL tendon from plantar to dorsal. Both FiberTape bands aim to recreate the native SLC anatomy. Full tension is applied to the tape branches and the FDL tendon, while maintaining the talonavicular joint in a reduced position. Finally, a 4.75-mm SwiveLock is inserted from plantar to dorsal to secure the construct (**Fig. 17**).

A removable boot is installed for 6 weeks to protect the FDL transfer. At this point, an intensive physiotherapy protocol is initiated to improve inversion strength. In cases of bony procedures that have been undertaken, the authors suggest maintaining the patient non–weight bearing for 3 weeks.

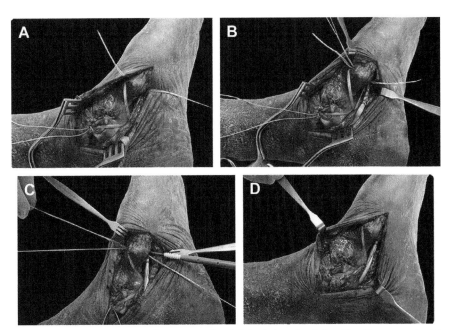

Fig. 17. SLC augmentation with FDL transfer. (*A*) Both bands of the FiberTape attached to the sustentaculum are passed through the navicular tunnel. (*B*) One of the bands is passed dorsal to plantar and the other together with the FDL tendon is passed from plantar to dorsal. (*C*) A 4.75-mm SwiveLock is inserted from plantar to dorsal to secure the whole construct. (*D*) Completed combined deltoid and SLC augmentation with FDL transfer.

SUMMARY

Currently, the biomechanical role of the SLC has been clearly elucidated as the main static restrain of the talonavicular joint. Isolated injury or secondary failure due to PTT dysfunction is responsible for midfoot abduction deformity and loss of the medial arch of the foot.

Even though there is a growing interest among orthopedic surgeons in including SLC repair or reconstruction as part of the flatfoot treatment plan, efficacy of such techniques has been difficult to quantify due to variable approaches and number of concomitant procedures carried out during flatfoot reconstruction.

Nevertheless, there is growing evidence that suggest that SLC reconstruction is capable of providing an excellent correction of the talonavicular deformity and re-establishment of the ligamentous structures of the midfoot arch, whereas bony procedures and tendon transfers alone commonly fail to do so.[5,17,32,34,42]

Myriad techniques for repairing, with and without augmentation or reconstructing the SLC, have been described, but no clinical evidence has shown superiority of any of these approaches. Comparative clinical studies with patient-reported outcomes are necessary to quantify the real effect of this techniques.

ACKNOWLDGMENTS

The authors want to acknowledge Ignacio Bielsa, MD and Promedon's Surgery Simulation Center at Clinica Universidad de los Andes for their help in specimen preparation.

REFERENCES

1. Omar H, Saini V, Wadhwa V, et al. Spring ligament complex: illustrated normal anatomy and spectrum of pathologies on 3T MR imaging. Eur J Radiol 2016; 85(11):2133–43.
2. Golano P, Fariñas O, Sáenz I. The anatomy of the navicular and periarticular structures. Foot Ankle Clin 2004;9(1):1–23.
3. Mousavian A, Orapin J, Chinanuvathana A, et al. Anatomic Spring Ligament and Posterior Tibial Tendon Reconstruction: New Concept of Double Bundle PTT and a Novel Technique for Spring Ligament. Arch Bone Jt Surg 2017; 5(3):201–5.
4. Davis WH, Sobel M, DiCarlo EF, et al. Gross, histological, and microvascular anatomy and biomechanical testing of the spring ligament complex. Foot Ankle Int 1996;17(2):95–102.
5. Steginsky B, Vora A. What to do with the spring ligament. Foot Ankle Clin 2017; 22(3):515–27.
6. Cromeens BP, Kirchhoff CA, Patterson RM, et al. An attachment-based description of the medial collateral and spring ligament complexes. Foot Ankle Int 2015; 36(6):710–21.
7. Taniguchi A, Tanaka Y, Takakura Y, et al. Anatomy of the spring ligament. J Bone Joint Surg Am 2003;85-A(11):2174–8.
8. Hintermann B, Golano P. The anatomy and function of the deltoid ligament. Tech Foot Ankle Surg 2014;13(2):67–72.
9. Vadell AM, Peratta M. Calcaneonavicular ligament: anatomy, diagnosis, and treatment. Foot Ankle Clin 2012;17(3):437–48.
10. Rule J, Yao L, Seeger LL. Spring ligament of the ankle: normal MR anatomy. AJR Am J Roentgenol 1993;161(6):1241–4.

11. Reeck J, Felten N, McCormack AP, et al. Support of the talus: a biomechanical investigation of the contributions of the talonavicular and talocalcaneal joints, and the superomedial calcaneonavicular ligament. Foot Ankle Int 1998;19(10): 674–82.

12. Masaragian HJ, Ricchetti HO, Testa C. Acute isolated rupture of the spring ligament: a case report and review of the literature. Foot Ankle Int 2013;34(1):150–4.

13. Tryfonidis M, Jackson W, Mansour R, et al. Acquired adult flat foot due to isolated plantar calcaneonavicular (spring) ligament insufficiency with a normal tibialis posterior tendon. Foot Ankle Surg 2008;14(2):89–95.

14. Nelson DR, Younger A. Acute posttraumatic planovalgus foot deformity involving hindfoot ligamentous pathology. Foot Ankle Clin 2003;8(3):521–37.

15. Deland JT, de Asla RJ, Sung IH, et al. Posterior tibial tendon insufficiency: which ligaments are involved? Foot Ankle Int 2005;26(6):427–35.

16. Deland JT. The adult acquired flatfoot and spring ligament complex: pathology and implications for treatment. Foot Ankle Clin 2001;6(1):129–35.

17. Deland JT. Spring ligament complex and flatfoot deformity: curse or blessing? Foot Ankle Int 2012;33(3):239–43.

18. Gazdag AR, Cracchiolo AC III. Rupture of the posterior tibial tendon: evaluation of injury of the spring ligament and clinical assessment of tendon transfer and ligament repair. J Bone Joint Surg Am 1997;79-A(5):675–81.

19. Pasapula C, Devany A, Magan A, et al. Neutral heel lateral push test: the first clinical examination of spring ligament integrity. Foot (Edinb) 2015;25(2):69–74.

20. Williams G, Widnall J, Evans P, et al. Could failure of the spring ligament complex be the driving force behind the development of the adult flatfoot deformity? J Foot Ankle Surg 2014;53(2):152–5.

21. Crim J. Medial-sided ankle pain: deltoid ligament and beyond. Magn Reson Imaging Clin N Am 2017;25(1):63–77.

22. Toye LR, Helms CA, Hoffman BD, et al. MRI of spring ligament tears. AJR Am J Roentgenol 2005;184(5):1475–80.

23. Mengiardi B, Pinto C, Zanetti M. Spring ligament complex and posterior tibial tendon: MR anatomy and findings in acquired adult flatfoot deformity. Semin Musculoskelet Radiol 2016;20(1):104–15.

24. Williams G, Widnall J, Evans P, et al. MRI features most often associated with surgically proven tears of the spring ligament complex. Skeletal Radiol 2013;42(7): 969–73.

25. Williams BR, Ellis SJ, Deyer TW, et al. Reconstruction of the spring ligament using a peroneus longus autograft tendon transfer. Foot Ankle Int 2010;31(7):567–77.

26. Zanolli DH, Glisson RR, Nunley JA 2nd, et al. Biomechanical assessment of flexible flatfoot correction: comparison of techniques in a cadaver model. J Bone Joint Surg Am 2014;96(6):e45.

27. Orr JD, Nunley JA 2nd. Isolated spring ligament failure as a cause of adult-acquired flatfoot deformity. Foot Ankle Int 2013;34(6):818–23.

28. Borton DC, Saxby TS. Tear of the plantar calcaneonavicular (spring) ligament causing flatfoot. A case report. J Bone Joint Surg Br 1997;79-B(4):641–3.

29. Lui TH. Endoscopic repair of the superficial deltoid ligament and spring ligament. Arthrosc Tech 2016;5(3):e621–5.

30. Deland JT, Arnoczky SP, Thompson FM. Adult acquired flatfoot deformity at the talonavicular joint: reconstruction of the spring ligament in an in vitro model. Foot Ankle 1992;13(6):327–32.

31. Thordarson DB, Schmotzer H, Chon J. Reconstruction with tenodesis in an adult flatfoot model: a biomechanical evaluation of four methods. J Bone Joint Surg Am 1995;77-A(10):1557–64.
32. Choi K, Lee S, Otis JC, et al. Anatomical reconstruction of the spring ligament using peroneus longus tendon graft. Foot Ankle Int 2003;24(5):430–6.
33. Toolan BC, Sangeorzan BJ, Hansen ST. Complex reconstruction for the treatment of dorsolateral peritalar subluxation of the foot. Early results after distraction arthrodesis of the calcaneocuboid joint in conjunction with stabilization of, and transfer of the flexor digitorum longus tendon to, the midfoot to treat acquired pes planovalgus in adults. J Bone Joint Surg Am 1999;81(11):1545–60.
34. Baxter JR, LaMothe JM, Walls RJ, et al. Reconstruction of the medial talonavicular joint in simulated flatfoot deformity. Foot Ankle Int 2015;36(4):424–9.
35. Jeng CL, Bluman EM, Myerson MS. Minimally invasive deltoid ligament reconstruction for stage IV flatfoot deformity. Foot Ankle Int 2011;32(1):21–30.
36. Lee WC, Yi Y. Spring ligament reconstruction using the autogenous flexor hallucis longus tendon. Orthopedics 2014;37(7):467–71.
37. Ryssman DB, Jeng CL. Reconstruction of the spring ligament with a posterior tibial tendon autograft: technique tip. Foot Ankle Int 2017;38(4):452–6.
38. Acevedo J, Vora A. Anatomical reconstruction of the spring ligament complex: "internal brace" augmentation. Foot Ankle Spec 2013;6(6):441–5.
39. Palmanovich E, Shabat S, Brin YS, et al. Anatomic reconstruction technique for a plantar calcaneonavicular (spring) ligament tear. J Foot Ankle Surg 2015;54(6): 1124–6.
40. Palmanovich E, Shabat S, Brin YS, et al. Novel reconstruction technique for an isolated plantar calcaneonavicular (SPRING) ligament tear: a 5 case series report. Foot (Edinb) 2017;30:1–4.
41. Nery C, Lemos AVKC, Raduan F, et al. Combined spring and deltoid ligament repair in adult-acquired flatfoot. Foot Ankle Int 2018;39(8):903–7.
42. Tan GJ, Kadakia AR, Ruberte Thiele RA, et al. Novel reconstruction of a static medial ligamentous complex in a flatfoot model. Foot Ankle Int 2010;31(8): 695–700.

Low-Energy Lisfranc Injuries in an Athletic Population

A Comprehensive Review of the Literature and the Role of Minimally Invasive Techniques in Their Management

Mario I. Escudero, MD, Michael Symes, MD,
Andrea Veljkovic, MD, MPH(Harvard), BComm, FRCSC,
Alastair S.E. Younger, MB,ChB, ChM, MSc, FRCSC*

KEYWORDS

- Lisfranc injuries management • Minimally invasive surgery • Arthroscopy
- Midfoot fusion • Open reduction and internal fixation

KEY POINTS

- The injury to the Lisfranc ligament can lead to substantial pain, midfoot arthritis, decreased function, and loss of quality of life.
- An accurate diagnosis of this pathology is mandatory. It is important to assess the inter-cuneiform distance to rule out a proximal Lisfranc's variant.
- Open reduction and internal fixation is the gold standard treatment modality for acute Lisfranc injuries.
- Minimally invasive surgery is a valid alternative in the management of Lisfranc injuries.

INTRODUCTION

The Lisfranc joint, also referred to as the tarsometatarsal (TMT) joint complex, is named after Jacques Lisfranc (1790–1847), a French surgeon who served in Napoleon's army and described an amputation through the TMT joint when a soldier fell

Disclosure Statement: Dr A. Veljkovic has research support and fellowship support from Acumed, Zimmer, Wright Medical, Synthes, and Arthrex. Dr A.S.E. Younger is a consultant with Zimmer, Cartiva, Wright Medical, and Acumed. He has research support from Acumed, Cartiva, Zimmer, Wright Medical, Synthes, and Bioventus. Drs M.I. Escudero and M. Symes have nothing to disclose.
Department of Orthopaedics, Division of Distal Extremities, University of British Columbia, Suite 221, 181 Keefer Street, Vancouver, BC V6B 6C1, Canada
* Corresponding author.
E-mail address: asyounger@shaw.ca

from a horse with his foot caught in the stirrup.[1,2] Injuries to the TMT joint complex occur in 1 per 55,000 persons each year in the United States, accounting for approximately 0.2% of all fractures.[3]

Up to 20% of these injuries are misdiagnosed or missed on initial radiographic assessment; therefore, a high index of suspicion is needed to accurately diagnose TMT joint injuries and avoid the late sequelae of substantial midfoot arthrosis, pain, decreased function, and loss of quality of life.[4]

Low-energy trauma, such as athletic injuries, accounts for approximately one-third of all Lisfranc injuries and lisfranc injuries have been shown to occur in up to 4% of American football players per season.[5–7] In contrast to injuries sustained during higher-energy trauma, such as motor vehicle accidents or falls from height, these type of Lisfranc injuries tend to be a distinct clinical entity that is often primarily ligamentous, rather than bony in nature. This review discusses the anatomy, diagnosis, and management of athletic Lisfranc injuries, including a detailed description of the preferred minimally invasive surgical techniques used by the senior author of this article.

Anatomy

The TMT joint complex represents the dividing line between the midfoot and the forefoot and is made up of bony and ligamentous elements that combine to add structural support to the transverse arch.[8] The bony architecture is composed of 9 bones: 5 metatarsals (MTs) and their respective articulations with the 3 cuneiforms medially and the cuboid laterally. The trapezoidal shape of the middle 3 MT bases and their associated cuneiforms produce a stable arch referred to as the transverse or Roman arch.[9] The keystone to the transverse arch is the second TMT joint, a product of the recessed middle cuneiform, which occupies a position 8 mm proximal to the medial cuneiform and 4 mm proximal to the lateral cuneiform.[5] On a cross-section, the midfoot forms a transverse plantar arch composed of asymmetrically shaped bones, with osseous and ligamentous anatomy providing a mortise configuration to the midfoot to support weight-bearing (WB) forces.[10,11]

In addition to the bony architecture, soft tissue and ligamentous stability is also important in the midfoot. Interosseous ligaments join the bases of the second through fifth MTs. The Lisfranc ligament runs on the plantar aspect of the foot from the lateral aspect of the medial cuneiform to the medial aspect of the second MT. It functions to stabilize the TMT articulation of the foot and plays a pivotal role, as there is no transverse MT ligament between the first and second MTs. Secondary stabilizers of the transverse arch of the midfoot include the plantar aponeurosis, peroneus longus tendon, and intrinsic muscles of the foot. The terminal branch of the dorsalis pedis artery and the deep peroneal nerve course between the bases of the first and second MTs. This site usually can be found directly under the extensor hallucis brevis muscle belly and tendon.[5,8]

Mechanism of Injury

TMT joint complex injuries can be caused by either direct or indirect injuries. Direct injuries are usually high-energy injuries, typically caused by a crush-type mechanism, and are often associated with significant soft tissue trauma, vascular compromise, and potentially compartment syndrome. Low-energy injuries often result from indirect mechanisms in which an axial load is applied to a plantar flexed foot or a twisting moment about the midfoot without an axial load.[6] Depending on the location of the force applied to the TMT joint complex, the MTs can undergo plantar or dorsal displacement.[12] However, because the plantar ligaments are stronger, Lisfranc injuries usually lead to dorsal (and mostly lateral) dislocation of the TMT, leading to midfoot instability.[13,14] These injuries often have a predominantly ligamentous pattern, with smaller avulsion-type fractures (the fleck sign) off the MT bases. The injury to the Lisfranc ligament can lead to substantial pain, midfoot arthritis, decreased function, and loss of quality of life.[3]

According to some investigators, the Lisfranc injury represents the second most common foot injury among college football players.[6] The force of injury can also extend proximally through the intercuneiform joint of the medial and middle cuneiforms and exit medially out the navicular-medial cuneiform joint. This variant injury pattern is often quite subtle but, if overlooked and untreated, may lead to a significantly increased risk of degenerative arthritis of the navicular-medial cuneiform joint.[6,10,15]

DIAGNOSIS

Patients will present with a history consistent with one of the injury patterns described earlier. Patients will often have generalized swelling over the midfoot. Plantar ecchymosis is a common finding but may not occur until several days after the injury (**Fig. 1**).[16] Patients typically are unable to bear weight on the affected limb and have significant pain with manipulation of the TMT joints. Patients with a proximal variant injury may have an unstable first ray with hypermobility and difficulty with a push off

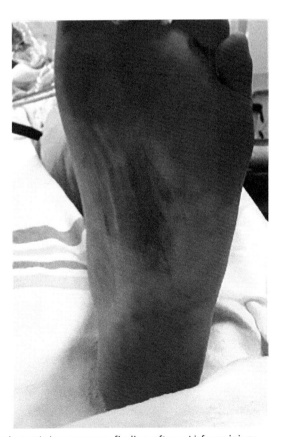

Fig. 1. Plantar ecchymosis is a common finding after a Lisfranc injury.

or heel rise.[10] Gentle stressing of the forefoot into plantarflexion and rotation may elicit significant pain during manipulation.

Imaging

Lisfranc injuries are a challenge to diagnose, partly because of the difficulty encountered with standard radiographic imaging. For example, many patients with so-called sprains present with non–WB (NWB) radiographs; although some investigators argue that midfoot instability, such as diastasis, avulsion, or subluxation, can be seen on NWB radiographs,[17] these films can be difficult to interpret. In the authors' opinion, a WB foot series is mandatory for the diagnosis of Lisfranc injuries and consists of an anteroposterior (AP) of both feet on the same film, a lateral, and a 30° oblique radiograph. It is important to explain to patients the importance of WB films for decision-making. If there is a high clinical suspicion for a Lisfranc injury but initial radiograph results are normal, it is recommended to obtain repeat WB radiographs in 7 to 10 days.[10] There are several important radiographic landmarks to rule out a Lisfranc injury:

1. On the AP view, the medial border of the second MT should align with the medial border of the middle cuneiform.
2. On the oblique view, the medial border of the fourth MT and the medial border of the cuboid should be aligned.
3. The lateral view should demonstrate alignment of the dorsal cortices of the MTs with their corresponding tarsal bones.
4. Avulsion fracture off the base of the second MT or medial cuneiform, known as the fleck sign, signifies disruption of the Lisfranc ligament.[18]
5. Assess the intercuneiform distance, comparing both feet, to rule out a proximal Lisfranc's variant (**Fig. 2**).

In 2002, Nunley and Vertullo[19] classified athletic midfoot injuries into 3 groups based on clinical findings, WB radiographs, and bone scintigraphy. Patients with stage I injury had pain only at the Lisfranc complex and increased uptake on bone scan, with negative radiographic findings. Stage II injuries exhibited diastasis between the first and second MT of 1 to 5 mm greater than that of the contralateral side, without loss of midfoot arch height. Diastasis greater than 5 mm and loss of midfoot arch height signified stage III injury. Nonsurgical treatment of stage I patients and surgical treatment of stage II and III patients led to an excellent result in 93% of cases.[19] One

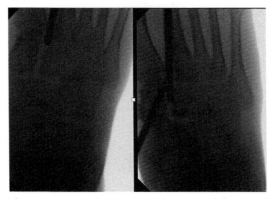

Fig. 2. Proximal Lisfranc's variant. The intercuneiform instability can be assessed by the arthroscope and fluoroscopy.

shortcoming of traditional classification systems is the lack of emphasis on the simple diastasis seen in low-energy athletic injuries. Also, no classification system has been published that takes in to account the intercuneiform or the navicular-cuneiform injury pattern.

Computed tomography (CT) scan is recommended in patients presenting with high-energy injuries, in which improved detection and delineation of fractures is required. However, subtle displacement may not be demonstrated on CT because this is a NWB study. It is useful to demonstrate fracture intra-articular involvement and comminution.

MRI can also be considered in patients with suspected Lisfranc injuries. Disruption of the plantar oblique component on MRI has been correlated with intraoperative instability on examination under anesthesia.[20] The investigators found that MRI demonstrating a rupture or grade 2 sprain of the plantar ligament between the first cuneiform and the bases of the second and third MTs is highly predictive of midfoot instability, and these patients should be treated with surgical stabilization.

MANAGEMENT

Lisfranc injuries represent a wide range of displacement from purely ligamentous to complex open fracture dislocations; therefore, a variety of nonsurgical and surgical management techniques and algorithms have been described. Hardcastle and colleagues[1] first reported their series of 69 patients with both high- and low-energy Lisfranc injuries in 1982 and found that the most important factor predictive of a successful outcome was the maintenance of an anatomic reduction, regardless of the inciting injury or the treatment modality used. Myerson's group,[12] in a review of 52 patients with 55 Lisfranc injuries, confirmed these findings. Although maintenance of anatomic alignment seems to be the critical factor in achieving a satisfactory result, it does not guarantee it. Other factors, such as the energy of the injury, cartilage damage, soft tissue injuries, and surgical technique, can compromise the outcome.

In cases whereby there is no documented instability or subluxation/diastasis on WB radiographs, patients are considered to have stable injuries and are managed nonoperatively. Initial treatment in this group usually consists of a period of 6 to 8 weeks of protected WB either in a short-leg cast or walker boot. According to Lewis and Anderson,[10] even a 1- to 2-week period of cast immobilization helps to speed recovery. Serial radiographs should be obtained to ensure there is no interval diastasis in the midfoot. Typically, patients recover in 8 to 16 weeks, although this varies widely among patients and respective injury patterns. Patients with minimal ambulatory ability, an insensate foot, or preexisting inflammatory arthritis may also be best treated nonsurgically. Reconstruction with midfoot arthrodesis can be performed later if pain persists.[5]

Most surgeons would agree that any TMT dislocation or fracture-dislocation leading to midfoot instability and/or malalignment, no matter how subtle, should be treated with operative stabilization.[4,10,13–15,21–23] However, debate remains as to the optimal surgical technique, with numerous surgical options described.

Closed reduction and internal fixation is one such technique; however, it is often unsuccessful secondary to interposed bone fragments or soft tissue structures and can be difficult not only to determine instability but also to achieve absolute anatomic alignment. Despite this, some investigators have reported good functional and radiological outcomes using this approach.[24] Open reduction and internal fixation (ORIF) is another option and can be performed via several different approaches. The traditional gold standard has been ORIF of the medial and middle columns with interosseous transarticular solid screw fixation to rigidly hold reduction while the ligaments heal.[10,11,18,19,21] Nevertheless, plating has become increasingly popular, as this technique avoids articular cartilage damage without the loss of fixation rigidity.[25–27] Recent biomechanical studies have shown similar rigidity between dorsal plates and transarticular screws in resisting TMT joint displacement with WB loads in cadaveric Lisfranc injury models.[27] The same model showed articular surface destruction of 2.0% in the medial cuneiform, 2.6% in the first MT, and 3.6% in the intermediate cuneiform and second MT created by a single 3.5-mm transarticular screw.[10,25,27] No significant differences regarding functional outcome, pain, and midterm arthritis have been shown between transarticular screws and joint-sparing plates.[26] Bridge plating has the additional advantage of avoiding broken hardware within the joint, which may be difficult to retrieve or lead to arthrosis. Long-term and prospective trials comparing transarticular screws versus dorsal plates are needed to define the best ORIF option.

Fusion Versus Open Reduction and Internal Fixation

No consensus exists regarding ORIF or primary arthrodesis (PA), in terms of which treatment leads to better function and less pain for Lisfranc injuries (**Table 1**). Some recent studies have suggested that PA may be a preferred technique for primarily ligamentous Lisfranc injuries. A small randomized prospective series of 41 patients with isolated primarily ligamentous Lisfranc joint injuries compared treatment with ORIF (n = 20) with PA of the medial 2 or 3 rays (n = 21).[28] In the ORIF group, 16 patients had hardware removal (HWR) at 6 months postoperatively and 5 patients underwent later midfoot arthrodesis for midfoot arthrosis. Four patients in the PA group had an HWR, and one patient (4.7%) required a revision fusion. The PA group rated their postoperative activity level at 92% of their preinjury level, compared with the ORIF group's rating of 65%. The investigators' conclusions were that PA provides a quicker recovery, superior function, and less secondary procedures compared with ORIF.

A recent study compared PA versus ORIF in low-energy Lisfranc injuries sustained by active-duty military personnel at a single institution.[29] Thirty-two patients were identified with the average age of 28 years. PA was performed in 14 patients and ORIF in 18. The implant removal rates, fitness test scores, return to military duty rates, and Foot and Ankle Ability Measure (FAAM) scores were compared. They concluded low-energy Lisfranc injuries treated with PA had a lower implant removal rate, an earlier return to full military activity, and better fitness test scores after 1 year; but there was no difference in FAAM scores after 3 years.[29] In contrast, another prospective randomized series of 32 patients comparing ORIF (n = 14) with PA (N = 18) showed no difference between groups at any time point in terms of postoperative 36-Item Short Form Health Survey and Short Musculoskeletal Function Assessment scores or final patient-reported satisfaction rates after surgery.[23] It is important to note that in this study, as a part of the investigators' standard protocol in the ORIF group, they removed the hardware in 11 of their 14 patients. Rammelt and colleagues[30] published a comparative cohort study over a period of 5 years comparing ORIF in 22 patients (23 feet) with secondary corrective arthrodesis (SCA) in 22 patients (22 feet) who presented with painful malunion at a mean of 22 months after injury. The mean American Orthopedic Foot and Ankle Society midfoot score was 81.4 after ORIF and 71.8 (35–88) after SCA. The investigators concluded that primary treatment by ORIF of TMT fracture-dislocations leads to improved functional results, earlier return to work, and greater patient satisfaction than SCA.

Smith and colleagues[3] performed a systematic review and a meta-analysis comparing ORIF with PA for acute Lisfranc injuries. In this level 1 therapeutic study, the investigators' objective was to determine if patients who sustain acute traumatic

Table 1
Comparison of Lisfranc Injuries treatment modalities

	Mulier et al,[33] 2002	Rammelt et al,[30] 2008	Henning et al,[23] 2009	Coetzee & Ly,[28] 2007	Cochran et al,[29] 2017
Patients (n)	12 PA, 16 ORIF	22 SCA, 23 ORIF	18 PA, 14 ORIF	20 PA, 21 ORIF	18 PA, 14 ORIF
Follow-up (mo)	30.1	36	24	42.5	36
Type of study	Retrospective	Retrospective	Prospective, randomized	Prospective, randomized	Retrospective
Return to work (mo)	NA	NA	NA	NA	PA 4.5, ORIF 6.7; $P<.05$
AOFAS midfoot score	NA	SCA 71.8, ORIF 81.0; $P = .031$	NA	PA 88.0, ORIF 68.6; $P = .005$	NA
SF-36	NA	NA	NS	NA	NA
FAAM	NA	NA	NA	NA	NS
Baltimore Painful Score	66% PA, 68% ORIF; NS	NA	NA	NA	NA
Additional surgery	17% PA, 12% ORIF; NS	NA	16.7% PA, 78.6% ORIF; $P<.05$	19% PA, 80% ORIF; $P<.05$	14% PA, 83% ORIF; $P<.05$
Maryland Foot Score	NA	SCA 76.2, ORIF 85.0; $P = .027$	NA	NA	NA
Radiographic anatomic reduction	Favor ORIF no P value reported	NS	94% PA, 100% ORIF; NS	NA	NA
SFMA	NA	NA	NS	NA	NA

Abbreviations: AOFAS, American Orthopedic Foot and Ankle Society; FAAM, Foot and Ankle Ability Measure; NA, not applicable; NS, not significant; SCA, secondary corrective arthrodesis; SFMA, Short Musculoskeletal Function Assessment; SF-36, 36-Item Short Form Health Survey.

Lisfranc injuries, either purely ligamentous or bony, achieve improved patient outcomes with PA compared with ORIF in terms of HWR, need for revision surgery, patient outcome measures, and anatomic reduction. They concluded that the ORIF group had a statistically significant higher rate of HWR compared with the PA group. There was no significant difference in patient-reported outcomes, revision surgery, and risk of nonanatomic alignment between the two groups. Of note, one of the studies analyzed regularly removed the hardware regardless of patient complaints. The investigators stated that surgeons should consider the increased risk of hardware removal, along with its associated morbidity, when considering ORIF for Lisfranc injuries treatment. Also, they report that each of the individual studies analyzed had design errors that may insert bias into the results of the meta-analysis. Therefore, they highlighted the importance of new randomized controlled trials to improve understanding of these interventions.[3]

Return to Sports Activities

As a result of Lisfranc injuries' considerable heterogeneity and injury mechanisms, there is a paucity of literature reporting the return to training for athletes who undergo surgery after a midfoot injury. A recently published study[31] of 28 National Football League (NFL) athletes who had a Lisfranc injury examined the length of time to return to play and tried to quantify the effect of the injury on the level of performance. More than 90% of the NFL players in the study returned to play at the professional level at an average of 11.1 months. Also, the investigators stated that although there was a trend toward decreased performance for both offensive and defensive players after the injury, this did not reach statistical significance. A similar study[32] of 17 professional soccer and rugby players with a follow-up of 2 years demonstrated that 94% of players who had a Lisfranc injury returned to training at 20 weeks and they were able to play at their prior level of sport at an average of 25 weeks. Another recently published study[29] retrospectively looked at low-energy Lisfranc injuries sustained by active-duty military personnel at a single institution. They compared return to full duty and outcomes during a fitness test for PA versus ORIF. The PA group returned to full duty at an average of 4.5 months, whereas the ORIF group returned at an average of 6.7 months ($P = .0066$). Also, the PA group ran the fitness test an average of 9 seconds per mile slower than their preoperative average, whereas the ORIF group ran it an average of 39 seconds slower per mile.

An important issue to consider is that current methods of treatment and fixation have serious potential postoperative complications, including wound complications, infection, and complex regional pain syndrome.[11,24] In an effort to minimize these soft tissue complications, techniques that minimize iatrogenic soft tissue trauma and dissection while still obtaining anatomic reduction of the TMT joint are needed. In the senior's author opinion, arthroscopically assisted surgery for Lisfranc injuries has a role in accomplishing a satisfactory joint reduction while minimizing soft tissue complications and possibly earlier return to daily and sports activities.

SENIOR AUTHOR'S PREFERRED SURGICAL TECHNIQUES

In younger, active patients the aim of management should be joint reduction and preservation. That being said, a comprehensive patient assessment and discussion about their expectations is required to make a surgical plan. Given that clear indications for each type of surgery are still evolving, the decision to operate and reduce, bridge plate, or fuse should be made on an individual patient basis.

JOINT REDUCTION AND FIXATION TECHNIQUE

Patients are placed on the operating table supine with a bump under the affected limb. A calf or thigh tourniquet is used depending on the method of anesthesia, and a 2.4-mm or 2.9-mm arthroscope and 3.5-mm shaver is used. The arthroscope is inserted into the first web space through an incision half way down the first MT shaft length (**Fig. 3**). The shaver is inserted more proximally and not used until it is clearly deeper than the neurovascular bundle. After debridement, the instability pattern is determined by visualization of the joints in the following order: the intercuneiform joint, the second TMT joint, the first TMT joint, and the space between the medial cuneiform and the second MT base (**Fig. 4**).

Percutaneous reduction is then achieved using a large fragment reduction or pelvic reduction forceps. The reduction is assessed via a combination of arthroscopy and fluoroscopy (**Fig. 5**). If the reduction is adequate, fixation is then achieved using full-thread screws or a suture anchor system depending on the instability pattern and fracture configuration, the age of patients, and their expectations. Ideally, if screws are to be used, they should be kept extra-articular. Screw fixation may be required from the second MT base to the medial cuneiform, between the cuneiforms, or across the first TMT joint if it is unstable using a headless screw.

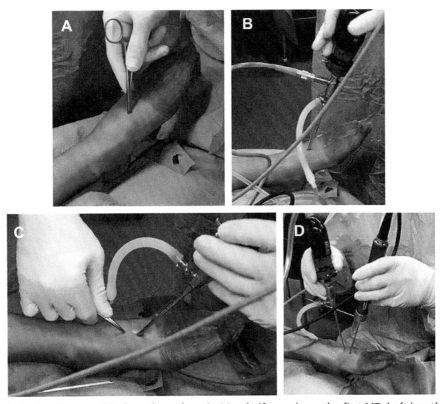

Fig. 3. (*A*) First portal is done through an incision half way down the first MT shaft length into the first web space. (*B*) The arthroscope is inserted. (*C*) The next portal is made more proximally, and the saver is not used until it is clearly deeper than the neurovascular bundle. (*D*) The arthroscope and the shaver can be used in both portals.

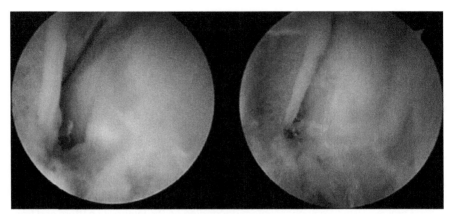

Fig. 4. After debridement the intercuneiform joint, the second TMT joint and the space between the medial cuneiform and the second MT base are visualized.

Alternatively, a suture anchor construct is used. In a similar manner, a percutaneous suture construct can be placed between the medial and intermediate cuneiforms and between the second MT base and the medial cuneiform (see **Fig. 5**). If the first MT is unstable, then a suture bridge technique may be required on the plantar medial aspect of the joint. Stress views and arthroscopy at the end of the procedure will determine if stability has been restored.

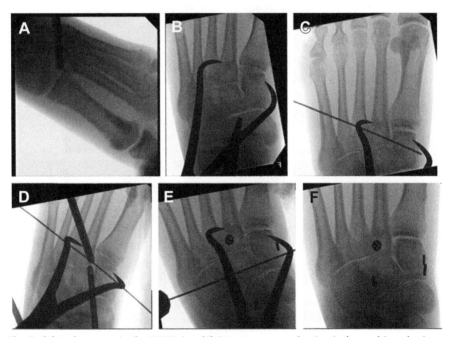

Fig. 5. (*A*) Arthroscope in the TMT joint. (*B*) Percutaneous reduction is then achieved using a large fragment reduction forceps or a pelvic reduction forceps. (*C, D*) The reduction is assessed using the arthroscope and fluoroscopy. (*E, F*) A percutaneous suture construct is placed between the medial and intermediate cuneiforms and between the second MT base and the medial cuneiform.

Postoperative care requires either 2 or 6 weeks NWB based on the stability of the construct. Patients are then remobilized with the assistance of physiotherapy and a walker boot. WB radiographs are obtained at 2, 6, and 12 weeks. Screw removal if required can be performed after 4 months.

FUSION TECHNIQUE

The senior author performs a TMT fusion for older patients, heavier patients, and patients with fractures of the bases of the MTs.

Procedure

The setup and instrumentation is similar to that outlined earlier; however, a 4.5 burr is also required. The space between the bases of the MTs and the cuneiforms is often easy to define due to the injury; however fluoroscopic guidance is recommended to confirm that the correct space is identified, of which particular care should be taken to identify the third TMT, which can often be challenging. If identification is difficult, further joint releases can also be performed with a small straight curette (**Fig. 6**). Once the correct joint spaces have been identified, using a burr, all the cartilage in the first, second, and third TMT joints is removed, as this may interfere with bone healing. After complete debridement, the joints are reduced percutaneously. The forefoot

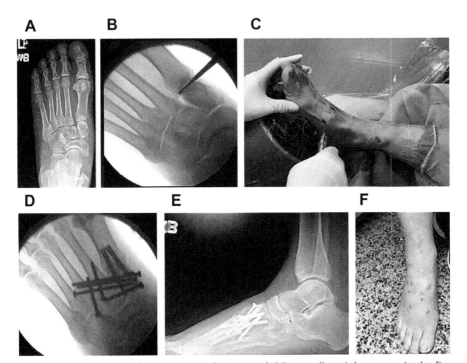

Fig. 6. TMT fusion. (*A*) Lisfranc injury can be assessed. (*B*) A small straight curette in the first TMT joint. (*C*) A 4.5 burr is placed in the TMT joint to remove remaining cartilage. (*D, E*) Headless full-threaded screws are required for the distal to proximal fixation of the first ray. The remainder of the fixation is performed using headed full-thread screws. (*F*) Clinical picture 6 weeks after TMT fusion.

should be corrected out of varus and external rotation, and the MT heads should be correctly aligned to ensure that none are plantar prominent.

Screw fixation is then achieved. Headless full-threaded screws are required for the distal to proximal fixation of the first ray. The remainder of the fixation can be performed using headed full-thread screws (see **Fig. 6**). Cannulated or noncannulated screws can be used depending on surgeon preference. A minimum of 2 screws should be placed across each joint to ensure stability. Bone graft can be added if the surgeon chooses.

At the end of the procedure the wounds are approximated with a nylon suture. Patients are placed in a below-knee slab and kept NWB for 6 weeks, with suture removal and wound review at 2 weeks. Radiographs are obtained at 6 and 12 weeks.

SUMMARY

Although considered relatively rare injuries, Lisfranc injuries of the TMT articulation must be promptly and correctly identified in patients presenting after a midfoot injury, as inadequate recognition and treatment result in substantial disability, deformity, and dysfunction. The diagnosis can usually be made with a routine history, a high index of suspicion, clinical examination, and WB radiographs. Outcomes after Lisfranc injuries strongly correlate with an anatomic and stable reduction and depend less on the severity of the injury, the amount of initial diastasis, or the pattern of displacement. There is not enough evidence to favor ORIF (with screws or plates) or PA; however, patients undergoing ORIF should be informed of the increased likelihood that they might subsequently require removal of hardware. In the authors' opinion, the minimally invasive arthroscopic technique is a reliable and valid therapeutic option to treat this severe type of injuries, which minimizes the risk of postoperative soft tissue complications and could have faster recovery time. The results of a well-designed, prospective randomized controlled trial will be required to confirm the authors' hypothesis regarding the effectiveness of this surgical technique.

REFERENCES

1. Hardcastle PH, Reschauer R, Kutscha-Lissberg E, et al. Injuries to the tarsometatarsal joint. Incidence, classification and treatment. J Bone Joint Surg Br 1982; 64(3):349–56.
2. Stavlas P, Roberts CS, Xypnitos FN, et al. The role of reduction and internal fixation of Lisfranc fracture–dislocations: a systematic review of the literature. Int Orthop 2010;34(8):1083–91.
3. Smith N, Stone C, Furey A. Does open reduction and internal fixation versus primary arthrodesis improve patient outcomes for lisfranc trauma? a systematic review and meta-analysis. Clin Orthop Relat Res 2016;474(6):1445–52.
4. Coetzee JC. Making sense of lisfranc injuries. Foot Ankle Clin 2008;13(4): 695–704.
5. Watson TS, Shurnas PS, Denker J. Treatment of lisfranc joint injury: current concepts. J Am Acad Orthop Surg 2010;18(12):718–28.
6. Meyer SA, Callaghan JJ, Albright JP, et al. Midfoot sprains in collegiate football players. Am J Sports Med 1994;22(3):392–401.
7. Curtis MJ, Myerson M, Szura B. Tarsometatarsal joint injuries in the athlete. Am J Sports Med 1993;21(4):497–502.
8. de Palma L, Santucci A, Sabetta SP, et al. Anatomy of the Lisfranc joint complex. Foot Ankle Int 1997;18(6):356–64.

9. Komenda GA, Myerson MS, Biddinger KR. Results of arthrodesis of the tarsometatarsal joints after traumatic injury. J Bone Joint Surg Am 1996;78(11):1665–76.

10. Lewis JS Jr, Anderson RB. Lisfranc injuries in the athlete. Foot Ankle Int 2016; 37(12):1374–80.

11. Benirschke SK, Meinberg E, Anderson SA, et al. Fractures and dislocations of the midfoot: lisfranc and chopart injuries. J Bone Joint Surg Am 2012;94(14):1–13.

12. Myerson MS, Fisher RT, Burgess AR, et al. Fracture dislocations of the tarsometatarsal joints: end results correlated with pathology and treatment. Foot Ankle 1986;6(5):225–42.

13. Eleftheriou KI, Rosenfeld PF. Lisfranc injury in the athlete. Foot Ankle Clin 2013; 18(2):1–18.

14. DeOrio M, Erickson M, Usuelli FG, et al. Lisfranc injuries in sport. Foot Ankle Clin 2009;14(2):169–86.

15. Myerson MS, Cerrato R. Current management of tarsometatarsal injuries in the athlete. Instr Course Lect 2009;58(2):583–94.

16. Ross G, Cronin R, Hauzenblas J, et al. Ovid: plantar ecchymosis sign: a clinical aid to diagnosis of occult lisfranc tarsometatarsal injuries. J Orthop Trauma 1996; 10(2):119–22.

17. Seo D-K, Lee H-S, Lee KW, et al. Nonweightbearing radiographs in patients with a subtle lisfranc injury. Foot Ankle Int 2017;38(10):1120–5.

18. Weatherford BM, Bohay DR, Anderson JG. Open reduction and internal fixation versus primary arthrodesis for lisfranc injuries. Foot Ankle Clin 2017;22(1):1–14.

19. Nunley JA, Vertullo CJ. Classification, investigation, and management of midfoot sprains: lisfranc injuries in the athlete. Am J Sports Med 2002;30(6):871–8.

20. Raikin SM, Elias I, Dheer S, et al. Prediction of midfoot instability in the subtle Lisfranc injury. Comparison of magnetic resonance imaging with intraoperative findings. J Bone Joint Surg Am 2009;91(4):892–9.

21. Welck MJ, Zinchenko R, Rudge B. Lisfranc injuries. Injury 2015;46(4):536–41.

22. Krause F, Schmid T, Weber M. Current Swiss techniques in management of lisfranc injuries of the foot. Foot Ankle Clin 2016;21(2):335–50.

23. Henning JA, Jones CB, Sietsema DL, et al. Open reduction internal fixation versus primary arthrodesis for lisfranc injuries: a prospective randomized study. Foot Ankle Int 2009;30(10):913–22.

24. Vosbikian M, O'Neil JT, Piper C, et al. Outcomes after percutaneous reduction and fixation of low-energy lisfranc injuries. Foot Ankle Int 2017;38(7):710–5.

25. Stern RE, Assal M. Dorsal multiple plating without routine transarticular screws for fixation of lisfranc injury. Orthopedics 2014;37(12):815–9.

26. Hu S-J, Chang S-M, Li X-H, et al. Outcome comparison of Lisfranc injuries treated through dorsal plate fixation versus screw fixation. Acta Ortop Bras 2014;22(6): 315–20.

27. Alberta FG, Aronow MS, Barrero M, et al. Ligamentous Lisfranc joint injuries: a biomechanical comparison of dorsal plate and transarticular screw fixation. Foot Ankle Int 2005;26(6):462–73.

28. Coetzee JC, Ly TV. Treatment of primarily ligamentous Lisfranc joint injuries: primary arthrodesis compared with open reduction and internal fixation. Surgical technique. J Bone Joint Surg Am 2007;89(Suppl 2 Pt.1):122–7.

29. Cochran G, Renninger C, Tompane T, et al. Primary arthrodesis versus open reduction and internal fixation for low-energy lisfranc injuries in a young athletic population. Foot Ankle Int 2017;38(9):957–63.

30. Rammelt S, Schneiders W, Schikore H, et al. Primary open reduction and fixation compared with delayed corrective arthrodesis in the treatment of tarsometatarsal (Lisfranc) fracture dislocation. J Bone Joint Surg Br 2008;90(11):1499–506.

31. McHale KJ, Rozell JC, Milby AH, et al. Outcomes of lisfranc injuries in the national football league. Am J Sports Med 2016;44(7):1810–7.

32. Deol RS, Roche A, Calder JDF. Return to training and playing after acute lisfranc injuries in elite professional soccer and rugby players. Am J Sports Med 2016; 44(1):166–70.

33. Mulier T, Reynders P, Dereymaeker G, et al. Severe Lisfranc Injuries: Primary Arthrodesis or ORIF? Foot Ankle Int 2002;23(10):902–5.

Turf Toe Injury - Current Concepts and an Updated Review of Literature

Tim M. Clough, FRCS (Tr&Orth)*,
Haroon Majeed, MRCS, MSC, FEBOT, FRCS (Tr&Orth)

KEYWORDS

• Turf toe • Plantar plate injury • Hallux MTP joint • Sesamoiditis

KEY POINTS

• Turf toe injuries can be a disabling if not recognized and treated early.
• A high index of suspicion, based on the mechanism of injury and appropriate imaging, helps in the timely diagnosis.
• These injuries are frequently known to occur on artificial playing surfaces, because of the increased traction at the shoe-surface interface.
• Stress and instability testing are key components to assess the need for surgical intervention.
• Accurate timely diagnosis and treatment can allow full return to physical activities for most athletes, back to their pre-injury level.

INTRODUCTION

Turf toe is a general term used to describe various injuries to the hallux plantar capsule, plantar muscles, and the sesamoid complex. Its current incidence and epidemiology remain unknown, as most of the literature describes small case series and addresses diagnosis and treatment rather than epidemiology.[1] It is frequently seen in elite American football players, and typically has been noticed to occur with the use of light-weight, flexible shoes on artificial turf.[2] The turf toe injury was originally described by Bowers and Martin in 1976. They noted an average turf toe injury incidence among American football players of 5 to 6 players per team per season, and speculated that this apparent increase in these soft tissue injuries to the hallux followed the introduction of firm artificial playing surfaces (Astroturf), and lighter more flexible running shoes.[3] The injury was further described by Rodeo and colleagues[4] in 1990, who found that in a survey of 80 active players, up to 45% had suffered

The authors have nothing to disclose.
Department of Foot & Ankle Surgery, Wrightington Hospital, Hall Lane, Appley Bridge, Wrightington, Lancashire WN6 9EP, UK
* Corresponding author.
E-mail address: tim.clough@doctors.org.uk

turf toe injuries in their professional careers, of which 83% occurred on an artificial turf. More recently however, George and colleagues[1] in 2014, reported the incidence of turf toe injuries to be much lower among collegiate American football players over a 5-year period (0.83% of all injuries reported – equating to 1 turf toe injury per team every other season), suggesting that this was due in part to the introduction of more modern artificial turf designs, with use of softer sand and/or rubber infill rather than concrete. Nevertheless, they still reported an 85% higher risk of turf toe injury when playing on artificial surfaces compared with grass.

In the United Kingdom, the incidence of turf toe in apparent similar elite level collision/contact sports (professional rugby) is much lower than these early American football figures, with Pearce and colleagues[5] reporting only 17 cases out of 147 foot and ankle injuries among 899 professional rugby union players from 14 English Premiership Rugby Union clubs over 4 seasons. This equates to around 1 turf toe injury per team every fourth season. The incidence in the United Kingdom, in the English Premier League (soccer), is even rarer, with only isolated case reports available.[6] These incidence differences across the sports are presumably because of differences in exposure to the precipitating injury mechanism, difference in pitch mechanics (with most pitches in the United Kingdom being grass rather than artificial), pitches in the United Kingdom being heavily watered before play for ball speed, and differences in the playing shoe mechanics across the sports.

Turf toe injury can easily be overlooked, and therefore, requires a careful assessment on initial presentation. This article aims to review the complex anatomy, clinical presentation, and current literature on management of turf toe injuries.

ANATOMY

The 2 hallux sesamoids lie within the flexor hallucis brevis (FHB) tendon and sit on the plantar surface of the forefoot, directly underlying the first metatarsal head. A bony ridge on the undersurface of the first metatarsal head, known as the crista, separates the sesamoids, delineating the medial and lateral metatarsal-sesamoidal joints.[7] The medial sesamoid is more frequently bipartite than the lateral sesamoid. A dense fibrous band, the plantar plate, connects the hallux sesamoids to the plantar base of the first proximal phalanx, forming the plantar aspect of the first metatarsophalangeal joint (MTPJ) capsule.[7] The abductor and adductor hallucis tendons insert on the medial and lateral bases of the proximal phalanx, respectively, and also give off small attachments to the sesamoids. Medial and lateral collateral ligaments, between the first metatarsal head and the proximal phalanx, provide valgus and varus stability.[8]

BIOMECHANICS

Primary stability of the first MTPJ is provided by the capsuloligamentous structures and short flexor complex, with a small contribution from the fairly shallow cavity of the proximal phalanx in which the metatarsal head articulates.[8] The medial sesamoid is larger and longer than the lateral sesamoid and tends to rest more distally. In addition, the medial sesamoid is situated more directly under the metatarsal head and sustains greater weight-bearing forces. The sesamoids function to reduce the friction and dissipate the force at the MTPJ.[9] Additionally, the sesamoids elevate the first metatarsal head and thereby increase the lever arm of the FHB, and indirectly, of the flexor hallucis longus (FHL) to mechanically augment flexion and push-off strength at the MTPJ.[10,11] The capsuloligamentous complex of the first MTP joint is a thick and strong soft tissue complex and is considered critical to maintain the normal function at this joint, especially during athletic activities. During normal gait, this complex withstands

40% to 60% of the body weight, which can increase to as much as 8 times body weight during running and jumping.[8]

MECHANISM OF INJURY

The usual mechanism of turf toe injury is an axial load of the first MTPJ in a fixed equinus foot. The 2 most common examples of this seen in American football players are with either violent explosive, but resisted, push-off from the stance position, or when the foot is fixed to the ground, with an elevated heel, and another player lands on the back of the foot. The load drives the hallux MTPJ into hyperextension, leading to attenuation or disruption of the plantar joint complex. This can potentially lead to a spectrum of injuries, ranging from a sprain of plantar structures to frank dorsal dislocation of the toe. With unrestricted extension, potential injury can occur to the articular surface or subchondral bone. Some variations of turf toe injury have also been described, the most common of which involves a valgus-directed force, resulting in greater injury to the medial ligamentous structures and tibial sesamoid complex. As a result, there is a relative contracture of the lateral sesamoid complex and adductor hallucis, leading to a traumatic hallux valgus deformity.[1,8]

CLINICAL PRESENTATION

Turf toe injury can be subtle. A high index of suspicion must be kept in a patient with an injury to the first MTPJ. The injury is a spectrum and can range from a mild sprain to complete disruption of the soft tissue structures. Patients with acute injury present with swelling, plantar bruising, and pain with weightbearing, especially during push-off phase.[12] Point tenderness can prove to be a critical part of the assessment, along with palpation of the collateral ligaments, dorsal capsule, and plantar sesamoid complex. Tenderness proximal to the sesamoids suggests a low-grade injury, and distal to the sesamoids suggests a more serious and often unstable injury. Range of motion should be screened through flexion and extension to assess the relevant tendons, careful varus and valgus stress assessing the collateral ligaments, and a dorsoplantar drawer test assessing the competence of the plantar plate.[9]

IMAGING

Obtaining appropriate imaging of the MTPJ is important to evaluate the extent of injury, formulate a treatment plan, and estimate the prognosis for the patient. As a part of initial assessment, weightbearing anteroposterior (AP) and lateral radiographs of the foot, along with axial sesamoid views, are recommended. This will help to identify various abnormalities including bony abnormalities, proximal migration of the sesamoid(s), bipartite sesamoid, or sesamoid diastasis.

There may not be an obvious bony abnormality, but a small fleck of bone may be visible, suggesting capsular avulsion. Location of the sesamoids under the metatarsal head is important to assess, and may require a comparison view of the other foot, to allow assessment of the sesamoid-to-joint distances on either side. The distal sesamoid-to-joint distance should be no greater than 3 mm (tibial) and 2.7 mm (fibular) compared with those on the contralateral side. Proximal migration of one, of both, sesamoids is suggestive of plantar plate rupture,[13] and a separation of 10.4 mm or more on the tibial side, or 13.3 mm on the fibular side, is 99% predictive of rupture of the plantar plate.[7] In these cases, a forced dorsiflexion view should be considered under local anesthetic, which would fail to show any distal tracking of the sesamoids with big toe extension. In a cadaveric study, Waldrop and colleagues[14] found that an increase of 3 mm or more in the distance from the sesamoid to the proximal phalanx, on a lateral-dorsiflexion stress radiograph, predicted a severe injury to the plantar plate that would require surgical intervention in a living subject.

Presence of a bipartite sesamoid on the plain radiograph is not uncommon, and again, comparative views of the other foot may help determine if this is a bipartite sesamoid, sesamoid fracture, or sesamoid diastasis. Favinger and colleagues,[15] in a review of 671 foot radiograph series, reported that in the appropriate clinical setting, sesamoid diastasis should be considered when the sesamoid interval in the bi- or mul-tipartitie sesamoid of the hallux exceeds 2 mm on a routine AP radiograph.

Establishing the diagnosis on plain radiography alone can often be difficult. A computed tomography (CT) scan may be obtained, to further evaluate the size and comminution of the fragments.[16] MRI is commonly performed to assess the extent of the injury (**Figs. 1** and **2**) and to help assess the soft tissue disruption.[17] MRI is also helpful to identify the presence of bone marrow edema or a loose body, which has been shown to be related to chronic stiffness, early MTPJ arthrosis, and ongoing pain at a later stage.[16] Even after radiographic imaging, fractures may be mistaken for bipartite sesamoids and therefore need to be clinically evaluated carefully (**Fig. 3**).

CLASSIFICATION

Clanton described a classification system, which was further modified by Anderson, and is based on the extent of injury.[8,9] Grade I injury is a sprain of the capsule without a loss of continuity, normal range of motion, no visible ecchymosis, ability to bear weight, normal plain radiographs, and intact soft tissues on MRI with surrounding edema. Grade II injury is a partial tear of the plantar plate and capsule, with obvious swelling and ecchymosis, painful range of motion, and difficulty in weight-bearing. Radiographs may still be normal, but MRI demonstrates soft tissue edema and high signal intensity that does not extend through the full thickness of the plantar plate. Grade III injury is a complete tear with loss of continuity of the plantar plate and

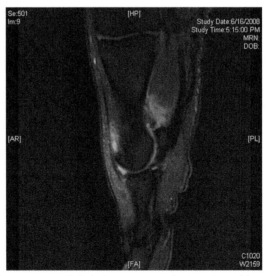

Fig. 1. Acute turf toe injury – full-thickness tear and retraction of lateral head of *Flexor Hallucis Brevis*.

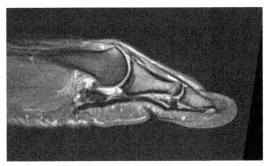

Fig. 2. Tear of plantar plate and intersesamoid ligament of D1.

capsule. Concomitant injuries may also be found, including sesamoid fracture and dorsal metatarsal articular impaction.[8]

TREATMENT

There are no prospective randomized controlled trials in the literature to compare the treatment options for turf toe injuries. Only a few retrospective case series exist, with level IV evidence primarily suggesting nonoperative management for grade I and II injuries, and most grade III injuries.[3,18,19] Only 1 case series is available that supports the operative treatment for some cases of grade III injuries.[20]

CONSERVATIVE TREATMENT

Regardless of the stage of injury, the initial treatment is similar and includes general measure of rest, elevation, ice packs, and pain management for first 48 to 72 hours. For the purpose of immobilization, a walking boot, short leg cast, or a toe spica extension in slight flexion is recommended, to keep the plantar soft tissues in a rested position.[8]

Grade I

In cases of grade I injuries, along with the initial supportive measures, the great toe usually gets benefit from taping in a slightly plantarflexed position, with the use of a stiff-soled shoe or individualized orthotics with a Morton extension. Care must be taken in using the tape, because it can potentially limit circulation because of swelling

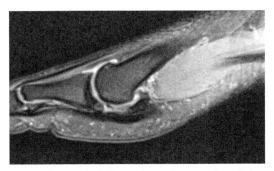

Fig. 3. Tear of D1 plantar plate and phalangeal attachment of medial sesamoid-phalangeal ligament with some proximal retraction to the sesamoid.

in the initial phase of injury.[18] In cases of medially based injury, a toe separator may be beneficial to prevent the development of traumatic hallux valgus. As the acute phase starts to settle, gentle range of motion may be commenced, with return to low impact activities in 3 to 5 days.[10] Athletes with grade I injury must be advised not to underestimate their injury. Rest is an important aspect of treatment, and athletic activity can worsen the sprain and its symptoms.

Grade II

In cases of grade II injuries, the supportive treatment is the same as for grade I injuries; however, the athlete is likely to lose about 2 weeks of playing time. After the resolution of acute pain and swelling, early gentle passive motion is started along with low-impact activities with the use of toe protection. When the toe is able to tolerate low-impact exercise, the athlete can gradually be allowed to progress to higher impact activities of running, push-off, jumping, and pivoting.

Grade III

In cases of grade III injuries, the treatment regime again is as previously described for grade I and II injuries; however, the athlete may require 8 weeks of immobilization for appropriate recovery. The first MTPJ should have 50° to 60° of painless passive dorsiflexion before considering returning to running or high-impact activities. It may take up to 6 months for complete resolution of symptoms in cases of a severe injury.[8]

SURGICAL TREATMENT

Surgery for turf toe injuries is rarely indicated. Anderson described indications for surgery in grade III injuries to include large capsular avulsions with an unstable MTPJ, diastasis of bipartite sesamoid, sesamoid fracture, retraction of sesamoid, traumatic hallux valgus, vertical instability, loose body in MTPJ, chondral injury, and failed conservative treatment with persistent pain.[20] The aim of surgery is to restore the normal anatomy and stability of the MTPJ. In case of isolated capsular disruption, the plantar soft tissue structures may be primarily repaired with end-to-end sutures. In case of a traumatic hallux valgus suggesting medial soft tissue injury, an adductor tenotomy is performed percutaneously to balance the MTPJ. The medial eminence may also require resection to allow a capsulodesis. In case of sesamoid fracture, care should be taken to preserve as much bone as possible.

Occasionally, complete sesamoidectomy becomes necessary,[21] although it is best avoided if at all possible. In these cases, some authors have suggested the interposition of the abductor hallucis tendon into the defect to provide collagen to the site of injury and allow the abductor to function as a plantar restraint to dorsiflexion.[8] Depending on the fragment size, some authors have suggested an open reduction and internal fixation, which although difficult, may be achievable using small screws (1.3 mm).[16]

Classically, acute repair or reconstruction of the plantar capsular ligamentous complex is performed through a medial incision or a J incision; however a 2-incision technique is also used for improved access to the lateral aspect of the plantar plate.[10] Depending on the pattern of the tear, it can be difficult to pass sutures through the disrupted capsuloligamentous complex without further damaging the tissue and without the need to further extend the surgical exposure in order to facilitate a repair.[22]

Following surgery, the foot is immobilized with a toe spica splint in plantarflexion, and the patient is kept nonweightbearing for 4 weeks. Gentle passive range of motion is commenced at 1 week, avoiding excessive dorsiflexion. At 4 weeks, protected weightbearing is commenced in a boot or heel-loading shoe, along with active range-of-movement exercises out of splint. At 8 weeks, a stiff-soled shoe and a turf toe plate are advised to prevent hyperextension, and weightbearing is advanced as tolerated with protective taping and shoe wear. Impact activities are introduced at around 12 weeks.[8,9,23]

DISCUSSION

Turf toe can be a debilitating sports injury for the athlete, because the first ray is pivotal in one's ability to jump, accelerate, and cut.[22] The plantar ligaments and tendons are the key structures in maintaining stability and congruent motion at the first MTPJ.[18] Turf toe injury represents a significant injury that requires early recognition and treatment, because a neglected injury can lead to long-term detrimental effects, including decreased athletic performance, restricted first MTPJ motion, degenerative arthritis, hallux valgus deformity, and potentially a premature end to one's sporting career.[24] It is critical to establish whether the injury is stable or unstable before planning management.

Bowers and Martin in their retrospective case-series review reported 27 grade I injuries in collegiate football players.[3] The patients were treated with ice packs 3 times a day until soft tissue edema resolved. They were allowed to return to sports, with the use of protective taping and a firm shoe insole when they had either minimal to no pain.

Coker and colleagues[19] reported a retrospective case series of 8 turf toe injuries in collegiate football players. Initial treatment included a period of rest with a plaster cast, crutches, and heel weightbearing. Players were allowed to progress on to walking, running, and high-impact activities when pain resolved, with the use of taping and modification of shoewear. A few patients underwent surgery, as pain remained a persistent problem beyond 3 weeks of injury; however, the demographics of these patients were not fully described in their study. The long-term problems reported in this series were pain and stiffness.

Clanton and colleagues[18] reported 56 turf toe injuries in their retrospective review over a 14-year period. Fifty-four injuries (96%) occurred in football players on synthetic turf. Players were initially treated with ice, compression, nonsteroidal anti-inflammatory medications (NSAIDs), and rest, followed by gradual mobilization and return to sports when pain resolved. A combination of taping and a stiff shoe was used in all players upon return to sports. Following this regimen, 53 of the 56 players (95%) were able to return to sports; however, half of these patients reported some level of ongoing pain and stiffness over a period of 5-year follow-up. In their series, only 1 patient required surgery. This patient had an avulsion fracture of the first metatarsal and required 56 days to return to play.

The only available study reporting the outcome of surgical intervention is a retrospective case series review by Anderson.[20] In this series, 9 patients underwent surgery for grade III injuries with radiographic evidence of sesamoid migration and disruption of the plantar soft tissue complex on MRI scans. The duration from injury to surgery ranged from 1 week to 7 months, with follow-up from 1 to 10 years, via questionnaires. Repair of the plantar plate complex was performed in all patients. In 4 patients (44%), sesamoidectomies were also performed because of fragmentation or degeneration, with abductor hallucis tendon transferred to fill in the defect in 3 of these patients. Seven patients (78%) were able to return to full level of activity with minimal pain. The remaining 2 patients were unable to return to full athletic activity, one because of persistent pain despite a stable toe; the other developed severe hallux rigidus.

George and colleagues[1] reviewed the data of 147 turf toe injuries among collegiate football players over 5 seasons. They reported that the athletes were nearly 14 times more likely to sustain the injury during games compared with practice/training sessions, with a mean loss of 10 days of athletic participation because of injury. There was a significantly higher injury rate on artificial surfaces, compared with natural grass. Most injuries occurred as a result of contact with the playing surface (35.4%) or contact with another player (32.7%). Nonoperative measures were the mainstay of treatment, leading to satisfactory recovery and return to sports. Fewer than 2% of these players required surgery.

SUMMARY

Turf toe injuries can be a disabling injury if not recognized and treated early. A high index of suspicion, based on the mechanism of injury and appropriate imaging, helps in the timely diagnosis. These injuries are frequently seen to occur on artificial playing surfaces, because of the increased traction at the shoe-surface interface. Stress and instability testing are key components to assess the need for surgical intervention. Accurate timely diagnosis and treatment can allow full return to physical activities for most of these athletes, back to their preinjury level. By contrast, a neglected injury can lead to long-term detrimental effects including decreased athletic performance, restricted 1st MTPJ motion, degenerative arthritis, hallux valgus deformity, and potentially a premature end to one's sporting career. The use of stiffer-soled shoes may help reduce these injuries, but also helps during the rehabilitation period. The choice of operative versus nonoperative treatment for these injuries requires more thorough research, to establish definitive guidelines for intervention.

REFERENCES

1. George E, Harris AH, Dragoo JL, et al. Incidence and risk factors for turf toe injuries in intercollegiate football: data from the National Collegiate Athletic Association injury surveillance system. Foot Ankle Int 2014;35(2):108–15.
2. Childs SG. The pathogenesis and biomechanics of turf toe. Orthop Nurs 2006; 25(4):276–80 [quiz: 281–2].
3. Bowers KD Jr, Martin RB. Turf-toe: a shoe-surface related football injury. Med Sci Sports 1976;8(2):81–3.
4. Rodeo SA, O'Brien S, Warren RF, et al. Turf-toe: an analysis of metatarsophalangeal joint sprains in professional football players. Am J Sports Med 1990;18(3): 280–5.
5. Pearce CJ, Brooks J, Kemp SP, et al. The epidemiology of foot injuries in professional rugby union players. Foot Ankle Surg 2011;17:113–8.
6. Roche AJ, Calder JD. An atraumatic turf toe in an elte soccer player - a stress related phenomenon? Foot Ankle Surg 2014;20:71–3.
7. Schein AJ, Skalski MR, Patel DB, et al. Turf toe and sesamoiditis: what the radiologist needs to know. Clin Imaging 2015;39(3):380–9.
8. Clanton TO, Ford JJ. Turf toe injury. Clin Sports Med 1994;13(4):731–41.
9. McCormick JJ, Anderson RB. Turf toe: anatomy, diagnosis, and treatment. Sports Health 2010;2(6):487–94.
10. McCormick JJ, Anderson RB. The great toe: failed turf toe, chronic turf toe, and complicated sesamoid injuries. Foot Ankle Clin 2009;14(2):135–50.
11. Aper RL, Saltzman CL,, Brown TD. The effect of hallux sesamoid excision on the flexor hallucis longus moment arm. Clin Orthop Relat Res 1996;(325):209–17.

12. Kadakia AR, Molloy A. Current concepts review: traumatic disorders of the first metatarsophalangeal joint and sesamoid complex. Foot Ankle Int 2011;32(8): 834–9.
13. Prieskorn D, Graves SC, Smith RA. Morphometric analysis of the plantar plate apparatus of the first metatarsophalangeal joint. Foot Ankle 1993;14(4):204–7.
14. Waldrop NE 3rd, Zirker CA, Wijdicks CA, et al. Radiographic evaluation of plantar plate injury: an in vitro biomechanical study. Foot Ankle Int 2013;34(3):403–8.
15. Favinger JL, Porrino JA, Richardson ML, et al. Epidemiology and imaging appearance of the normal Bi-/multipartite hallux sesamoid bone. Foot Ankle Int 2015;36(2):197–202.
16. Drakos MC, Fiore R, Murphy C, et al. Plantar-plate disruptions: "the severe turf-toe injury." three cases in contact athletes. J Athl Train 2015;50(5):553–60.
17. Crain JM, Phancao JP, Stidham K. MR imaging of turf toe. Magn Reson Imaging Clin N Am 2008;16(1):93–103, vi.
18. Clanton TO, Butler JE,, Eggert A. Injuries to the metatarsophalangeal joints in athletes. Foot Ankle 1986;7(3):162–76.
19. Coker TP, Arnold JA,, Weber DL. Traumatic lesions of the metatarsophalangeal joint of the great toe in athletes. Am J Sports Med 1978;6(6):326–34.
20. Anderson RB. Turf toe injuries of the hallux metatarsophalangeal joint. Tech Foot Ankle Surg 2002;1(2):102–11.
21. Richardson EG. Injuries to the hallucal sesamoids in the athlete. Foot Ankle 1987; 7(4):229–44.
22. Doty JF,, Coughlin MJ. Turf toe repair: a technical note. Foot Ankle Spec 2013; 6(6):452–6.
23. McCormick JJ, Anderson RB. Rehabilitation following turf toe injury and plantar plate repair. Clin Sports Med 2010;29(2):313–23.
24. Coughlin MJ, Kemp TJ, Hirose CB. Turf toe: soft tissue and osteocartilaginous injury to the first metatarsophalangeal joint. Phys Sportsmed 2010;38(1):91–100.

Plantar Plate Injury and Angular Toe Deformity

Craig C. Akoh, MD[a],*, Phinit Phisitkul, MD[b]

KEYWORDS

- Lesser toe deformity • Plantar plate • Crossover toe

KEY POINTS

- Lesser toe plantar plate injuries at the metatarsophalangeal (MTP) joint are a common source of metatarsalgia.
- The fibrocartilaginous plantar plate is the most important static stabilizer of the MTP joint.
- Plantar plate tears found on MRI imaging are typically lateral full-thickness tears at the proximal phalanx insertion.
- The goals of surgery should be to restore a plantigrade position of the lesser toes during the static stance position and to correct angular deformity.
- Combined Weil osteotomy and plantar plate repair yields favorable pain relief and angular deformity correction for patients who fail conservative treatment.

INTRODUCTION

Lesser toe plantar plate injuries and angular deformity at the metatarsophalangeal (MTP) joint are a common source of metatarsalgia.[1] Coughlin[2] first described crossover toe deformity in 1987, with the second MTP joint being the most commonly affected.[3] Chronic lesser toe deformities are most commonly seen in women older than 50 years.[3–5] In Kaz and Coughlin's[6] series of 169 patients, 86% of patients with second toe instability were female and the mean age at the time of surgical intervention was of 59 years old. Similarly, Nery and colleagues[3] found in their series of 28 patients (55 lesser MTP joints) that 73% of the study cohort were women. They also found that the second MTP joint was most commonly affected (63% of cases), followed by the third MTP (32%) and fourth MTP (4%).[3] The most common cause of lesser toe plantar plate instability is chronic attritional wear of the plantar

Disclosure Statement: The authors report the following potential conflicts of interest or sources of funding: P.P. is a paid consultant for Arthrex and Restor 3D, receives royalties from Arthrex; and has stock/stock options in First Ray and Mortise Medical. Full ICMJE author disclosure forms are available for this article online, as supplementary material.
^a Orthopaedic Department, University of Iowa Hospital and Clinics, 200 Hawkins Drive, Iowa City, IA 52242, USA; ^b Orthopaedic Surgery, Tri-State Specialist, LLC, Suite 300, 2730 Pierce Street, Sioux City, IA 51104, USA
* Corresponding author.
E-mail address: ccakoh@gmail.com

Foot Ankle Clin N Am 23 (2018) 703–713
https://doi.org/10.1016/j.fcl.2018.07.010
1083-7515/18/Published by Elsevier Inc.

capsuloligamentous structures.[3] Chronic synovitis is another potential cause and is commonly seen in individuals with rheumatoid arthritis.[7,8] In rare cases, lesser toe instability can be associated with acute athlete injuries.[3,9–14] Other extrinsic factors for lesser toe plantar plate instability include overloading of the lesser toes due to tight shoe wear, hypermobile first ray, and a long second metatarsal.[3]

ANATOMY

The MTP capsuloligamentous complex of the lesser toes is a complex structure composed of static and dynamic stabilizers.[15] The most important static stabilizer is the fibrocartilaginous plantar plate, which represents a rectangular confluence of the plantar synovium and periosteum of the metatarsal bone. The plantar plate's main functions are to resist dorsal instability of the MTP joint, to act as a cushion to offload compressive forces during gait, and to support the windlass mechanism through its attachments with the longitudinal fibers of the plantar fascia.[16–18] In Johnston and colleagues'[17] cadaveric study, they found that the average thickness of the plantar plate ranged from 2 to 5 mm.[16,17] Deland and colleagues[16] also performed a cadaveric study and found that the average length of the plantar plate was 20 mm for the second and third toes and 17 mm for the fourth and fifth toes. The intraarticular portion of the plantar is composed of longitudinally oriented fibrocartilage tissue that resists tensile forces. Conversely, the extraarticular portion of the plantar plate is composed of a loose meshwork of connective tissue.[16] The collateral ligaments are another important structure in maintaining coronal plane stability of the lesser MTP joints. The collateral ligaments originate from the lateral tubercle of the metatarsal head and travel in an oblique orientation to insert onto the plantar base of the proximal phalanx. The accessory ligaments are fan shaped and attach directly onto the dorsal aspect of the plantar plate. The lateral collateral ligaments tend to be thicker and stronger than the medial ligaments. Several additional structures attach to the dorsal aspect of the plantar plate, including the transverse lamina of the extensor hood and interossei muscles. Plantar attachments to the plantar plate include the deep transverse intermetatarsal ligament and the flexor tendon sheath.[15,16] Dynamic stabilizers of the lesser toes serve an important role in the formation of angular instability of the lesser toes. At the MTP joint, the lumbrical muscles pass plantar to the deep transverse metatarsal ligament and the interossei muscles travel dorsal to the deep transverse metatarsal ligament.[19] Other dynamic structures include the flexor digitorum tendon sheath, transverse head of the adductor hallucis, and vertical fibers of the plantar aponeurosis. Muscle imbalance of these structures can also exacerbate MTP joint deformity.

BIOMECHANICS

The forefoot plays a significant role in load bearing during locomotion.[20,21] During the heel-off phase, the forefoot can experience up to 120% of the total body load, predisposing the MTP joint to sheer injuries.[22] The plantar plate serves as the most important checkrein to resist dorsal displacement of the proximal phalanx during gait. Chronic attritional wear of the plantar plate structures from high loading can ultimately lead to dorsal MTP joint subluxation.[2,3] As the damage to the plantar plate becomes more severe, an imbalance between the static and dynamic stabilizers leads to medial displacement and crossover deformity. Ford and colleagues'[23] cadaveric study showed that sectioning of the plantar plate increases dorsal instability of the MTP joint by 74%. Chalayon and colleagues[24] showed that plantar plate sectioning led to a 33% increase in sagittal plane instability. In regard to the collateral ligament's contribution in MTP joint stability, Barg and colleagues[18] showed that sectioning of both accessory collateral ligaments or both proper collateral ligaments resulted in 41.6% and 26.1% increased instability during dorsal subluxation of the MTP joint, respectively. They postulated that the accessory collateral ligament is more important than the proper collateral ligament for MTP joint stability because of its broad insertion onto the plantar plate. The deep transverse metatarsal ligament may also contribute to dorsal stability of the MTP joint. In Wang and colleagues'[25] study, sequential sectioning of one side or both sides of the deep transverse metatarsal joint at its insertion on the plantar plate led to 16.1% and 23.7% more dorsal instability. Biomechanically, the intrinsic foot musculature also plays a role in dorsal displacement of the MTP joint. When the MTP joint is in a plantigrade position, the lumbricals and interossei muscles travel plantar to the axis of rotation at the MTP joint. However, during the heel off phase of gait, hyperextension of the proximal phalanx forces the interossei to be oriented dorsal to the axis of rotation at the MTP joint, rendering it ineffective at flexing the toes.[20] This dynamic imbalance can lead to worsening of dorsal displacement of the MTP joint.

CLINICAL PRESENTATION

The most common presentation of lesser toe instability is malalignment and pain at the second MTP joint aggravated by weight bearing.[2,6] Women older than 50 years present often with chronic pain lasting several months before presentation.[6,8] Kaz and Coughlin's[6] cohort of 169 subjects showed that 92% presented with second MTP joint pain and 98% presented with dorsomedial deviation of the second toe.[6]

A thorough physical examination is paramount to precisely diagnose and define the potential cause of lesser plantar plate instability. Inspection of the forefoot in patients with early second MTP joint synovitis often is marked by the V-sign.[26] The V-sign represents subtle separation of the second and third rays and typically occurs before frank MTP joint instability occurs (**Fig. 1**). As plantar capsuloligamentous attritional wear continues, dorsal subluxation and cock-up deformity of the proximal phalanx occurs. Instability at the collateral ligaments can lead to a medial crossover of the second toe and the disappearance of the V-sign. Chronic plantar plate instability can lead to soft tissue contractures involving the extensor tendons, leading to claw and hammer toe deformities.[6,27] Careful examination of the skin will often show callus formation at the plantar aspect of the affected MTP joint.[5,6]

One of the most important examination maneuvers in distinguishing plantar plate instability is the drawer test. First described by Thompson and Hamilton[28] in 1987,

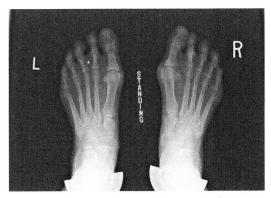

Fig. 1. *Radiographic V-sign.* Anteroposterior bilateral standing feet radiographs reveal bilateral lateral deviation of the third MTP joint (*asterisk*), indicating plantar plate instability.

the test is performed by applying a dorsal vertical force on the proximal phalanx while holding the metatarsal head in the neutral position. Another physical examination test is the paper pullout test, which is used to evaluate the dynamic plantar force of the affected toe.[29] The test is performed by placing a narrow strip of paper between the affected toe and the ground. Patients attempt to grasp the piece of paper by plantar flexing the affected digit while the examiner pulls the paper from underneath the toe. A positive examination occurs when patients are unable to resist the examiner from pulling out the paper. Klein and Coughlin's[30] retrospective diagnostic study of 90 patients with lesser toe plantar plate instability found that pain at the second metatarsal head (98.0%), gradual onset of pain (93.0%), and positive drawer sign (80.6%) were highly sensitive examination findings. They also found that the positive drawer test (99.8%) and crossover toes (88.9%) were highly specific tests. The investigators concluded that 95% of patients with surgically treated plantar plate injuries presented with gradual onset of forefoot pain, MTP joint edema, and a positive drawer sign.

Although careful examination often yields a correct diagnosis, there are often other pathologies that occur concomitantly with lesser toe plantar plate instability. Kaz and Coughlin's[6] study showed the following associations with crossover second toe deformities: second hammer toe (44.0%), second mallet toe (5.3%), hallux valgus (49.0%), hallux rigidus (14.2%), and hallux varus (6.5%).[6] Patients with hammer toe deformity often have slowly progressing deformity without pain and a negative drawer test. Morton neuroma often presents with paresthesias over the third interspace and a positive Mulder sign without MTP joint edema. Coughlin and colleagues[31] found that in their cohort of 121 patients with Morton neuromas, 20% had concomitant instability of the second MTP joint. Kaz and Coughlin's[6] study found that 7.6% of subjects with crossover deformity of the lesser toes had a coexisting Morton neuroma.[6] Although isolated hallux deformities are common, they are rarely painful. A history of previous hallux surgery is associated with developing plantar plate instability.[30] Patients with rheumatoid arthritis have a unique presentation of plantar plate instability, presenting with erosive changes that preferentially involving the fourth and fifth toes.[32,33]

IMAGING

Plain radiographs are typically less helpful than clinical evaluation in diagnosing plantar plate instability. Plain radiographs can be used to assess the degree of osseous malalignment, length of the second metatarsal, degree of MTP joint arthritis, and articular erosions. Anteroposterior (AP) radiographs of the foot can reveal splaying of the second and third MTP joints that can often be seen in patients with lesser plantar plate instability. Kaz and Coughlin[6] found that the mean medial deviation of the second MTP joint angle and lateral deviation of the third MTP joint angle were 3° and 6°, respectively.[6] Klein and colleagues[34] similarly found that the presence of second and third MTP joint splaying (64.9%) was significantly correlated with the presence of plantar plate deformity (mean 8.8°). Lateral plain radiographs can reveal dorsal subluxation of the MTP joint.[6,35] Kaz and Coughlin[6] also found a high radiographic association with both hallux rigidus (28%) and hallux valgus (49%) and plantar plate instability. Conversely, Kaz and Coughlin[6] found that plantar plate instability had no significant radiographic association with first ray hypermobility and pes planus deformity.

When plain radiographs do no reveal osseous abnormalities, soft tissue imaging can be used to assess plantar plate tears. Yao and colleagues[36] first described the use of MRI for plantar plate injuries. Patients with normal plantar plates had smooth low-intensity signal on T1 images at the plantar aspect of the metatarsal head. Patients with plantar plate disruption typically have a discontinuity of the hypointense plantar plate on T1 imaging[37] (**Fig. 2**) and increased T2 signal that extends toward the plantar plate distal insertion on the proximal phalanx. There is often isointense synovitis seen in conjunction with plantar plate abnormalities. Plantar plate tears found on MRI are typically lateral full-thickness tears at the proximal phalanx insertion.[1] Other MRI findings include pericapsular fibrosis, flexor tenosynovitis, and neuromas.[1] Sung and colleagues'[37] study compared MRI findings with interoperative findings with plantar plate instability in 45 feet. The investigators found that MRI was highly sensitive (96%), specific (95%), and accurate (91%) in determining plantar plate injuries.[37] MRI severity grading moderately correlates with intraoperative anatomic grading of plantar plate injuries.[37] Dinoa and colleagues[1] found that the addition of gadolinium contrast improves the visualization of plantar plate lesions by 30%.

Some clinicians have advocated the use of ultrasound imaging as a useful tool to evaluate plantar plate injuries.[38] Although ultrasound grading moderately correlates with MRI grading of plantar plate tears,[38] more recent studies have refuted the diagnostic accuracy of ultrasound imaging.[39] Klein and colleagues[39] found, in their study of 42 patients with metatarsalgia, that although ultrasound imaging was more sensitive than MRI (91.5% vs 73.9%), MRI was more specific than ultrasound (100% vs 25%). They also noted that four collateral ligament injuries were missed on ultrasound that were discovered on MRI. The investigators concluded that ultrasound should not replace MRI as the gold standard imaging modality for plantar plate injuries.

CLASSIFICATION

Haddad and colleagues[40] first described a clinical staging system in 1999 based on static alignment of patients with second toe instability.[3] Stage 1 deformity was

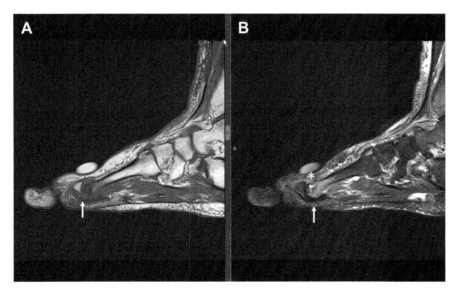

Fig. 2. *MRI of second MTP plantar plate injury.* Sagittal T1 (*A*) and T2-weighted (*B*) sequences of the second ray reveals significant synovitis and thickening of the plantar plate (*arrows*). There is also a large osteochondral lesion of the dorsal second metatarsal head (*asterisk*).

marked by synovitis and mild medial MTP joint deviation. Stage 2 deformity was marked by dorsomedial subluxation at the MTP joint. Stage 3 deformity was marked by overlapping of the hallux onto the second toe. Stage 4 deformity was marked by the complete dislocation at the MTP joint.[40] Coughlin and colleagues,[4] in 2011, combined static alignment and degree of dynamic instability to stage MTP joint instability (**Table 1**). In 2012, Coughlin and colleagues[41] described an anatomic grading system for plantar plate injuries in a cadaveric study. Grade 0 injuries were characterized by plantar plate attenuation. Grade 1 injuries had a less than 50% distal tear or a less than 50% midsubstance tear. Grade 2 injuries had a transverse distal tear greater than 50% and a midsubstance tear less than 50%. Grade 3 injuries had an extensive transverse or longitudinal tear that involved the collateral ligaments. Lastly, grade 4 tears involved an extensive transverse and longitudinal plantar plate tear with dislocation of the MTP joint.

The severity of plantar plate injury has been found to correlate with clinical deformity severity. Nery and colleagues[3] found in their prospective study of 68 patients with 100 lesser plantar plate instabilities that intraoperative higher-grade plantar plate instability correlated with increased medial deviation of the affected digit. Grade 3 lesions were most common in the study cohort, accounting for 33% of cases, followed by grade 0 (23%) and grade 4 (17%).

NONOPERATIVE TREATMENT

The natural history of untreated plantar plate instability can lead to stiffness, rigid hammer toe, and rigid mallet toe deformities.[2] Unfortunately, patients often do not seek treatment until the later stages of the disease.[6,8] Patients who present in the early stage of the disease can benefit from nonoperative treatment. The use of well-fitting shoes can decrease the pressure of adjacent toes and risk of crossover toe deformity.[5] Also, decreasing the heel height can reduce the amount of forefoot overload during gait. In Coughlin's[2,9] original studies, MTP joint taping of the affected side can aid in the stabilization and scarring of the unstable MTP joint. If irretractable keratosis develops along the plantar aspect of the affected digit, the use of metatarsal pads and extradepth shoes can alleviate discomfort.[5]

Table 1
Coughlin clinical staging system for second metatarsophalangeal joint instability

Grade	Static Alignment	Dynamic Physical Examination
0	Normal MTP joint alignment	MTP joint pain with swelling, reduced toe purchase, negative drawer
1	Mild MTP malalignment, positive V-sign, medial deviation	MTP joint pain with swelling, loss of toe purchase, positive drawer (<50% subluxation)
2	Moderate MTP malalignment, dorsomedial deformity, toe hyperextension	MTP joint pain, reduced swelling, no toe purchase, positive drawer (>50% to 100% subluxation)
3	Severe malalignment, dorsomedial deformity, crossover toe, flexible hammer toe	MTP joint pain, little swelling, no toe purchase, positive drawer
4	Dorsomedial dislocation, fixed hammer toe	MTP joint pain, little swelling, no toe purchase, positive drawer (fixed dislocation)

Trepman and Yeo,[42] in 1995, studied 13 patients with isolated MTP synovitis treated conservatively with intra-articular injections and rocker-bottom shoes to reduce passive dorsiflexion. At a mean follow-up of 18 months, 97% of patients were near asymptomatic. In 1997, Mizel and Michelson[43] described their nonoperative protocol for 13 patients (14 feet) with monoarticular synovitis that included oral antiinflammatories, intra-articular corticosteroids, and stiff steel sole modification. At a mean 6-year follow-up, 70% of patients had resolution of symptoms.[43] Although these previous studies show good pain relief with intra-articular corticosteroid injections, there are concerns that these injections can lead to iatrogenic MTP joint instability.[44] Furthermore, there are concerns that nonoperative treatment only temporarily relieves pain and does not address the underlying pathologic condition.

OPERATIVE TREATMENT

Operative intervention is the final option for chronic plantar plate instability after conservative treatment has failed. The goals of surgery should be to restore the plantigrade position of the lesser toes during the static stance position and to correct angular deformity.[3] The severity and rigidity of the deformity dictates the treatment options used. Plantar plate instability can be addressed by synovectomy, plantar plate repair, bony decompression, extensor tendon lengthening, or tendon transfers.[23,43,45–51]

The dorsal surgical approach to the plantar plate is performed by making a longitudinal incision over the web space of the corresponding digit.[45] A capsulotomy is then performed at the interval of the long and short extensor tendons. The capsule is released both medially and laterally at the level of the metatarsal head. During the release of the metatarsal head, the surgeon must be careful to avoid the vascular supply to the metatarsal head. Contractures of the extensor tendons, if present, should be released to help gain access to the plantar plate. After this, an elevator can be used to release the scarred plantar plate from the metatarsal neck to aid in mobilization and repair. Recently, Phisitkul and colleagues[52] described a minimally invasive dorsal approach that limited dissection through the lateral plantar plate and collateral ligament to reduce the amount of destabilization from more extensile dorsal approaches. They found that 6 mm of joint distraction could be achieved and that adequate suture passage was possible during this approach. Watson and colleagues[50] published a technique guide for direct repair of the plantar plate via the dorsal approach using a Mini Scorpion DX 0-Fiberwire kit (Arthrex, Naples, FL). A mattress repair is performed to tag the injured plantar plate, and then 2 oblique holes are drilled to tie the sutures onto the dorsum of the metatarsal head and secured with the MTP joint held in 15° of plantarflexion.

The plantar approach for plantar plate repair involves making a longitudinal incision between the metatarsal heads.[29,45,53] The longitudinal fibers of the plantar fascia are divided, and the dissection is carried through the plantar fat pad. Sharp dissection of the plantar fat pad should be used to avoid postoperative scarring.[53] Although avoiding the plantar neurovascular bundle, the long and short flexor tendon sheaths are retracted to gain access onto the plantar plate. If a transverse plantar plate tear is encountered, direct repair using 3-0 sutures are performed. If an avulsion injury is found at the proximal phalanx, Mitek (Depuy, Raynham, MA) suture anchors can be used to reapproximate the insertion site of the plantar plate.[29] The flexor tendon sheath is not repaired in order to avoid stenosis unless significant bowstringing is present. Usually skin repair is adequate to restore the stability of the flexor tendon. If needed, provisional K-wire stabilization of the MTP joint can be used. Plantar scarring from the disruption of the fat pad is a potential downside to this approach.[53]

OUTCOMES

Historical surgical treatment of plantar plate instability has included flexor to extensor tendon transfers. Chalayon and colleagues[24] showed in their biomechanical cadaveric study that adding a 3-mm shortening Weil osteotomy to a flexor tendon transfer restored sagittal plane stability during dorsiflexion and dorsal subluxation forces when compared with intact plantar plates. Plantar plate repairs with and without Weil osteotomy continued to have 28% more plantarflexion instability when compared with control specimens. Despite the biomechanical benefits of the classic flexor tendon transfer, there are concerns about stiffness and poor patient outcomes.[49,54] Myerson and Jung[54] reported their results of 64 MTP flexor tendon transfers in 59 patients. At a mean follow-up of 45 months, they found that 27% of patients had residual pain and 22% of patients were unsatisfied with their outcome.

Ford and colleagues,[23] in 1998, described the anatomic direct repair of the plantar plate as being as effective as flexor tendon transfers in restoring MTP joint stability. Nery and colleagues[3] performed a retrospective clinical study of 40 Weil osteotomies and plantar plate repairs (22 patients) via the dorsal approach. Nery and colleagues proposed a treatment algorithm using the dorsal approach based on the anatomic grading system. Grade 0 and 1 injuries were treated with an arthroscopic synovectomy, radiofrequency shrinkage, and Weil osteotomy. Grade 2 and 3 lesions were treated with a Weil osteotomy and direct repair of the plantar plate. Grade 4 lesions lacked sufficient plantar plate to undergo a direct repair; a flexor to extensor tendon transfer was, thus, performed. He found that the visual analog pain score (VAS) improved from 8 to 1 postoperatively. Additionally, there was no correlation between anatomic severity of the plantar plate lesion and pain scores. In a follow-up clinical study of 100 MTP joint repairs, Nery and colleagues[46] found that at a mean 2-year follow-up, grade 4 lesions had less postoperative improvement in their VAS pain score (2.3) and American Orthopedic Foot and Ankle Surgery (AOFAS) scores (72 points) compared with lower-grade lesions. Grade 1 to 4 lesions all had reduced MTP stability and plantigrade toe purchase postoperatively. In Flint and colleagues'[47] clinical prospective series of 97 feet with 138 lesser plantar plate tears, a dorsal approach was used to perform a Weil osteotomy and direct plantar plate repair.[47] The study found that 68% of patients regained the plantigrade position of the affected toes. Eighty percent of patients had good or excellent outcome results at 1 year, improving from 49 to 81 points on the AOFAS score. However, this study group was heterogeneous; several secondary procedures were performed at the time of surgery, including hammer toe correction, hallux valgus correction, extensor tendon lengthening, and neuroma excisions. In elderly patients with plantar plate instability and rigid MTP joint arthritis, a resection arthroplasty of the metatarsal head may be a viable option for pain relief.[51]

SUMMARY

Lesser toe plantar plate injuries at the MTP joint are a common source of metatarsalgia. The second MTP joint is the most commonly affected digit. The fibrocartilaginous plantar plate is the most important static stabilizer of the MTP joint, and high loading with weight bearing can lead to attritional plantar plate injuries. Chronic pain with weight bearing is the common presentation of lesser toe instability. Untreated plantar plate instability can lead to rigid hammer toe and mallet toe deformities. Combined Weil osteotomy and plantar plate repair yields favorable pain relief and angular deformity correction for patients who fail conservative treatment.

REFERENCES

1. Dinoa V, von Ranke F, Costa F, et al. Evaluation of lesser metatarsophalangeal joint plantar plate tears with contrast-enhanced and fat-suppressed MRI. Skeletal Radiol 2016;45:635–44.
2. Coughlin MJ. Crossover second toe deformity. Foot Ankle 1987;8:29–39.
3. Nery C, Coughlin MJ, Baumfeld D, et al. Lesser metatarsophalangeal joint instability: prospective evaluation and repair of plantar plate and capsular insufficiency. Foot Ankle Int 2012;33:301–11.
4. Coughlin MJ, Baumfeld DS, Nery C. Second MTP joint instability: grading of the deformity and description of surgical repair of capsular insufficiency. Phys Sportsmed 2011;39:132–41.
5. Coughlin MJ. Subluxation and dislocation of the lesser metatarsophalangeal joint. Mann's surgery of the foot and ankle. 9th edition. Philadelphia: Mosby Elsevier; 2014.
6. Kaz AJ, Coughlin MJ. Crossover second toe: demographics, etiology, and radiographic assessment. Foot Ankle Int 2007;28:1223–37.
7. Mann RA, Coughlin MJ, DuVries HL. The rheumatoid foot: review of literature and method of treatment. Orthop Rev 1979;8:105–12.
8. Mann RA, Mizel MS. Monarticular nontraumatic synovitis of the metatarsophalangeal joint: a new diagnosis? Foot Ankle 1985;6:18–21.
9. Coughlin MJ. Second metatarsophalangeal joint instability in the athlete. Foot Ankle 1993;14:309–19.
10. Brunet JA, Tubin S. Traumatic dislocations of the lesser toes. Foot Ankle Int 1997; 18:406–11.
11. Hynes D, D'Souza LG, Stephens M. Irreducible dislocation of the fifth metatarsophalangeal joint: a case report. Foot Ankle Int 1994;15:625–6.
12. Rao JP, Banzon MT. Irreducible dislocation of the metatarsophalangeal joints of the foot. Clin Orthop Relat Res 1979;(145):224–6.
13. Tung TS. Metatarsal shaft fracture with associated metatarsophalangeal joint dislocation. Case Rep Orthop 2016;2016:9629585.
14. Leung WY, Wong SH, Lam JJ, et al. Presentation of a missed injury of a metatarsophalangeal joint dislocation in the lesser toes. J Trauma 2001;50:1150–2.
15. Sarrafian S. Ligaments of metatarsophalangeal joints and proximal phalangeal apparatus. Anatomy of the foot and ankle: descriptive, topographic. Philadelphia: Lippincott Company; 1993. p. 207–10.
16. Deland JT, Lee KT, Sobel M, et al. Anatomy of the plantar plate and its attachments in the lesser metatarsal phalangeal joint. Foot Ankle Int 1995;16:480–6.
17. Johnston RB 3rd, Smith J, Daniels T. The plantar plate of the lesser toes: an anatomical study in human cadavers. Foot Ankle Int 1994;15:276–82.
18. Barg A, Courville XF, Nickisch F, et al. Role of collateral ligaments in metatarsophalangeal stability: a cadaver study. Foot Ankle Int 2012;33:877–82.
19. Sarrafian S. Intrinsic muscles of the lesser toes. Anatomy of the foot and ankle: descriptive, topographic, functional. 2nd edition. Philadelphia: Lippincott; 1993. p. 268–79.
20. Sarrafian S. Forces during gait. Anatomy of the foot and ankle: descriptive, topographic, functional. Philadelphia: Lippincott; 1993. p. 582–90.
21. Hutton WC, Dhanendran M. A study of the distribution of load under the normal foot during walking. Int Orthop 1979;3:153–7.
22. Stokes IA, Hutton WC, Stott JR. Forces acting on the metatarsals during normal walking. J Anat 1979;129:579–90.

23. Ford LA, Collins KB, Christensen JC. Stabilization of the subluxed second meta-tarsophalangeal joint: flexor tendon transfer versus primary repair of the plantar plate. J Foot Ankle Surg 1998;37:217–22.

24. Chalayon O, Chertman C, Guss AD, et al. Role of plantar plate and surgical reconstruction techniques on static stability of lesser metatarsophalangeal joints: a biomechanical study. Foot Ankle Int 2013;34:1436–42.

25. Wang B, Guss A, Chalayon O, et al. Deep transverse metatarsal ligament and static stability of lesser metatarsophalangeal joints: a cadaveric study. Foot Ankle Int 2015;36:573–8.

26. Panchbhavi VK, Trevino S. Clinical tip: a new clinical sign associated with meta-tarsophalangeal joint synovitis of the lesser toes. Foot Ankle Int 2007;28:640–1.

27. Myerson MS, Shereff MJ. The pathological anatomy of claw and hammer toes. J Bone Joint Surg Am Vol 1989;71:45–9.

28. Thompson FM, Hamilton WG. Problems of the second metatarsophalangeal joint. Orthopedics 1987;10:83–9.

29. Bouche RT, Heit EJ. Combined plantar plate and hammertoe repair with flexor digitorum longus tendon transfer for chronic, severe sagittal plane instability of the lesser metatarsophalangeal joints: preliminary observations. J Foot Ankle Surg 2008;47:125–37.

30. Klein EE, Weil L Jr, Weil LS Sr, et al. Clinical examination of plantar plate abnor-mality: a diagnostic perspective. Foot Ankle Int 2013;34:800–4.

31. Coughlin MJ, Schenck RC Jr, Shurnas PS, et al. Concurrent interdigital neuroma and MTP joint instability: long-term results of treatment. Foot Ankle Int 2002;23: 1018–25.

32. Siddle HJ, Hodgson RJ, Hensor EMA, et al. Plantar plate pathology is associated with erosive disease in the painful forefoot of patients with rheumatoid arthritis. BMC Musculoskelet Disord 2017;18:308.

33. Siddle HJ, Hodgson RJ, Redmond AC, et al. MRI identifies plantar plate pathol-ogy in the forefoot of patients with rheumatoid arthritis. Clin Rheumatol 2012;31: 621–9.

34. Klein EE, Weil L Jr, Weil LS Sr, et al. The underlying osseous deformity in plantar plate tears: a radiographic analysis. Foot Ankle Spec 2013;6:108–18.

35. Yu GV, Judge MS, Hudson JR, et al. Predislocation syndrome. Progressive sub-luxation/dislocation of the lesser metatarsophalangeal joint. J Am Podiatr Med Assoc 2002;92:182–99.

36. Yao L, Cracchiolo A, Farahani K, et al. Magnetic resonance imaging of plantar plate rupture. Foot Ankle Int 1996;17:33–6.

37. Sung W, Weil L Jr, Weil LS Sr, et al. Diagnosis of plantar plate injury by magnetic resonance imaging with reference to intraoperative findings. J Foot Ankle Surg 2012;51:570–4.

38. Gregg J, Silberstein M, Schneider T, et al. Sonographic and MRI evaluation of the plantar plate: a prospective study. Eur Radiol 2006;16:2661–9.

39. Klein EE, Weil L Jr, Weil LS Sr, et al. Magnetic resonance imaging versus muscu-loskeletal ultrasound for identification and localization of plantar plate tears. Foot Ankle Spec 2012;5:359–65.

40. Haddad SL, Sabbagh RC, Resch S, et al. Results of flexor-to-extensor and extensor brevis tendon transfer for correction of the crossover second toe defor-mity. Foot Ankle Int 1999;20:781–8.

41. Coughlin MJ, Schutt SA, Hirose CB, et al. Metatarsophalangeal joint pathology in crossover second toe deformity: a cadaveric study. Foot Ankle Int 2012;33: 133–40.

42. Trepman E, Yeo SJ. Nonoperative treatment of metatarsophalangeal joint synovitis. Foot Ankle Int 1995;16:771–7.

43. Mizel MS, Michelson JD. Nonsurgical treatment of monarticular nontraumatic synovitis of the second metatarsophalangeal joint. Foot Ankle Int 1997;18:424–6.

44. Reis ND, Karkabi S, Zinman C. Metatarsophalangeal joint dislocation after local steroid injection. J Bone Joint Surg Br Vol 1989;71:864.

45. Doty JF, Coughlin MJ. Metatarsophalangeal joint instability of the lesser toes and plantar plate deficiency. J Am Acad Orthop Surg 2014;22:235–45.

46. Nery C, Coughlin MJ, Baumfeld D, et al. Prospective evaluation of protocol for surgical treatment of lesser MTP joint plantar plate tears. Foot Ankle Int 2014; 35:876–85.

47. Flint WW, Macias DM, Jastifer JR, et al. Plantar plate repair for lesser metatarsophalangeal joint instability. Foot Ankle Int 2017;38:234–42.

48. Thompson FM, Deland JT. Flexor tendon transfer for metatarsophalangeal instability of the second toe. Foot Ankle 1993;14:385–8.

49. Steensma MR, Jabara M, Anderson JG, et al. Flexor hallucis longus tendon transfer for hallux claw toe deformity and vertical instability of the metatarsophalangeal joint. Foot Ankle Int 2006;27:689–92.

50. Watson TS, Reid DY, Frerichs TL. Dorsal approach for plantar plate repair with weil osteotomy: operative technique. Foot Ankle Int 2014;35:730–9.

51. Gallentine JW, DeOrio JK. Removal of the second toe for severe hammertoe deformity in elderly patients. Foot Ankle Int 2005;26:353–8.

52. Phisitkul P, Hosuru Siddappa V, Sittapairoj T, et al. Cadaveric evaluation of dorsal intermetatarsal approach for plantar plate and lateral collateral ligament repair of the lesser metatarsophalangeal joints. Foot Ankle Int 2017;38:791–6.

53. Blitz NM, Ford LA, Christensen JC. Plantar plate repair of the second metatarsophalangeal joint: technique and tips. J Foot Ankle Surg 2004;43:266–70.

54. Myerson MS, Jung HG. The role of toe flexor-to-extensor transfer in correcting metatarsophalangeal joint instability of the second toe. Foot Ankle Int 2005;26: 675–9.

UNITED STATES POSTAL SERVICE ® **Statement of Ownership, Management, and Circulation (All Periodicals Publications Except Requester Publications)**

1. Publication Title	2. Publication Number	3. Filing Date
FOOT AND ANKLE CLINICS OF NORTH AMERICA	016 – 368	9/18/2018

4. Issue Frequency	5. Number of Issues Published Annually	6. Annual Subscription Price
MAR, JUN, SEP, DEC	4	$326.00

7. Complete Mailing Address of Known Office of Publication (Not printer) (Street, city, county, state, and ZIP+4®)

ELSEVIER INC.
230 Park Avenue, Suite 800
New York, NY 10169

Contact Person: STEPHEN R. BUSHING
Telephone (Include area code): 215-239-3688

8. Complete Mailing Address of Headquarters or General Business Office of Publisher (Not printer)

ELSEVIER INC.
230 Park Avenue, Suite 800
New York, NY 10169

9. Full Names and Complete Mailing Addresses of Publisher, Editor, and Managing Editor (Do not leave blank)

Publisher (Name and complete mailing address)

TAYLOR E. BALL, ELSEVIER INC.
1600 JOHN F KENNEDY BLVD. SUITE 1800
PHILADELPHIA, PA 19103-2899

Editor (Name and complete mailing address)

LAUREN BOYLE, ELSEVIER INC.
1600 JOHN F KENNEDY BLVD. SUITE 1800
PHILADELPHIA, PA 19103-2899

Managing Editor (Name and complete mailing address)

PATRICK MANLEY, ELSEVIER INC.
1600 JOHN F KENNEDY BLVD. SUITE 1800
PHILADELPHIA, PA 19103-2899

10. Owner (Do not leave blank. If the publication is owned by a corporation, give the name and address of the corporation immediately followed by the names and addresses of all stockholders owning or holding 1 percent or more of the total amount of stock. If not owned by a corporation, give the names and addresses of the individual owners. If owned by a partnership or other unincorporated firm, give its name and address as well as those of each individual owner. If the publication is published by a nonprofit organization, give its name and address.)

Full Name	Complete Mailing Address
WHOLLY OWNED SUBSIDIARY OF REED/ELSEVIER, US HOLDINGS	1600 JOHN F KENNEDY BLVD. SUITE 1800 PHILADELPHIA, PA 19103-2899

11. Known Bondholders, Mortgagees, and Other Security Holders Owning or Holding 1 Percent or More of Total Amount of Bonds, Mortgages, or Other Securities. If none, check box ▸ ☐ None

Full Name	Complete Mailing Address
N/A	

12. Tax Status (For completion by nonprofit organizations authorized to mail at nonprofit rates) (Check one)
The purpose, function, and nonprofit status of this organization and the exempt status for federal income tax purposes:
☒ Has Not Changed During Preceding 12 Months
☐ Has Changed During Preceding 12 Months (Publisher must submit explanation of change with this statement)

PS Form **3526**, July 2014 [Page 1 of 4 (see instructions page 4)] PSN: 7530-01-000-9931   PRIVACY NOTICE: See our privacy policy on www.usps.com

---

13. Publication Title				14. Issue Date for Circulation Data Below
FOOT AND ANKLE CLINICS OF NORTH AMERICA				JUNE 2018

15. Extent and Nature of Circulation				Average No. Copies Each Issue During Preceding 12 Months	No. Copies of Single Issue Published Nearest to Filing Date
a. Total Number of Copies (Net press run)				288	373
b. Paid Circulation (By Mail and Outside the Mail)	(1)	Mailed Outside-County Paid Subscriptions Stated on PS Form 3541 (Include paid distribution above nominal rate, advertiser's proof copies, and exchange copies)		174	210
	(2)	Mailed In-County Paid Subscriptions Stated on PS Form 3541 (Include paid distribution above nominal rate, advertiser's proof copies, and exchange copies)		0	0
	(3)	Paid Distribution Outside the Mails Including Sales Through Dealers and Carriers, Street Vendors, Counter Sales, and Other Paid Distribution Outside USPS®		70	91
	(4)	Paid Distribution by Other Classes of Mail Through the USPS (e.g., First-Class Mail®)		0	0
c. Total Paid Distribution (Sum of 15b (1), (2), (3), and (4))			▸	244	301
d. Free or Nominal Rate Distribution (By Mail and Outside the Mail)	(1)	Free or Nominal Rate Outside-County Copies included on PS Form 3541		32	57
	(2)	Free or Nominal Rate In-County Copies Included on PS Form 3541		0	0
	(3)	Free or Nominal Rate Copies Mailed at Other Classes Through the USPS (e.g., First-Class Mail)		0	0
	(4)	Free or Nominal Rate Distribution Outside the Mail (Carriers or other means)		32	57
e. Total Free or Nominal Rate Distribution (Sum of 15d (1), (2), (3) and (4))			▸		
f. Total Distribution (Sum of 15c and 15e)			▸	276	358
g. Copies not Distributed (See Instructions to Publishers #4 (page #3))			▸	12	15
h. Total (Sum of 15f and g)			▸	288	373
i. Percent Paid (15c divided by 15f times 100)			▸	88.41%	84.08%

* If you are claiming electronic copies, go to line 16 on page 3. If you are not claiming electronic copies, skip to line 17 on page 3.

16. Electronic Copy Circulation		Average No. Copies Each Issue During Preceding 12 Months	No. Copies of Single Issue Published Nearest to Filing Date
a. Paid Electronic Copies	▸	0	0
b. Total Paid Print Copies (Line 15c) + Paid Electronic Copies (Line 16a)	▸	244	301
c. Total Print Distribution (Line 15f) + Paid Electronic Copies (Line 16a)	▸	276	358
d. Percent Paid (Both Print & Electronic Copies) (16b divided by 16c × 100)	▸	88.41%	84.08%

☒ I certify that 50% of all my distributed copies (electronic and print) are paid above a nominal price.

17. Publication of Statement of Ownership
☒ If the publication is a general publication, publication of this statement is required. Will be printed
in the DECEMBER 2018 issue of this publication.   ☐ Publication not required.

18. Signature and Title of Editor, Publisher, Business Manager, or Owner   Date

Stephen R. Bushing   9/18/2018

STEPHEN R. BUSHING - INVENTORY DISTRIBUTION CONTROL MANAGER

I certify that all information furnished on this form is true and complete. I understand that anyone who furnishes false or misleading information on this form or who omits material or information requested on the form may be subject to criminal sanctions (including fines and imprisonment) and/or civil sanctions (including civil penalties).

PS Form **3526**, July 2014 (Page 2 of 4)   PRIVACY NOTICE: See our privacy policy on www.usps.com

Moving?

Make sure your subscription moves with you!

To notify us of your new address, find your **Clinics Account Number** (located on your mailing label above your name), and contact customer service at:

Email: journalscustomerservice-usa@elsevier.com

800-654-2452 (subscribers in the U.S. & Canada)
314-447-8871 (subscribers outside of the U.S. & Canada)

Fax number: 314-447-8029

Elsevier Health Sciences Division
Subscription Customer Service
3251 Riverport Lane
Maryland Heights, MO 63043

*To ensure uninterrupted delivery of your subscription, please notify us at least 4 weeks in advance of move.

Printed and bound by CPI Group (UK) Ltd, Croydon, CR0 4YY

08/05/2025

01864735-0001